TREATMENT OF BEHAVIOR PROBLEMS IN DOGS AND CATS

D1289387

DATE DUE

APR 20 1999

TREATMENT OF BEHAVIOR PROBLEMS IN DOGS AND CATS

A Guide for the Small Animal Veterinarian

Henry R. Askew
PhD
Experimental Psychologist, Munich

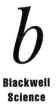

Blackwell Science

© 1996 German language edition by
Blackwell Wissenschafts-Verlag
© 1996 English language edition by
Blackwell Science
Editorial Offices:
Osney Mead, Oxford OX2 0EL
25 John Street, London WC1N 2BL
23 Ainslie Place, Edinburgh EH3 6AJ
238 Main Street, Cambridge
    Massachusetts 02142, USA
54 University Street, Carlton
    Victoria 3053, Australia

Other Editorial Offices:
Arnette Blackwell SA
    224, Boulevard Saint Germain
    75007 Paris, France

Blackwell Wissenschafts-Verlag GmbH
    Kurfürstendamm 57
    10707 Berlin, Germany

    Zehetnergasse 6
    A-1140 Wien, Austria

All rights reserved. No part of this publication
may be reproduced, stored in a retrieval system,
or transmitted, in any form or by any means,
electronic, mechanical, photocopying,
recording or otherwise, except as permitted
by the UK Copyright, Designs and Patents Act
1988, without the prior permission of the
publishers.

First published 1996

Set in 8.5/11 pt R Concorde Roman
by SiB, 10969 Berlin
Printed and bound in Austria

The Blackwell Science logo is a trade mark of
Blackwell Science Ltd, registered at the United
Kingdom Trade Marks Registry

SF
433
A75
1996

DISTRIBUTORS

Marston Book Services Ltd
PO Box 269
Abingdon
Oxon OX14 4YN
(*Orders*: Tel: 01235-465500
         Fax: 01235-465555)

USA
Blackwell Science, Inc.
238 Main Street
Cambridge, MA 02142
(*Orders:* Tel: 800 215-1000
              617 876-7000
         Fax: 617 492-5263)

Canada
Copp Clark, Ltd
2775 Matheson Blvd East
Mississauga, Ontario
Canada, L4W 4P7
(*Orders:* Tel: 800 263-4374
              905 238-6074)

Australia
Blackwell Science Pty Ltd
54 University Street
Carlton, Victoria 3053
(*Orders:* Tel: 03 9347-0300
         Fax: 03 9347-5001)

A catalogue record for this title is available from
the British Library.

ISBN 0-632-04108-0

Preface

Owners, veterinarians, and reporters often ask why dog and cat behavioral problems are so much more common now than they used to be. Is it a symptom of something wrong in our modern society - the crowded conditions in our big cities or the excessive demands placed on pets by their lonely or neurotic owners? Are animals being used by their owners as surrogates for the friends or children which many people don't have? Or are they simply being neglected more than they used to be? Are they being left too long alone or kept in tiny apartments that don't provide them with the minimum amount of space they require?

There are no statistics one can use to compare the frequency of pet behavior problems nowadays with that of 50 or 100 years ago. However, I suspect that things have not changed as much as these kinds of questions assume. The problems are probably the same ones that some dog and cat owners have always had with their pets. It is our response to them that has changed.

This book describes the new, scientific approach to treating dog and cat behavior problems which first began to develop in earnest in the United States two decades ago and is now in the process of rapidly spreading to all of the world's developed countries where dogs and cats are kept in the home in much the same way as in North America or Western Europe. In writing it, I have tried to use a combination of my experimental psychology training and years of intensive experience helping Munich pet owners cope with their animals' behavior problems to advance in small ways the field which pioneers such as Voith, Borchelt, Hart, Houpt, Beaver, and Campbell in the United States, Brunner in Austria, and Mugford and O'Farrell in England have worked so tirelessly to develop. Although in some places in the book, I am sharply critical of certain views expressed by these and other well-known pet behavior problem specialists, my criticisms are uttered against a background of respect and full acknowledgment of the debt all of us who now work in this field owe to them. Without their work, there would be no foundation to build on and none of us would be as far along as we are today.

This book is primarily addressed to small animal veterinarians and veterinary students who rightly regard the development of the pet behavior problem field as a natural extension of veterinary medicine into a new treatment domain which has the potential not only of providing new, much-needed services to clients, but also of saving the lives of the millions of cats and dogs that are euthanized for behavior problems throughout the world every year. For the behavioral scientist, however, writing for veterinarian readers is considerably different than writing for either pet owners or other behavioral scientists and their students. On the one hand, veterinarians are highly-trained professionals with a strong academic background in the biological and medical sciences and a great deal of hands-on experience with pets, pet behavior, and dealing with pet owners. But on the other hand, they have had little or no behavioral science training.

The problem is therefore how to impart behavioral science concepts, principles, and analytic approaches to such an audience. In this connection, my approach in this book is to basically tell it like it is - or how it appears to the behavioral scientist to be - using terms normally used by behavioral scientists when dealing with similar topics. While I have made a conscious effort to introduce, define, and exemplify technical concepts more clearly and carefully than would be necessary, for example,

HOLYOKE COMMUNITY COLLEGE
ELAINE NICPON MARIEB LIBRARY

if addressing a psychology graduate student audience, I have tried very hard to avoid talking down to readers by simplifying to the point of oversimplifying as is sometimes the case in the presently available books on pet behavior problems. To be an effective pet behavior counselor within or outside of a small animal practice, one must be able to conceptualize and view the animal's behavior and its relationship to the surrounding environment from the behavioral scientist's perspective. And there is simply no way to assist the reader in developing these kinds of conceptual, perceptual, and analytic skills without freely making use of all the theoretical and conceptual „thinking tools" which have been developed by ethologists and experimental psychologists over the course of nearly a century of intense scientific study of the behavior of animals.

Accordingly, this book has several unusual features which bear some mention here. Firstly, rather than listing example recommendations within the context of particular case histories, I have opted for summarizing them in the form of *sample recommendations boxes* describing the various types of recommendations experienced behavior problem counselors give clients in such cases. Trying to avoid the „simple tips" approach at all cost, I have chosen instead to describe the types of recommendations which are helpful both in more detail and in a way which requires the veterinarian to select from the potentially available approaches and recommendations those which are best for the individual case involved. Often this means presenting various common scenarios or forms in which problems like dominance aggression in dogs are seen and then suggesting the types of recommendations which are appropriate for each form. The recommendations listed are, however, specific. Each was taken from letters I have written to clients summarizing the recommended treatment a few days after the consultation.

Secondly, for each of the major dog and cat problems, a *problem overview diagram* is presented. It summarizes and briefly annotates both the *possible causal factors* which the behavior problem counselor must bear in mind

when questioning owners and the *possible treatment elements* which basically represents the whole treatment method arsenal which is available when treating cases of this sort. As well as providing a summary overview which complements the accompanying discussion, it is hoped that these diagrams will be especially useful to veterinarians later when the book is again taken down from the bookshelf for guidance in dealing with specific cases. My intention in preparing these overview diagrams was to provide the veterinarian with enough „at a glance" information to stimulate recall of the salient features of such problems and treatments without having to reread the chapter again in its entirety. If some rereading is necessary, section headings directly corresponding to the various items listed in the diagrams facilitate quick location of the required information.

Thirdly, rather than separating explanations of technical animal behavioral science principles and concepts from the rest of the text as is common in other books, I have opted for providing such explanations as an integral part of the discussion of specific problems. The advantages of this approach are considerable. One can deal teach the necessary lessons in small doses, bring in technical concepts and provide technical explanations in a context in which their relevance and value are clear, and repeatedly illustrate the most critical among them as they become relevant to each of the various problems. In short, it is a way of presenting the various behavioral science principles and concepts which can help to make thinking about and perceiving pet behavior problems in such terms almost second nature to the reader.

And last but not least, I devote considerable space early in the book to discussing the phenomenon of pet ownership, the nature of the relationship between owners and pets, and the general nature and goals of the pet behavior problem counseling process. Aside from the fact that these topics are interesting in and of themselves, it is hoped that such discussions will provide the reader with insights which are helpful to understanding owners, their family situations, and the role the animal and its problem behavior is playing in the family. Understanding such phenomena are crucial when it comes to analyzing behavioral problem situations and envisioning realistic solutions within the complex and dynamic family context. In the last analysis, such insights help the counselor deal with pet behavior problems in a way which tends to maximize clients' compliance with the treatment recommendations. As will be considered in a number of places in the book, inducing owners to diligently follow the treatment recommendations is the most difficult and critical problem faced by any pet behavior problem counselor.

Cautionary note: In providing drug and dosage information throughout this book, I am essentially only reporting what is recommended by well-known veterinary behavior specialists like Voith, Marder, Hart, Burghardt, Overall, and others. As an experimental psychologist, I am not qualified or competent to prescribe drugs or provide drug-related or associated medical information to any greater extent than this. When including such information at various places, I have been careful to provide the veterinary reference(s) from which the recommendation was taken. I would urge the veterinarian who is contemplating the prescribing drug therapy not to rely solely on the information provided in this book, but rather to first consult the accompanying references as well as those referred to in the section on drug therapy in Chapter 8 which provide discussions of drugs, dosages, side effects, and associated medical issues related to the use of drugs to treat pet behavior problems.

Finally, a few brief acknowledgments. First and foremost, heartfelt thanks to my wife, Eva-Maria, to whom this book is dedicated, for her encouragement and firm support for the course I had chosen since the day I decided to specialize in the pet behavior area. She has provided invaluable help over the last several years with everything from translating and client relations to critically examining and rethinking the most difficult of conceptual and treatment-related issues. Secondly, thanks are due to Rebecca Holmes DVM for editing the English edition and to Dr. Andreas Müller DVM, my editor at Blackwell Wissenschaft in Berlin, for his strong support, sound advice, and untiring assistance throughout all phases of the project. Thirdly, many thanks to the well-known English painter, Peter Unsworth, an old family friend, for agreeing to allow a photograph of his painting, Napoleon, to be reproduced on the cover of this book. And finally, my sincere thanks are also extended to the many Munich small animal veterinarians who have supported my pet problem practice over the years by referring clients with problem animals to me. Without this basis of extensive treatment experience, I would never have been in a position to contribute something like this book to the young and rapidly-developing pet behavioral problem field.

September 1995
Munich, Germany

To Eva

Table of Contents

Part I

Pet Behavior Counseling

1 Introduction to Pet Behavior Counseling

Families who take a new puppy into their home know that some problems with its behavior are to be expected. It may whine and disturb the house during its first night. It will urinate and defecate in the home many times before it finally becomes housebroken. It may chew up shoes and other items, become unruly during walks, bark or growl at guests, or steal food from the table and therefore require a certain amount of behavioral training if it is to become the kind of pet the family wishes it to be. While cat owners expect fewer problems with the behavior of their new kitten, it comes to them as no great surprise when the cat occasionally eliminates outside of the litter box, scratches furniture, eats house plants, or pounces on a hand that happens to be loosely dangling over the arm of an easy chair. Based on a survey of several hundred dog and cat owners, Voith (1985) reported that 42 % of the dog owners and 47 % of the cat owners indicated that their pet "engaged in a behavior they considered to be a problem".

Such "normal" behavior problems are therefore common. Most are minor. They may occur only occasionally or be relatively easy to live with. Some are problems common in young animals which either disappear as the animal matures or are easily solved by giving the pet a little training or by making minor changes in the household like, for example, where a plant is placed, where the animal is fed, or whether a particular door is left open or closed.

However, pet behavior problems can be much more serious than this. Cats may begin urine marking in the home and persist in this behavior in spite of the application of corrective measures. Dogs may begin viciously attacking other dogs, unfamiliar adults, children, or family members causing serious injuries which require medical attention. Keeping dogs

and cats as pets would not be as popular as it is today if such serious behavior problems were common. Statistically speaking, they are relatively uncommon. The overwhelming majority of cats do not mark in the home and the overwhelming majority of dogs never bite people. Throughout the long domestication process, strong selection pressures have acted on domestic cat and dog species to keep the probabilities of such behaviors low. In the past, animals that displayed serious behavioral problems were killed without hesitation. And even today, many ultimately meet this same fate.

Underlying the development of modern pet keeping practices in the highly developed Western societies are attitudes which have essentially acted to make owners more reluctant to simply dispose of problem animals as was routinely practiced in times past. Companion animals are regarded as family members which are valued as individuals rather than merely for the protection or other behavioral services they perform. They are loved and people feel in some sense bound to them and responsible for their physical and emotional well-being much as if they were human children. It is therefore not surprising that pet owners are often willing to expend considerable time and energy, and go to considerable expense, to solve serious behavior problems before considering euthanasia, finding a new home for their pet, or surrendering it to an animal shelter.

The existence of severe dog and cat behavior problems can create disturbances which are serious enough to outweigh the positive contributions the pets are making to family life. But even in such cases, most modern family members are extremely attached to their pets and willing to exert a considerable effort to keep them healthy and happy and part of the family. This has led to the development of the new pet behavior problem treatment specialty of *pet behavior counseling* – also commonly referred to as *clinical animal behavior* or *animal behavior therapy*. Modern pet owners have been seeking advice for decades from those who possess special knowledge about pets and their behavior such as breeders, dog trainers, and veterinarians. But it is only within the last two decades that knowledge from the animal behavioral sciences began to be consciously and systematically employed with the aim of developing a new applied scientific specialty focused on the treatment of pet behavior problems.

After rudimentary beginnings prior to the turn of the century, a new concern among American experimental psychologists and European zoologists with focusing on the behavior of animals as a phenomenon worthy of scientific study in its own right resulted in two thriving scientific disciplines, experimental psychology and ethology. Within the space of a only a few decades, workers in these fields have produced a new and deeply-satisfying understanding of animal behavior. It is natural for scientific knowledge of all kinds to be applied in the society at large whenever there is the need and opportunity to do so. And it was therefore natural that sooner or later this new animal behavior knowledge would be applied to understand and counteract the problems people have always had with the behavior of their domestic animals.

The applied animal behavior science specialty focused on treating behavior problems in domestic animals has essentially developed along two lines. The first involves domestic animals that are bred and kept in large numbers for economic purposes like food and pelt production, or for research or educational purposes. *Farm, laboratory,* and *zoo animals* frequently exhibit behavior problems such as self-mutilation, behavior that injures other animals, disturbances of normal behavioral functioning (e.g. sexual behavior, care of young), and abnormal reactivity which are now basically understood as consequences of unnaturally crowded, impoverished, confined, or otherwise inadequate living conditions. The ethological approach, with its primary emphasis on understanding the natural behavioral repertoire and associated environmental requirements of each species, has helped us to understand why these behavior problems occur and how the environmental conditions to which animals are subjected must be improved to eliminate or prevent them. Thus, the occurrence of behavioral problems in the farm, laboratory, or zoo environment is usually regarded as a sign of *environmental deficiencies*. Accordingly, it indicates the need for making some kind of modification of the conditions under which the animals are kept by, for example, reducing group sizes to ease overcrowded conditions, keeping formally isolated animals in groups, separating animals from conspecifics at certain times, allowing more access to outdoor areas, or changing feeding methods, bedding materials, diets, etc.

The second animal behavior problem field is focused on *companion animals* – domesticated animals which receive personal attention from owners, remain in close proximity to and are part of the daily life of owners, and are kept primarily for noncommercial purposes (Young, 1985). These are mainly dogs and cats that live as animal members of human families and are usually kept unconfined with few if any movement restrictions in the home. While originally invited into human settlements and family dwellings for utilitarian reasons (e.g. defense, rodent control), companion animals are now kept mainly because of various rewarding effects which their presence and behavior have on family members.

Some of the problem behaviors displayed by dogs and cats are similar to those exhibited by farm and zoo animals. However, most are quite different due to the fact that the animals move freely about within the human home and interact with human family members on a more or less full-time basis. With farm animals, house-soiling, for example, is never an issue. And large animals which are especially aggressive to human beings may simply be handled more carefully or kept in a somewhat different way than less aggressive animals.

An *environmental modification* approach is often successfully used to treat some behavioral problems in dogs and cats as well. With housesoiling in cats, for example, it is often the only method employed: additional litter boxes are added, new types of litter are used, the location of litter boxes in the home are changed, or preferred surfaces for elimination are covered with plastic or some other material. There are, however, a variety of other types of methods that can be applied to solve companion animal behavior problems. Dogs have always been subjected to extensive *training* to keep their behavior within acceptable limits and promote the kinds of behavioral skills (e.g. hunting) which might be required of them. Intensive training measures based on the same principles may also be applied to correct behavioral problems like aggression towards human strangers. Finally, where dogs or cats are extremely fearful, a version of the *systematic behavior therapy* approach developed to treat this problem in human beings may be applied.

Recognition began to develop as early as the 60s that veterinarians' behavior-related advice to clients could and should be based on knowledge derived from the scientific study of animal behavior. During the 70s, it came to be increasingly recognized that it was not only possible to use knowledge from the animal behavioral sciences to develop special methods to correct the various kinds of problems pet owners often have with their pets, but indeed that the treatment of such problems had the potential of developing into a new specialty within veterinary medicine. Fueled at the grass roots by the practicing veterinarian's great interest in learning more about what to tell the many clients who ask for advice in how to cope with pet behavior problems, the number of papers published in veterinary journals and given at veterinary meetings by pet behavior problem specialists increased rapidly during the next two decades.

Two scientific disciplines are of primary importance to the field of pet behavior counseling. The first is *ethology,* the biological study of animal behavior. To successfully treat animal behavioral problems, one must have a good understanding of the normal behavior of the species concerned. Ethologists believe that to understand the behavior of any complex animal species, one must know how it normally behaves in its natural environment. Although complicated by the fact that further evolution has occurred during the domestication process making domestic dogs and to a lesser extent domestic cats dissimilar in many ways to their wild-living ancestors, this simply adds another dimension to the task of understanding the normal and natural behavior of the two species. In addition to understanding how the domestic animals' wild-living ancestors lived and behaved, one must also strive to understand how (and why) this behavior has been modified during the domestication process.

Solving pet behavioral problems means changing the animals' behavior in situations in which problems occur. Particularly with dogs where behavior often must be modified by the application of training measures, the general principles or laws of learning derived from decades of laboratory research by *experimental psychologists* – behavioral scientists who study the nature of and factors affecting the various learning processes in complex animal species like rats and pigeons – have turned out to be highly relevant and useful.

Due to the parallels between, for example, fear problems in pets and those experienced by some fearful or anxious human beings, a third, applied scientific field has also made an important contribution to the pet behavior therapy area: *human behavior therapy,* a branch of clinical psychology which regards human behavioral disturbances as basically "learned habits" which are most effectively treated by applying training methods derived from the application of animal learning principles. First developed in the 50s, it was soon clear that this new behavior therapy approach was extremely effective in treating problems such as human phobias which were often impossible to treat successfully using traditional "talk psycho-therapy" methods. That analogous behavior therapy methods could be applied to treat similar problems in companion animals was first made clear in Tuber et al. (1974) which reported on their successful application to treating dog phobia, fear-aggression, and separation anxiety problems within the household setting.

Most behavior problems cannot presently be eliminated or improved with drug therapy. Progestins and psychotropic drugs like diazepam, amitriptyline, buspirone, and a number of others are however playing a useful role in the treatment of problems like urine marking and stereotypies. While many veterinary behavior specialists hope along with Voith (1991) that "veterinary behavior medicine is on the edge of an exciting new frontier in the pharmaceutic area", it is probably fair to state that few animal behavioral scientists who are well-acquainted with the whole gamut of dog and cat behavioral problems would anticipate that drugs could ever be helpful in coping with the overwhelming majority of behavioral problems for which some combination of behavioral training and/or environmental modification measures are obviously required.

As this short overview makes clear, pet behavior counseling is essentially an interdisciplinary field which involves the application of knowledge and experience from veterinary medicine, human medicine, ethology, experimental psychology, and clinical psychology. Family veterinarians are generally the first type of specialist to which the pet owner turns for help in coping with behavioral problems. And they alone are in a position to identify and treat cases where a behavior problem is symptomatic

of some pathophysiological condition. When no disease condition exists, they may choose to treat the problem as purely a behavioral problem themselves or refer the client to a pet behavior problem specialist. And finally, in cases where a behavior specialist is contacted, the specialist may refer the client back to his/her family veterinarian for drug therapy or castration as the sole treatment, or more commonly, as an adjunct to behavioral treatment methods.

During the course of the last two decades, pet behavior counseling has become an increasingly international field. Although it developed in the United States, it has been well-established for years in England, it is developing rapidly in other Western European countries such as Germany and France, and knowledge of and interest in the field is growing in all of the world's other developed and developing countries.

Even in the United States where it is now an officially recognized veterinary specialty, the pet behavior problem field has yet to win the kind of full acceptance by the veterinary profession which translates into adequate numbers of university courses and programs, faculty members specializing in this area, companion animal behavior clinic facilities, and associated research opportunities in university veterinary schools. But these developments are bound to

---

Terminological note:

Behavior specialist: *a qualified person with a <u>pet behavior counseling referral practice</u> to which pet problems are referred by family veterinarians. The behavior specialist may be a veterinarian or a person with some other kind of academic background such as an ethologist or psychologist.*
Behavior counselor: *a qualified person who <u>carries out pet behavior counseling</u> as it is described throughout this book. Here too, the behavior counselor can be either a veterinarian or non-veterinarian. And if he/she is a veterinarian, the behavior counseling activities can be carried out as one of the services offered by the veterinarian's own practice (i.e. family veterinarian) or in the context of a referral practice to which pet problems are referred by other veterinarians.*

As used throughout this book, the terms "veterinarian", "behavior specialist", and "behavior counselor" are therefore not mutually exclusive. Indeed, most well-known behavior specialists and behavior counselors are veterinarians.

come. For companion animal behavior problems are widespread and severe, creating much stress and suffering within pet-owning families, causing many serious injuries to owners and other human and animal members of our communities, filling the world's animal shelters with unwanted animals, and representing a leading cause of death of the millions of cats and dogs which are euthanized throughout the world every year. In short, the magnitude of the societal problem that needs to be addressed is enormous and, correspondingly, the need for the pet behavior counseling area to develop further in the direction of becoming a respected and thriving discipline is acute. A few animal behavioral scientists are attempting to play a role in this development process. However, it is clear to them and all others who work in this area that the field ultimately represents a natural and much-needed extension of the veterina-

rian's traditional role of primary advisor to pet owners concerning anything and everything which affects their animals' health, welfare, and life within the human family environment.

References

Tuber, D.S., Hothersall, D., and Voith, V.L. (1974): Animal clinical psychology: a modest proposal. *American Psychologist* **29**, 762–766.

Voith, V.L. (1985): Attachment of people to companion animals. *Veterinary Clinics of North America: Small Animal Practice* **15**, 289–295.

Voith, V.L. (1991): Applied animal behavior and the veterinary profession: a historical account. *Veterinary Clinics of North America: Small Animal Practice* **21**, 203–206.

Young, M.S. (1985): The evolution of domestic pets and companion animals. *Veterinary Clinics of North America: Small Animal Practice* **15**, 297–309.

2 Pets in the Human Family

Biologically speaking, the first type of relationship between human beings of several thousand years ago and the ancestors of modern domestic dogs and cats was probably a *commensal* one – a type of association between two species where only one of them benefits and the other is not harmed. Food possibilities would have attracted wolf scavengers to the vicinity of hunter-gatherer campsites, and cats would have been drawn to early agricultural settlements by the large rodent population which such settlements supported. However, once young wild wolves were being regularly being adopted into and allowed to breed in hunter-gatherer bands, and cats had become welcome residents of agricultural communities, the interspecies relationships had evolved into a form of *mutualism* – a type of symbiosis in which *both* species benefit from associating with one another.

The benefits provided to animals in the earliest mutualistic associations between humans and the ancestors of modern dogs and cats were obvious: primarily food but also shelter and protection (e.g. against predators and perhaps hostile conspecifics). But as is common in mutualistic relationships in the animal world, there would have been a certain degree of asymmetry in these early relationships, with the animals obtaining primarily food and human beings profiting mainly from other benefits associated with tame wolves as campsite guardians and hunting assistants and cats as rodent controllers. In considering the relationship between human families and their pets today, it is the nature of these "other benefits" provided to human beings which is the interesting question. For while farm cats are still valued by farmers for their ability to hold down the rodent population and city watchdogs still protect the human members of their family against poten-

tially harmful strangers, these benefits which were crucial during the early stages of the development the human-pet mutualistic relationship have become increasingly less important. So much so that in today's modern industrialized societies, they are best regarded as additional benefits which pet keeping provides to some owners.

Why do people in our modern society world who don't feel the need for protection or have a rodent pest problem still keep dogs or cats as household pets? The survey of the German pet-owning population described in detail in the next chapter confirms the results of a survey of American pet owners reported by Voith (1985): most modern society pet owners view their animals not as useful servants, but rather as *family members* whose primary benefit is social and not economic. In the German pet-owning population too, people talk to their pets every day. Almost half of them confide in their pets "about important matters at least once a month". They take their pets with them (particularly dogs) on vacations. They share snacks with them. They allow animals (particularly cats) to sleep in their beds and use all areas of the home at will. And the animals are often touched and petted and sometimes even hugged and kissed in much the same way as human children.

Interviewing pet owners at length – as behavior problem counselors must always do – is revealing, for it makes it clear just how much pets mean to their owners and how strongly owners feel emotionally attached to them. Why keep a pet which is making so many problems? If asked this, most owners of problem pets will unhesitatingly reply "because I love him". Obviously, it is the socially rewarding aspects of pet ownership that have become most crucial to the human side of the human-pet relationship. This in turn is often explained by pointing to the therapeutic role pets play as surrogate children or friends for lonely people suffering under the somewhat "inhuman" social conditions which prevail in our modern societies. But there is surely more to it than this. For as anyone who has a lot to do with pet owners knows, pets provide precisely the same kind of social benefits with precisely the same powerful impact in big, healthy, happy human families in which no one seems to be lonely or suffering at all. The socially impoverished conditions under which many modern society residents live may indeed play a role in the formation and maintenance of strong bond relationships between particularly lonely owners and their pets. However, their role is at most contributory – only one of the factors which help account for modern pet-keeping practices.

The human parental behavior system

The primary thesis which will be developed in this section to help account for modern pet-keeping practices is that the behavior of modern pet owners towards their dogs and cats not only resembles human parental behavior, it *is* parental behavior – in this case directed not towards a human child, but rather towards the member of another species displaying evolutionary modifications of its ancestral behavioral characteristics whose primary function is to effectively elicit human parental behavior. The biological term for the evolution of physical and/or behavioral resemblances to other species – or objects, in the case of insects which have evolved to look like leaves or sticks – is *mimicry*. It would be going too far to describe the modern domestic dog or cat as a child-mimic. However, a similar kind of evolutionary development as that which produces mimicry in the animal world may have been involved. Of course, dogs and cats don't look anything like children, but their puppy-like or kitten-like playfulness, non-aggressiveness and submissiveness, desire for physical contact with us, frequent following, food-begging, and attention- and play-soliciting behavior, looking to-

wards us for protection and reassurance in anxiety-arousing situations, and apparent total dependence on us and distinctly personal relationship with us as individuals are all characteristics which have obvious parallels in the behavior of a child towards its parent.

Of course, some of these general pet behavioral characteristics like following us and begging for food might be seen in any wild animal raised from birth by human beings. However, direct comparisons of wolves and dogs, as well as what can be inferred concerning differences between domesticated and wild cats, indicate that certain behavioral characteristics have evolved during the domestication process which, in effect, have made these animals not only easier to keep and manage, but also turned them into more appealing and emotionally satisfying companions for human beings. One of the major findings of the comparative research project described in detail in Chapter 7 (Zimen, 1988), for example, was the identification of many ways in which the behavior of adult dogs resembles the behavior of juvenile rather than adult wolves. In effect, direct support was provided for the hypothesis that one of the outcomes of the domestication process which turned wolves into domestic dogs was *neoteny* – the retaining into adulthood of juvenile behavioral characteristics.

While not nearly as marked as in dogs, some evolutionary changes in cat behavior which are thought to be domestication-related such as continuing to display kitten-like playfulness into adulthood, head and flank rubbing against owners' legs, kneading with forepaws when being held on owners' laps, and frequent physical contact-seeking and food-soliciting behavior resembling that which kittens or juveniles might direct towards their mother can be viewed in the same way: as reflecting neotenous evolutionary adaptations which primarily function to make animals into more appealing pets.

Assuming that no new behavioral system has evolved during the past several thousand years of human history to account for human pet-keeping behavior – which is tantamount to making the biologically reasonable assumption that our behavior towards our pets is a reflection of the operation of behavioral systems which were designed for other purposes – the question of which of our basic behavioral systems is involved arises.

Human beings display several types of relationships with the members of other animal species. They kill predators to protect themselves when attacked, they hunt and kill animals for food, they kill animals like rats, wolves, etc. which compete with them for food, and modern farmers first raise and then kill animals for food. This latter case presents some interesting variants. Consider, for example, large-scale ranchers with thousands of head of cattle. Their animals are treated by them with a combination of the systems of behavior human beings use to defend and care for their possessions as well as to locate and kill prey. But what about the small peasant farmer family which raises one single pig each year to provide the year's supply of sausage. This animal too is cared for and defended like any other valuable possession, and then killed and eaten. But here the relationship the family has with the pig is more personal. They may feel a certain amount of affection for it. They may feel it has its own personality, a unique one which makes it noticeably different from the pigs of previous years. And when the time comes for the slaughter, they may feel a tinge of sadness because after all, for many months now the pig has been almost like a member of the family.

As mentioned previously, virtually all pet owners answer with an immediate and unqualified yes to the question of whether they consider their pet to be a member of the family. This is, in fact, part and parcel of the phenomenon of pet keeping in families which seek help from pet behavior problem counselors: taking animals into the family home and caring for them and treating them to some extent as if they were human members of the family. Most owners also claim to love their pets dearly and say they would be heartbroken if they died or ran away. And like relationships between human family members, the relationship between owner and pet is extremely personal on the part of the owner. The attachment is to one particular dog or cat individual, one with its own distinctive appearance and personality. Replacing a dog which has died with another may help a pet owner to more quickly get over the loss of a much-loved pet, but in the first days and perhaps weeks after the loss, the new animal does not really function as an effective substitute the way, for example, that a new car would function as a fully adequate and possibly superior replacement after the family's car has been stolen.

In short, the family dog or cat *is* a member of its human family. And if you ask owners to think about the relationship they have with their pet, and kinds of feelings they have for it, and then decide what kind of family member it is most like in human terms, they were surely say it's most like a child rather than, for example, husband, brother, or any other human family relationship possibility.

Our pet's dependence on us for everything it needs is indeed child-like. And we take a similar kind of responsibility for *nurturing* it, *protecting* it, providing it with *leadership, teaching* or training it, and confirming and strengthening its special *bond relationship* to us (e.g. by responding positively to its approaches and encouraging physical contact with us) as we do with our own children. We feel emotionally attached to our pets too. So much so that we love them, grieve when they are ill, and unselfishly expend our time, energy, and financial resources to try and keep them not only healthy but also happy in much the same way as we do with our own children. Finally, the fact that childless people often openly admit that their pets function as life-enhancing child-substitutes which they can cuddle, fuss over, take on vacations, talk to, etc. also provides support for the hypothesis that it is the *parental behavioral system* which primarily determines modern society pet owners' behavior and feelings towards their pets.

Pets as children

The parallels between how parents behave towards their children and pets are certainly close enough to suggest that our behavior towards our pets is essentially parental behavior. But in comparing human behavior towards children and pets, another rather obvious conclusion can be drawn. Namely, that behavior towards pets is most definitely a *modified* form of human parental behavior which varies from normal parental behavior towards children in some very crucial ways.

In the first place, what could be termed the strength of motivation differs. While most people would give up their fortunes or risk their lives to save the lives of their children, few people would do the same for their pets. Indeed when it comes to a choice between preserving the family's carpets or keeping a dog with an apparently insoluble housebreaking, even the most loving owner normally decides that the dog must go. Such "selfish" behavior towards one's own child is of course unthinkable. The motivation to protect and nurture children at all costs is far too strong. It seem clear therefore that pets are comparatively much weaker elicitors of human parental behavior than human children – biologically speaking, not at all surprising given the great physical appearance and behavioral differences between a pet and a human child.

In addition, there are also obvious differences in the specific behaviors shown by human beings when nurturing, protecting, training, leading, etc. their pets and children. Dogs are fed different sorts of food on a different kind of schedule than children. Dogs are not covered by their owners in their beds at night. Few owners dress their dogs in clothes even on the coldest days. And even though dogs may be talked to, bathed, petted, hugged, and taken on trips like a child, the actual sequences of behavior performed by human beings differ drastically both qualitatively (e.g. most owners find kissing their dogs somewhat repulsive) and quantitatively from the similar types of behavior directed towards children. Here too, these differences in the specific behaviors towards children and dogs aren't surprising. Saying that human beings treat their dogs to some extent like they treat their children is of course not at all to say that people don't notice the differ-

ence, or that this difference isn't crucial to determining specific features of their behavior. People know and indeed behave as if dogs are dogs and not children. But it is nevertheless also true that in terms of biological fundamentals, it is modified parental behavior rather than behavior from one of the other major behavioral systems found in our species' ethogram (i.e. catalogue of characteristic behavior patterns) which human beings are displaying towards their pets.

Particularly interesting differences between behavior towards children and dogs are found in the area of teaching. On the most general functional level, teaching or training children and dogs is the same. The adult *monitors* the behavior of child or dog, *compares* this behavior to some sort of "cognitive model" or internal representation of what this behavior should *ideally* be like, and then does whatever is required to *modify* the behavior to make it correspond more closely to this cognitive model by using the various teaching/training strategies.

Of course, an obvious major child-versus-pet difference in this area involves the detailed features of the cognitive model of desirable or normal behavior. No one tries to train their dog to behave like a child. But what one does try to do is modify the dog's behavior when disparities between one's conception of *ideal* dog behavior (e.g. a good dog should come immediately when called) and *real* dog behavior (e.g. Fido comes only when he's good and ready) indicate that such an effort is needed. In other words, it is at the level of the owner's cognitive conception of normal or desirable dog behavior versus normal or desirable child behavior where the major difference in the teaching/training area is seen.

There are obviously great differences in what specifically is taught to dogs and children. Consider, for example, the language, cultural customs, and tool-use behaviors which must be taught to children. But there are some very close parallels too. Both child and dog are taught to cross streets in particular ways, to come without delay when called, and to otherwise react obediently when commanded. And they are taught in a somewhat similar way. They are scolded for misbehavior, rewarded or can avoid punishment for correct behavior, and shown – via demonstration or symbolic language with the child, and by physically moving or manipulating the dog – what kind of behavior is required when this helps the training process. Essentially, the general behavioral modification tactics used in managing the behavioral development of the child and dog are similar in a number of respects.

However, the fact that one can use symbolic language to instruct a child obviously makes a big difference when trying to shape complex behavior like, for example, how to operate tools. Information concerning the target behavior and where present behavioral shortcomings lie can be easily transmitted to the child. This in turn has the effect of directly modifying the internal processes that control the child's behavior so that errors can be reduced and behavior improved without the kind of step-by-step training process required for animals. With animals, the trainer can only "describe" what he wants indirectly, by the timing of rewards and punishments – or by physically manipulating the animal in some way. Thus, training a dog to perform even a simple behavior such as lying down in response to a verbal command can be relatively laborious compared to what is necessary to first elicit a similar behavioral response from, say, a 3-year-old child.

Interestingly, even though one can't really explain to a dog in words how exactly it should behave when it hears "down", observe the frustrated owner who is having trouble getting this message through to the dog using hand gestures, pushing down on the dog's back, or trying to coax it to lie down by dangling a tidbit in front of its nose. Even though the owner knows perfectly well that the dog isn't a human being and doesn't understand the meaning of the words it is hearing, the verbal explanation tendency which is a major component of human parental teaching behavior often surfaces: "Oh come on! Just move your front paws a little forward like this. That's right. Good! Now just...". Here, as in many other contexts in which owners talk to their dogs, the fundamental *hu-man-to-human* nature of the social behavior exhibited is obvious.

Implications for the treatment of behavior problems

The hypothesis that pet owners display parental behavior towards their pets which parallels in many ways that which is elicited by human children is of paramount importance to the veterinary pet behavior problem counselor. The remainder of this chapter illustrates the relevance of this view to both understanding the family context in which pet behavior problems occur and determining the specific type of advice which is required to help owners cope with their pets' problem behaviors.

Why pet owners put up with so many minor behavior problems

Given the many minor behavior problems which awkward, unskilled, untrained young children bring with them such as spilling milk, eliminating in the wrong place at the wrong time, destroying things, and not doing what they're told, it is not surprising that the basically "parental" owner is not at all daunted by a pet's minor behavior problems like stealing food, disobedience, or scratching or chewing on valuable household objects. One might even argue that being a problem in minor, basically tolerable ways helps make pets even more child-like. Certainly most owners take minor problems as a matter of course and are very patient in this regard. And in talking with pet owners, one sometimes gets the feeling that these minor faults are viewed almost positively – as signs that the pet is indeed a unique individual in its own right, with its own unique personality, its own unique strengths, and its own unique problems – just like the rest of us.

Why the world is full of "experts" on how owners should treat their pets

This is of course one of the behavior counselor's major problems. For not only do owners themselves have strong ideas about how people should treat their pets, but they are surrounded by countless relatives, immediate family members, friends, neighbors, pet book writers, animal breeders, and helpful assistants in veterinary practices or animal shelters who also regard themselves as born experts on this topic. The contradictory and often astonishingly bad advice owners receive from these other sources is one of the primary reasons why people may not entirely accept the behavior counselor's explanation and comply with his/her advice.

The interesting question here is this: where exactly does all of this "expertise" come from? What is the source of this great fountain of wisdom? And how is it that all who eagerly offer such advice can do so with such complacent self-confidence?

One reason is that having had pets before which exhibited no serious problems may fuel people's conviction that they are one of those unusual people that have that special knack – that instinctive something that tells them what to do and what not to do – of how best to handle pets. That they were one of the lucky ones who just happened by chance to obtain a pet which, like the overwhelming majority of pets, can adjust to all of the demands of our human-oriented world without showing serious problems never occurs to them. Indeed, it is highly experienced pet owners who are most shaken when one of their pets turns out to be a problem in spite of their confident feeling of having done what they have always known with something approaching absolute certainty were the right things all along.

The second reason for the boundless self-confidence of the world's many millions of amateur behavior problem experts is more subtle but probably much more powerful. In behaving "instinctively" towards animals by doing what comes entirely naturally, owners are essentially relying on their parental behavioral system and therefore reacting similarly to how they might react towards a young child in similar circumstances. If a dog shows fearful behavior in a new situation, they talk to it, pick it up, pet it, and try to comfort and reassure it as one would a small child. And when the

counselor points out to them that such reactions may be rewarding and hence, in the long run, increase the animal's fearful behavior, they are at first shocked that what feels to them at the time to be obviously the right thing to do may do more harm than good.

Essentially, in treating pets like children, people are employing a behavioral system which is as ancient as the human species itself and – with regard to children at least – has withstood the evolutionary test of time and proven itself to be highly effective and efficient. It is therefore no wonder that such basically parental behavioral reactions "feel right". Given these powerful feelings of instinctively knowing what is the right thing to do, and the virtually reflexive nature of many of the associated responses to the animal's behavior, it's no wonder that people tend to feel so confident in this regard.

Why owners sometimes try to reason with problem animals

This may or may not be verbal. Watch an owner of a stubborn dog which is fearful of crossing a street and refuses to budge even when the owner tugs on its leash. In such a situation, it is likely that at some point the owner will resort to a strategy which might well be effective with a young child by trying to convince the dog that there is nothing to be afraid of – by telling it just that in words, by pointing, by walking into the street to demonstrate how safe it is, and perhaps even by pleading a little. Owners laugh about this. They know it's silly. But they admit that they do or have done such things now and then all the same. Thus, here too is another example of how the fundamental parent-to-child character of many owner-pet interactions can surface in spite of the owner's intellectual realization that this is probably a rather foolish way to deal with the problem.

Why applying certain kinds of corrective treatment measures feels cruel to owners

How often do counselors see owners' mouths gape adding surprise to the look of alarm on their faces when the counselor recommends, for example, that their dog should no longer be allowed on the furniture ("Not even on *his* chair?") or worse, that it should be totally ignored whenever it comes to be petted. While people may not express their reservations openly, and although one may apparently convince them during the consultation that this kind of treatment measure would be extremely helpful, whether or not they will follow the advice later is another matter. Some owners do indeed do so, but they must harden themselves somewhat to do it. For treating their pet this way *feels wrong* – as heartless and cruel as it would feel to ignore a young child who comes running up with outstretched arms to be picked up and hugged.

In giving such advice to owners of dominant aggressive dogs, for example, it is especially important that the counselor deal openly with owners' feelings in this regard, for compliance with the recommended treatment can only be assured by convincing owners to "go against their instincts" and treat their dogs in ways in which it would indeed be heartless and cruel to treat their young child.

Why certain kinds of behavioral interactions with pets feel so pleasurable to owners – and why they don't want to give them up

Why should it feel good to pet a dog or a cat? The answer is not just the tactual stimuli which are involved, for let's face it: holding an old fur coat on one's lap and petting it while watching TV isn't quite as satisfying.

When instructed by the behavior counselor to pet their animal only very briefly as a reward for following commands, some owners may very well not comply; for fondling their animal is one of the joys of owning a pet which owners are often very reluctant to give up entirely or even partially. Biologically speaking, the self-rewarding quality of such stroking, patting, fondling, etc. behavior is only understandable if one assumes that parental behavior is involved – that petting a dog feels good because of whatever makes it feel good to "pet" one's child. That it's indeed right and natural to pet

one's child is beyond dispute. But treating one's pet like a child in this respect may not at all be desirable for some problems like dominance aggression in dogs where such owner behavior may give the dog the wrong message concerning its position in the family social structure. When this is the case and one must try to convince owners to stop doing what comes so naturally and feels so right and good to them, behavior counselors only stand a chance when they know what they are up against: the owner as loving parent to the family's furry, four-legged child.

How this parental behavior conception helps to explain the course of development of some behavioral problems

Some people have trouble saying no to their pets in much the same way – and for much the same reason – as they have trouble saying no to their children. Biologically speaking, responding positively to a child's request is often tantamount to meeting its need for some important resource or behavioral assistance – and meeting such needs too is basically self-rewarding parental behavior. But when elicited by pets, such laudable parental behavior can cause problems. When owners just can't seem to say no to a pet and mean it, having to get up in the middle of the night to keep a bored cat company, or having to constantly interrupt a conversation with another person to keep a dog quiet by playing with it, may be the result.

The development of these kinds of begging or attention-getting problems as well as certain other dog disobedience and dominance-related problems seems to be at least partially explainable in terms of the effects of such inappropriate parental behavior where owners are just trying to be good and fair to their animal by unselfishly complying with its requests much the way they always do or did with their own children.

Why owners take criticism so personally

If is assumed that behavior towards pets is essentially human parental behavior, then it is easy to understand why owners tend to be especially sensitive to criticism in this regard; for by explaining that behavior problems are the result of mistakes on their part, one runs the risk of implying that they have been bad parents – which tends to hit people about as hard as they can be hit.

In problem cases, the counselor should avoid making blanket condemnations of owners for treating their pets like children for two reasons. In the first place, such treatment usually does no harm to the animal at all. It's the owner who suffers the consequences, not the pet. And secondly, one stands a far better chance of eliciting the cooperation (i.e. compliance) of owners if, instead of essentially implying "you have been a bad parent", one says something like "It's not always easy to know what is the right thing to do with a somewhat difficult animal like you have". Besides, it's far closer to the truth in most cases. Most commonly, behavioral problems are the result of an inherently "difficult" animal's reaction to prevailing conditions which are more or less normal in modern families. If treating animals like children was really as undesirable and harmful as some critics of this practice maintain, the problem pet would be the rule rather than the exception.

Eliciting the support of the parent in the owner

As a general rule, it can probably be stated that treatment recommendations which are designed to enlist and essentially take advantage of human parental motivation are superior to those which attempt to counteract or weaken it. For example, arguing that castrating a male dog to control intermale aggression or urine marking will also probably have positive effects on the quality of its life – by reducing sexual motivation and thereby reducing frustration stemming from its being prevented from engaging in normal mating activities – is an argument which may help to convince some owners who initially find the idea of castration distasteful. Another example is the advice given with fear problems in dogs. In trying to convince owners of fearful dogs to ignore their pitiful shivering,

shaking, crouching animals on the street, it helps to emphasize that the owners' well-meaning attempts to reassure and comfort their dog are actually making the dog's problem worse by in some sense telling it that there is indeed something to be afraid of. And finally, by being what owners initially often regard as heartless or cruel to the dominant-aggressive dog by turning it off the furniture, banning it from the family bedrooms, and ignoring it when it comes for attention and petting, one is likely to end up with a more relaxed, less nervous, less restless, and seemingly happier dog. Therefore, the message to get across to owners in this case is that if they want to *really* do what's best for their dog (i.e. be a good parent), they must change their ways even though they are not so comfortable about doing it.

Dealing with owners is like dealing with parents

As a pet behavior problem counselor, one is in a better position to understand the dynamics of the family situation and provide effective help to owners when one understands that they are highly motivated to be good parents to their animals whether we like it or approve of it or not. To simply sit back and criticize their behavior and related feelings as if they represented some kind of human frailty or egotistical vice which should be vigorously combated is naive and counterproductive. For human parental motivation is the driving force behind and very reason for existence of the human-pet relationship. And practically speaking, such a critical viewpoint is a luxury the behavior problem counselor simply can't afford. One can't tell owners to change their basic instincts any more than one can tell them to move to a larger apartment. It's part and parcel of the set of prevailing conditions within which the behavior counselor must operate.

References

Grier, J.W., and Burk, T. (1992): *Biology of Animal Behavior.* 2nd edition. St. Louis, Missouri, Mosby – Year Book, Inc.

Voith, V.L. (1985): Attachment of people to companion animals. *Veterinary Clinics of North America: Small Animal Practice* **15**, 289–295.

Zimen, E. (1988): *Der Hund.* München, C. Bertelsmann Verlag

3 Nature of Dog and Cat Behavior Problems

The view of dog and cat behavioral problems which is common among members of the general public and echoed in the press, popular pet books, and by people who try to use the pet behavior phenomenon to advance the animal rights cause is that such problems are a reflection of owner mistreatment, either direct mistreatment or indirect mistreatment by forcing the animal to live in an impoverished or stressful environment.

The function of this chapter is to examine both the element of truth and the more significant element of untruth in this view with the aim of developing a more balanced and productive general perspective from which to view the range of fascinating animal behavioral phenomena and family problems with which the pet behavior problem counselor is confronted.

Can one identify certain general types of pet behavior problems? This is not an easy task, for a simple ethological classification system which focuses solely on the biological function of the problem behavior is not as helpful to understanding the general nature of pet behavior problems as the ethologist might assume. The major difficulty in this regard is that the notion of a pet behavioral problem is a relative one: pet behavior problems can only be characterized and understood relative to the human environmental context in which they occur. As a simple example, take the case of a dog with a high activity level. For an elderly owner whose top walking speed is about 1/2 mph, whose maximum range is a few city blocks, and who gets nervous when his/her dog restlessly paces around in the home, the dog's high activity level is a serious problem. Not so, however, for the hobby marathon runner who takes the dog along on his/her daily 20-mile jaunt. Here the problem might be quite the opposite: the dog is too lazy to keep up. Obviously, in both cases "the problem" is not the animal's behavior per se, but rather *the problem that this behavior poses for its owner.*

Take another example: urine marking in cats. Here too, it's the human being who has the problem, not the cat. Or more precisely, the cat is performing some species-typical behavior that is fully normal and natural but which nevertheless is so unacceptable to owners that they may have the cat euthanized because of it. As a final example, consider territorial aggression in dogs. In one very common scenario, the young puppy barks at strangers and is rewarded for this by its owner who likes the idea that it will turn out to be a good watchdog later. A time comes, however, when the dog begins becoming more aggressive to strangers, barking and snarling menacingly and perhaps even attacking them. But for a combination of reasons related to the people's lack of experience training and controlling animals, their personalities, their beliefs about the rights and wrongs of treating animals in particular ways, the dog's level of aggressiveness generally, its tendency to accept or resist owner authority in a variety of circumstances, and the extent to which it has been trained to follow commands and inhibit aggression in the past, the owners do not know how to bring the behavior under control. Commonly, their control attempts may even make the problem worse; for example, when owners use petting, food tidbits, or ball throwing to distract the dog in problem situations and thereby inadvertently reward the aggressive behavior. In this example too, the problem is not aggression towards strangers per se, for aggression directed towards a threatening stranger is desirable behavior and therefore not a problem for owners. In this latter case, it would be *not* aggressively defending home and family against a hostile intruder that would be the problem.

In Parts II and III of this book, the conventional way of classifying dog and cat behavior problems in functional categories such as defensive aggression, elimination behavior, and sexual behavior will be followed. This is indeed the most logical organizational structure for discussing the various types of dog and cat behavior problems. But when it comes to this chapter's aim of understanding the general nature of pet behavior problems, another sort of classification scheme is required which stresses the various factors which cause such problems to develop.

One approach to the question of the etiology of behavior problems is presented by Borchelt and Voith (1982). They present a diagram in which behavior is classified as "normal" or "abnormal", with normal behavior classified as "instinctive" and "learned" and abnormal behavior is classified into "pathophysiologic" and "experiential". The latter two categories are then broken down further into "hereditary" vs. "acquired" and "early experience" vs. "psychosomatic" respectively. This system contains major elements which must be represented in any etiological classification system. Namely, that some problem behaviors are a reflection of hereditary or acquired disease conditions, learned as a result of particular environmental experiences, reflect a lack of learning because of inadequate early experience, or are genetically-preprogrammed or "instinctive" in the sense that they develop no matter what kind of experiences the animal has had.

While sound as far as it goes, this relatively simple classification scheme does not take us very far when trying to characterize the general nature of pet behavior problems. The reason it falls short is that it focuses almost exclusively on the animal's behavior alone and therefore strictly equates the question of the etiology of the problem to that of the etiology of the pet's behavior problem. However, to understand the nature of behavior problems, the problem behavior must be conceptualized from the start in a way which does not separate and isolate it from its *environmental context*; for this is a crucial dimension in characterizing behavior problems and understanding why they develop.

While it may be obvious that an animal's fear of strangers has been learned – in the sense that the animal would not have been this way had it been exposed to other sorts of environmental conditions during its lifetime – the animal may be this way because of mistreatment suffered at the hands of strangers, lack of experience with strangers early in life, or the occurrence of some frightening event in the presence of a stranger. In effect, specifying *how* and *why* the fear has developed must also be considered in any descriptive or etiological account of the behavior.

The environmental context is relevant in another, entirely different sort of way as well. A cat's killing birds that its owner lovingly feeds may represent a major problem. The behavior is fully normal, instinctive cat behavior, but simply saying so is not enough; for "the problem" here may be basically the owner's lack of understanding of normal cat behavior or the incompatibility of the cat's normal behavior with the demands of its present human-oriented environmental context.

In short, what is required is to focus not only on the descriptive and etiological characterization of the animal's behavior per se, but also on the descriptive and etiological characterization of the associated *problem situation* as well – and therefore on how and why the animal's behavior has become a problem for its owners.

Nature of pet behavior problem situations

The following paragraphs describe the most common types of problems in a way which emphasizes physiological, genetic, and/or environmental etiological factors. The aim here is to give the reader a preliminary overview of the diverse nature of the types of problems and related problem situations which are subsumed under the general rubric of pet behavior problems.

Problems symptomatic of a pathophysiological disorder

Pathophysiological disorders like toxicoses, neurological disease, cardiovascular disease, inflammatory and infectious disease, metabolic disease, parasite infestations, trauma, etc. can lead to minor or serious behavior problems such as lethargy, anorexia, hyperexcitability, excessive grooming, aggression, elimination in the home, self-mutilation, and others (Reisner, 1991; Voith, 1989). Such problems are suspected when the behavior problem is of recent origin, does not appear to be an understandable response to the prevailing environmental conditions, involves what appears to be a "personality change" in the animal, and shows some major symptoms which are inconsistent with any of the usual, purely behavioral problems.

Problems symptomatic of restricted early experiences

Several common types of behavior problems are symptomatic of the lasting, only partially irreversible effects of a young animal's spending the first two or three months of life in an environment which is limited in some crucial way. Although similar effects are sometimes seen in cats, this early experience effect is most common in dogs which (1) had little experience with human strangers or children during the second and third months of life and therefore react fearfully towards them their whole life long, (2) were taken away from their litter much too early and later fear other dogs, or behave as if they do not recognize them as conspecifics, or (3) have spent the first few months of their life in quiet, secluded rural locations and later cannot comfortably adjust to life in the bustling, noisy city environment.

Problems symptomatic of present environmental deficiencies/stress

As is the case with similar behavior problems in farm and zoo animals, excessive grooming (sometimes to the point of self-mutilation), various repetitive, stereotyped behaviors like pacing, snapping at imaginary flies, staring at the wall, tail chasing, repetitive barking, and many others are sometimes revealed to be a reaction to some present environmental deficiency associated with inadequate opportunities for phy-

sical exercise or interactions with conspecifics, continuous exposure to aversive stimuli of any sort, or other aspects of the surrounding environment such as a lack of stability or features arousing conflicting motivations.

Problems symptomatic of past exposure to intense aversive environmental stimuli

Conditioned fear and defensive aggression problems which do not stem from overly restricted early experience are very common in companion animals. Cats may come to fear owners who punish them, young children who make too much noise or chase and catch them, or other cats which have attacked them. And dogs often become fearful when too harshly punished, teased by children, inadvertently mistreated by very young children, attacked by other dogs, involved in a traffic accident, or exposed to loud, frightening noises like fireworks or thunderstorms.

Problems primarily resulting from a lack of required behavioral training

Some dogs become very unruly and difficult to control during walks, steal food, chew shoes and other household objects, direct aggressive play towards owners, or continue eliminating in the home if not properly trained. Such problems may be minor or secondary to other behavior problems, or they may be major and the reason for contacting a behavior problem specialist.

Problems primarily resulting from unintentional owner fostering/reinforcement

In direct contrast to problems stemming from a lack of training, some owners unintentionally "train" their dogs or cats to perform problem behaviors. Most common are problem situations in which begging (for food, playing, or attention) and other pushy, demanding forms of dog or cat behavior have been so often rewarded that they have developed into well-entrenched habits which are extremely difficult to eliminate. Other types of problems falling into this general category are where owners encourage or tolerate basically harmless aggression towards human strangers in a young dog which develops into a severe problem later, exacerbate dominance-related disputes between family dogs by giving preferential treatment to the underdog, or inadvertently turn their baby or small child into a conditioned aversive stimulus by paying much less attention to the dog whenever the child is present.

Problems involving unacceptable forms of species-typical behavior

Normal species-typical behavior a problem for owner

Normal species-typical behavior which is not unusual (e.g. overly intense, inappropriate to the situation) in any way can nevertheless be a problem for some owners. Examples are problems with predatory behavior, playful aggression towards humans, and furniture scratching in cats, and chewing problems, coprophagia, intermale aggression between animals in the same home, and high activity levels in dogs.

Intensity of species-typical behavior inappropriate

Animals may essentially be showing normal species-typical behavior which is unusually intense and a problem for this reason. This is sometimes the case, for example, with territorial aggression in dogs and playful aggression in both dogs and cats.

Species-typical behavior elicited by inappropriate stimuli

Many problems involve cases of species-typical behavior which is a problem because it is being elicited in inappropriate situations or directed towards inappropriate stimuli. Urine marking in both cats and dogs, for example, is acceptable outdoors but a problem inside the home. Another example is dominance aggression towards human family members in dogs. Here, the dog's dangerously aggressive behavior

would be fully understandable and appropriate if directed towards another dog.

Summary comments

Three aspects of this general characterization of the nature of the major types of dog and cat problems/problem situations require special comment. The first is that there are many different types of problems or problem situations which essentially have nothing in common with one another beyond the mere fact that they involve behavior on the part of the pet which poses a problem for owners. This in turn implies that theories concerning the nature and causes of pet problems must necessarily be confined to specific problem types. Popular notions of the nature and causes of pet behavior problems such as those discussed later in the chapter are therefore doomed to failure from the start.

The second aspect requiring comment is that these various types of problems and problem situations are not mutually exclusive. While the source of an animal's fear of strangers may be lack of experience with strangers during the first few weeks of life, owners may inadvertently strengthen fearful behavior by exposing the animal to strangers or trying to combat the fear by comforting or distracting the animal when it reacts fearfully. Similarly, conditioned fear may be increased by an owner who uses excessively intense or frequent punishment to attempt to control the animal's behavior. Additionally, the animal's fearful behavior – while a problem – may be a normal, species-typical behavior which is fully appropriate to the environmental circumstances. It is clear, therefore, that these types of problems or problem situations differ mainly in terms of what kinds of factors seem to be the primary, root causes which give problems of one type or another their own distinctive character.

And finally, while it is always true that some type of animal behavior that represents a problem for owners is involved, the nature of *the problem* which must be addressed by treatment recommendations differs considerably from problem to problem. Sometimes the problem is best conceptualized in a way which places more emphasis on the owner's rather than the pet's behavior as is the case with behavior problems caused by unintentional owner fostering/reinforcement. With behavior problems symptomatic of present environmental deficiency/stress, the animal's present environment is the problem which must be addressed. In the case of behavior problems related to physiological disorders or reflecting conditioned fear or restricted early experience, the problem which must be addressed by the treatment lies in the animal's body – either in terms of some pathophysiological disorder or some long-term effect of past experience now stored or represented in some way in the animal's nervous system. And finally, the last major type of problem, unacceptable species-typical behavior, is again quite different from the others. Here, the problem essentially involves a combination of factors which is best characterized by focusing on the relationship between the animal's behavior and its human-oriented environmental context. Most commonly, the animal displays some undesirable (for people) behavioral tendency, the owner fails to respond correctly, and the undesirable behavior worsens instead of improves. Thus, it is a case here of an animal requiring a relatively special kind of owner treatment or surrounding environment – compared to that given to the average pet – if its behavior is to be kept within acceptable bounds. To accomplish this objective, changes in the owner's behavior towards the animal, changes in the animal's environment, and/or direct changes in the animal's behavioral tendencies themselves via special training procedures, castration, or drugs may be required. Many pet behavioral problems fall into this latter category where the pet's natural behavioral tendencies, the owner's treatment of the pet, and the environment in which the problem behavior occurs all fall within the range of the normal, and where the problem which needs to be addressed and remedied is somehow associated with a *complex interaction of all of these factors*.

Particularly this latter case highlights the fact that it is the problem situation as a whole and not merely the animal's problem behavior which the pet behavior counselor must address. In discussing with owners the various problems they are having with their pets, one is necessarily dealing with a real-world situation involving highly intricate relationships between the members of two different species occurring within the context of a complex, changeable, sometimes unpredictable social and physical environment. This is the dynamic, exceedingly complex, and often emotionally-charged situation which the pet behavior counselor confronts in every problem case. And it is the pet behavior counselor's skill in identifying aspects of this complex situation that are causally related to the animal's behavior problem and recommending practically feasible ways the owner can modify or counteract them which determine the degree to which the counselor can provide the client with the help required.

Specific causal factors

In analyzing these complex, real-world problem situations, many specific features are often identified as being causally connected with the pet's problem behavior. What follows is a brief listing of those will be referred to again and again throughout the book. The purpose of doing so at this time is simply to round out this discussion of the general nature of dog and cat behavior problem situations by briefly summarizing the various specific ways in which a behavior problem may reflect the interaction of the animal's distinctive (genetically preprogrammed or experience-determined) behavioral tendencies, physiological state, and state of health with detailed features of the complex human-dominated environment in which it lives.

As mentioned above, there is a suspicion of a *pathophysiological disorder* in some cases, particularly where the onset of the problem is sudden and inexplicable on other grounds. *Inherited predispositions* and *hormonal influences* often need to be considered as possible causative factors in cases where animals seem usually highly motivated to perform problem behavior. *Past experience* plays an obvious role in most problem cases: animals may have been subjected to overly *restricted early experiences* with humans or environmental stimuli early in life, they may show a clear *lack of proper training* that most animals are given, they may have been subjected to *traumatic experiences* or subjected to frequent *mistreatment* which causes them to react fearfully or aggressively to their owners, they may have been *unintentionally rewarded* for problem behaviors by owners, or owners may have been doing something else to *unintentionally foster* the development of behavior problems. Often *erroneous beliefs* lead owners to react incorrectly to developing behavior problems. And the *care/maintenance conditions* provided by owners may be inadequate (e.g. dog not given needed opportunities for exercise) causing various kinds of deprivation, stress, or conflict effects. Sometimes animals show *social facilitation* effects, barking and becoming aggressive as a kind of imitative response to conspecifics. The general *nature of the owner-animal relationship* itself may be exerting a adverse effect on the animal in a variety of circumstances. And finally, the animal may be simply showing *normal species-specific behavior* which is a problem because it is incompatible with its surrounding human-oriented environment. This kind of basic incompatibility between normal animal behavior on the one hand, and the various requirements and demands of a human-oriented environment on the other, is a characteristic feature of many cases.

Critique of popular views on the causes of pet behavioral problems

Owners are *egotistical* and *self-centered*: they care too much about themselves and too little about the welfare of their pets. Owners are *exploitive*: they view their pet as means to satisfy their own needs and desires, and they do not hesitate to subject it to various hardships to get the satisfaction they are seeking. Owners are *ignorant* or they lack *common sense*: they don't understand what their pet needs and they

do the opposite of what they should do to cope with its problem behaviors. Owners are *irresponsible*: they don't try hard enough to give their pet what it needs, and they don't hesitate to dispose of it as soon as it becomes a liability.

That is one *human nature-related* view of why so many pets show behavior problems. The following is another view which regards a presumed epidemic-like increase in pet behavioral problems as a kind of *sociological* consequence of our problem-ridden modern society world. Our modern society environment is becoming increasingly impersonal and inhuman. More and more people are living alone in cramped, big city apartments, and they try to combat the resulting loneliness and alienation with pets which they can talk to, cuddle, sleep with, baby, etc. But for the pets, this situation can be disastrous. They are locked away alone in the home all day while their owners are at work. They are often left home alone in the evening and on weekends. They often cannot go outside, interact with other animals, or get the daily exercise they require. And when they begin to show problems in response to the stressful and impoverished environment to which they are being subjected, this only precipitates punishment, coldness, and other reactions from their neurotic owners, which make matters even worse.

Interestingly, I don't know of one pet behavior problem specialist anywhere in the world who subscribes to either of these two popular views in anything like the form or with anything like the critical emotional tone they are expressed here. Essentially, first-hand experience observing and dealing with the realities of the problem situations with which behavior counselors are confronted leads them to other conclusions.

In the first place, most animals seen by behavior counselors don't seem to be suffering in any obvious way, which is a major underlying premise of both of the above views. Although there are exceptions, most problems are highly specific to certain kinds of situations. Outside of these, the animals are indistinguishable from those in the normal pet population. They behave normally, they live the same kinds of lives as other pets, and they don't look or act any less happy or satisfied than other pets. Some individual pets may indeed be suffering (e.g. fearful animals), but as a whole, the population of problem pets appears to the behavior counselors who know it well to be not much different than the remainder of the pet population. And even if some differences could be established such as, for example, problem pets tending on average to be more anxious or excitable than members of the normal pet population, this would still be a far cry from the picture of the abused, suffering animals which the two popular views conjure up.

Secondly, behavior counselors do indeed run across owners who are unusually self-centered, exploitive, or irresponsible. Such people do exist and sometimes an animal's problem behavior is related to these owner characteristics. But this is certainly not the rule. By and large, the owners who contact behavior counselors seem to be more or less a cross-section of the general population. While one cannot completely rule out the possibility that there may be differences between the populations of owners of problem and non-problem pets in terms of selfishness, irresponsibility, and so on, such differences are certainly not as great as would be expected if these negative human personality or attitude characteristics were indeed the major cause of pet behavioral problems.

Essentially, to the pet behavior problem counselor, the vilification of the owners of problem pets inherent in the first popular view seems unjustified. Counselors tend to be sympathetic towards rather than critical of their clients. At worst, these owners have made mistakes in their treatment of their animals. But the mistakes they have made are basically the ones that all owners tend to make under similar circumstances such as petting a frightened animal or punishing a pet long after it has eliminated in the home.

The second popular view deserving of criticism is that of the would-be sociologist who argues that the increasing number of pet behavior problems is another symptom of what is wrong with our modern society environment. However, to my knowledge there is no evidence confirming the facts this view takes as self-evident: namely, that the pet behavioral problems are now much more common than they used to be, and that they are much more common in big cities than elsewhere. Although one hears more about pet behavioral problems than one used to, the whole idea of consulting pet problem specialists and treating pet behavioral problems is a new and rather fashionable one which receives a lot of press. In terms of basics, the second view doesn't differ all that much from the first in that it simply tries to explain why owners tend to end up mistreating animals the way the first view criticizes them of doing. If there is an element of truth in this popular view, however, it is probably not that there are more problems nowadays – or more in cities – but rather that people who live in cities may tend to be more educated and progressive and, hence, not as ready to simply do away with a problem pet as those who live in rural communities.

If general views of pet behavioral problems and their causes are to appear in the press, then the following would be far closer to the truth:

- It is not known whether the incidence of dog and cat behavior problems is higher now than it was several decades ago. If it is, it is probably because people nowadays tend more to try and cope with and live with problem animals than they used to.
- It is not known whether the incidence of such problems is higher in big cities than in rural areas. If such differences were detected, however, they might also reflect more enlightened and humane attitudes towards pets and their problem behaviors by city residents.
- Most pet behavioral problems are caused by a complex combination of the genetic and environmental factors which vary enormously from case to case and are otherwise not easy to characterize on the rather simple level in which matters are discussed in the popular press. Perhaps the most common scenario is an inherently difficult pet whose owners require the help of a behavior counselor to learn how to give it the special treat-

ment or training required to keep undesirable behavioral tendencies in check.

- Behavior counselors who have had a great deal of contact with the owners of problem pets do not notice any obvious differences between them and owners of normal, non-problem pets.

The results of two studies are relevant to this last point. Voith et al. (1992) analyzed responses of 711 dog owners to a questionnaire given to owners awaiting medical treatment for their animals in a university veterinary hospital. The questions asked how often dogs could sleep in bed with a member of the family, if they were allowed on a piece of furniture, how often they were given tidbits from the table while the family was eating, how often people shared snacks with them other than at mealtimes, how often they were taken on errands, how often owners took their dogs with them when they were going to be gone one night or longer, did they celebrate their dogs' birthdays, did they confide in their dogs by talking to them about problems or important events, did they con-

sider their dogs to be a member of the family, had the dogs been to obedience school or been trained by a professional obedience trainer, and did their dogs engage in any behavior which they considered to be a problem. If this latter question was answered affirmatively, the questionnaire asked the owner to explain what kind of problems these were.

This quote from the abstract of the Voith et al. (1992) study summarizes the major conclusion:

"...dogs whose owners interacted with them in an anthropomorphic manner, 'spoiled' them in certain ways, or did not provide obedience training were no more likely to engage in behaviors considered a problem by the owners than were dogs not viewed anthropomorphically, spoiled by their owner, or given obedience training." (p. 263)

Given that this sample was from the normal population of pets, it leaves open the possibility that there might be a difference in anthropomorphic attitudes and spoiling between this population – where behavior problems tend to be minor or easy to live with – and the popula-

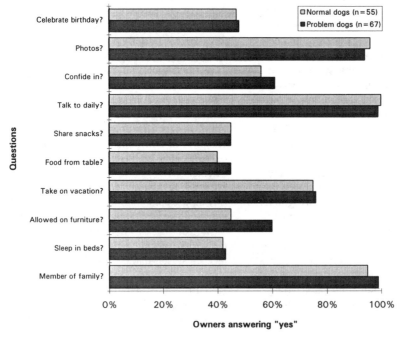

Figure 3.1: Comparison of answers to questions concerning anthropomorphizing and "spoiling" behavioral practices given by the owners of problematic and non-problematic (normal) dogs.

tion of problem dogs from which the animals seen by pet problem counselors come. To examine this possibility, I administered a questionnaire containing similar questions to the owners of 67 problem dogs and the owners of 55 normal, non-problem dogs whose owners were waiting for medical treatment for their animals in the waiting rooms of a number of Munich small animal practices. Figure 3.1 summarizes the results for the 10 questions presented in brief form along y-axis to which the owners were instructed to reply with "yes" or "no".

Problem dogs are allowed more often than normal, non-problem dogs on the furniture (15% higher). However, the profile of the answers to the remaining nine questions is remarkably similar given the widespread popular belief in both Germany and the United States that anthropomorphizing and spoiling dogs is the leading cause of behavior problems. Basically, this small-scale comparison of the owners of problem and normal dogs confirms the results of the Voith et al. (1992) study. In terms of these anthropomorphic attitudes and spoiling treatment practices, the two groups of owners do not differ to any noticeable degree.

This does not mean, however, that it makes no difference whether the owners of problem dogs spoil them or view and treat them anthropomorphically, as if they were human children.

To the contrary, the conventional, often very effective treatment for dominance aggression (see Chapter 10), for example, requires owners to abandon such treatment practices. But this in itself does not contradict the results of the above two surveys. Rather, it simply says that the normal, spoiling, anthropomorphizing treatment which many or most owners of problem *and* non-problem dogs tend to give their pets is contraindicated for dogs with this particular problem. If you will, that these are very special kinds of dogs which require a very special kind of treatment to reduce the seriousness of their behavior problems.

References

Borchelt, P.L., and Voith, V.L. (1982): Classification of animal behavior problems. *Veterinary Clinics of North America: Small Animal Practice* **12**, 571–585.

Reisner, I. (1991): The pathophysiologic basis of behavior problems. *Veterinary Clinics of North America: Small Animal Practice* **21**, 207–224.

Voith, V.L. (1989): Chapter 43: Behavioral disorders. In Ettinger, J.S. (ed): *Textbook of Veterinary Internal Medicine*. Philadelphia, W. B. Saunders Company.

Voith, V.L., Wright, J.C., and Danneman, P.J. (1992): Is there a relationship between canine behavior problems and spoiling activities, anthropomorphism, and obedience training? *Applied Animal Behaviour Science* **34**, 263–272.

4   The Consultation

Figure 4.1 represents a schematic diagram of the pet behavior problem counseling process. As the diagram suggests, the consultation represents an interchange between owner and counselor whose goal is to prepare owners to deal effectively with their animals' behavior problems in the following days, weeks, and months. While changing the animal's behavior is the ultimate goal of the pet behavioral counselor's efforts, the proximate goal and indeed the only means of ultimately resolving the problem is to *change the owner's behavior* and the various attitudes and beliefs which underlie it. Effectiveness as a pet behavioral counselor depends not only on the counselor's ability to understand and change animal behavior, but equally importantly on his/her ability to understand and change human behavior. In effect, not only the animal behavioral scientist's skills are required, but also those of the psychologist or family counselor called in to help people cope with family problems whose solution require behavioral changes on the part of some or all of the family members.

Regardless of whether the consultation takes place in the client's home or the counselor's office, or whether it is the only contact between client and counselor or the first of a series of contacts taking place over a number of weeks, the structure of the consultation is the same.

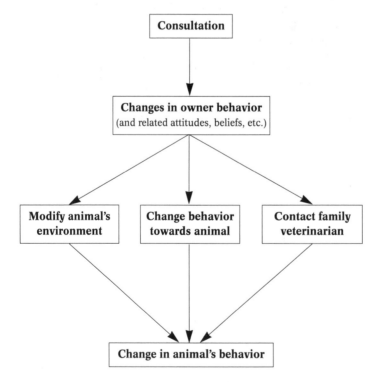

Figure 4.1: Schematic diagram of the pet behavior problem counseling process. For family veterinarians treating behavior problems, the "contact family veterinarian" feature of the model obviously doesn't apply.

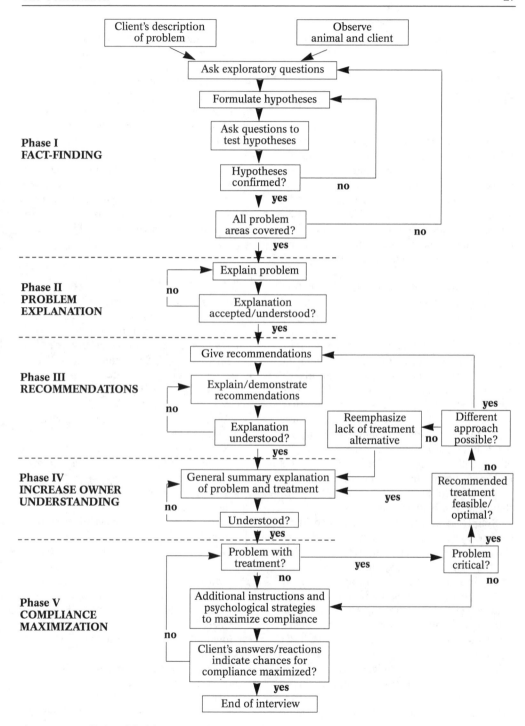

Figure 4.2: Detailed model of the course of a pet behavior problem consultation

Figure 4.2 presents a detailed model of a pet behavior problem consultation describing the course of the meeting between client and counselor.

Phase I: Fact-finding

This phase begins as soon as clients enter the counselor's office or open the front door and invite the counselor inside their home; for observations of the behavior of the client, the pet, the general home situation – and the manner in which client and pet interact with one another – provide one major source of information required to achieve the goal of this initial, fact-finding phase: *understanding the detailed nature of the problem clients are having with their pet.*

The counselor's first step is to ask clients to describe the present problem and when and how it developed. As Danneman and Chodrow (1982) point out, it is important that the counselor only listens at this stage and doesn't interrupt unnecessarily with questions while the clients are telling their story. And it usually is a story of sorts because in comparison to medical patients who might need do little more than simply point to their shoulder and say "it hurts there" to their doctor, describing the nature of a pet behavior problem takes time. Normally, clients will not only describe what the animal does and under what circumstances, but also why this represents such a big problem for them and how it affects their lives.

Simply listening until clients have had a chance to say everything they have prepared themselves to say is also an extremely important first step from the psychological viewpoint of establishing the right kind of relationship with clients from the start. Listening demonstrates to clients that the counselor is sincerely interested in understanding their problem – and by implication – helping them solve it. It's the first step in fostering the image of him/herself as a concerned, credible, ethical, and competent specialist, which encourages clients to be open and honest during the interview and to have enough confidence in his/her advice to follow it diligently later.

As soon as clients have given what they regard as an adequate initial description of the problem and its impact on family life, the lengthy questioning process begins. The goal of this phase is to obtain a detailed picture of the nature of the problem or problems. This can be extremely time-consuming because the client's initial description of the problem contains only a small fraction of the information the counselor requires to be able to understand all of the relevant details of the case. Much of what the counselor must know is summarized in the following types of questions which are invariably asked in one form or another during this active, history-taking stage:

Problem-related questions:

- What is the main problem?
- Are there other problems?
- How serious is each problem?
- How frequently does each occur?
- Under what specific circumstances?
- Describe step-by-step what happened during the last few problem incidents:
  - Where was the animal?
  - What was it doing before it showed the problem behavior?
  - What exactly did the animal do?
  - What people and other animals were present?
  - How did they react to the animal's problem behavior?
  - How did the animal react to these reactions?
  - Was the animal punished? How? How did it react to that?
  - Did you do anything else in response to the animal's problem behavior?
  - What specifically did you do at that moment?
- How and when did the problem occur the very first time?
- Did you have other problems with the animal at that time or previously?
- What are the various methods you have used until now to try and control the problem behavior(s)?

- How diligently and consistently did you apply each method?
- With what kind of results?

Other relevant general question areas:

- Questions concerning the general care/ maintenance conditions under which the animal is kept.
- Questions concerning the family's daily routine.
- Questions concerning the animal's daily routine and prior medical and life history.
- Questions concerning relevant opinions, attitudes, wishes, intentions, etc. of family members.

Considering the fact that these questions basically represent only starting points which often open up extended discussions of related aspects of each topic, it is not surprising that this fact-finding phase may require more than a half an hour in cat cases and well over an hour in dog cases. In effect, there is a lot that must be talked about before counselors have learned what they need to know to give competent advice.

The feature of the model dealing with hypothesis formulation and testing – with further questioning either confirming the counselor's tentative hypothesis or indicating that a new hypothesis needs to be formulated – highlights a second time-consuming aspect of the fact-finding phase of the interview. Excessive barking, for example, can be symptomatic of many different problems – several different types of aggression problems, fear problems, separation anxiety, an effect of environmental stress, or normal behavior in response to external eliciting stimuli. The diagnostic category to which a given behavior problem belongs may be clear from the start. But this is not certainly not always the case. It may take some time, for example, to determine why a dog which is kept downstairs away from the family bedroom is barking during the night. Is it responding to outside eliciting stimuli like barking dogs or other noises from outside? Is it demanding the attention it will get when the owner finally gets out of bed and comes down to quiet it down?

Is it expressing its discomfort at being alone? Many kinds of detailed questions often must be asked to assess alternative hypotheses concerning the nature of the problem.

Towards the end of this fact-finding phase, I always ask clients to fill out the *client information form* presented in Chapter 6. It asks for information about the animal and family situation, and it includes a behavior problem checklist and the set of questions described in the last chapter asking about owner attitudes and behavior towards the pet. Aside from recording important information about the case which may be useful for research activities later, giving the questionnaire at this time is a good way to make sure that nothing has been left out – perhaps another type of problem which the client has forgotten to mention.

Phase II: Problem explanation

Once the counselor fully understands the nature and causes of the problem, these must be explained to the client. This is not only because the client expects this and has a right to the counselor's opinion, but helping the client to understand the problem is vital to laying the groundwork for later treatment.

In the complex problem of dominance aggression of dogs towards family members, for example, one explains to the client that dogs in a pack often show this kind of aggression towards one another, and thus the dog's aggressive behavior would be perfectly normal if it were directed towards another dog. Furthermore, one explains that the existence of the problem indicates that the dog doesn't have the right kind of relationship with family members: namely, a relationship in which the dog is so clearly submissive to family members that it would never dream of threatening and attacking them in the kinds of circumstances where it might do so to establish or confirm its dominance over another dog. And this is just the beginning. For the counselor then must explain why it is that the dog is like this by pointing out, for example, the problem-producing effect that certain owner practices such as always giving in to the dog's demanding behavior or giving it too many privileges (e.g. sleeping in family members' beds and climbing on furniture) can have on a dog with a predisposition towards developing a dominance-related problem. Finally, the counselor might also suggest at this point how, in very general terms, this kind of problem must be treated; for example, by avoiding eliciting aggression while treating the dog much differently than before in a number of specific ways.

The loop in the model in Figure 4.2 asking whether the explanation is accepted or understood – and then directing the counselor to spend additional time explaining the problem when it is not – is especially important at this point for two reasons. The first is that clients come to the interview with their own theories about the nature and causes of the problem behavior which they must be persuaded to abandon. This could be something simple like, for example, that the animal has something wrong with its brain. Or it might be more complicated. The animal is jealous perhaps, and making problems as a kind of protest in response to a new person who has joined the family. As will be considered later in the chapter, compared to diagnosing and treating medical problems, the behavior problem counselor is in a curious position. For the client, other family members, the client's relatives, neighbors, and other owners encountered during walks have already pronounced their own diagnoses and given their own detailed explanations of the reasons for the development of the problem. Therefore the explanation offered by the counselor must essentially compete with those offered by all of these amateur animal behavior problem experts. And in order to succeed, the counselor must convince the client that his/her more genuinely scientific explanation is the only correct one. It is critical, therefore, that the counselor be on the lookout at this point for any obvious or subtle signs indicating that the client is skeptical, for there can be no mistakes here. The client must be completely convinced that the counselor knows exactly what he/she is talking about; for this is an indispensable precondition for the client's later compliance with the treatment recommendations.

The second reason for this "explanation accepted/understood?" loop in the model has to do with the logical connection between the problem explanation and treatment recommendations. Namely, clients are only in a position to grasp the logic behind the various treatment recommendations if they fully understand and accept the counselor's explanation of the nature of the problem. This too is critical, for one is often asking clients to treat animals in rather unnatural ways or invest a great deal of time training animals using special procedures. And clients may only be willing to do this if they understand the logical connection between the nature of the problem and the various recommendations which are needed to combat it.

Phase III: Treatment recommendations

When the time comes to give the specific treatment recommendations, each must be very clearly stated and explained in terms of exactly what the owner must do in various specific situations. One might, for example, recommend that the owner ignore the dog every time it comes to be petted. By this, the counselor must explain, is meant that one must pretend that one doesn't even notice the dog when it comes; one mustn't look at it and certainly not talk to it or pet it, and one must make sure not to react in any way no matter what it does. While it might seem strange to have to explain this to owners in such a childishly simple way, sometimes owners are not quite sure what exactly they should do or not do when they are being asked to ignore the dog whenever it comes to them.

In addition to explaining *what* clients must do in various situations, the counselor must also explain *why* they should do this; that is, the dog should be ignored at this time to, in effect, teach it the lesson 50 times a day that now it is the owner who is controlling all of the attention and petting in this pack. With this recommendation in particular, compliance is often a problem. Owners don't like treating their dogs this way. It feels unnatural and cruel to them. And so they are obviously only going to do it if they are convinced that it is necessary for solving the problem.

In some cases, recommendations must be demonstrated as well as explained. For example, with owners who have never trained a dog, I always show them how to teach their dog to sit, lie down, come, and stay on command. They are asked to prepare a plate with 30 or so very small food tidbits of cheese or something else the dog really loves. And then they simply watch while I quickly train the dog to perform these behaviors with the method discussed in Chapter 8. As soon as the dog begins reliably sitting, lying down, coming, and staying, I ask the client to take over while I watch and make sure that he/she understands when to give rewards, when not to, what to do if the dog comes before it is called, and so on.

Demonstrations can also be in the form of acting out what one should do in some imagined situation. Counselors often find themselves getting up and actively miming such things as how to react on the street when the dog sits down and refuses to go father. Often a certain kind of attitude can be communicated here as well. During such acting-out demonstrations, the determined, no-nonsense look on the counselor's face may help convey to the clients that they can't just go through the motions, but must also really feel determined if they hope to accomplish anything.

Phase IV: Increase owner understanding

The treatment recommendations may seem strange and unappealing to the client. The behavioral science-oriented explanation of the problem may seem foreign and quite unlike the way the client has previously viewed the animal and its behavior. Essentially, one is asking owners to give up their old ideas about their animal's behavior, ignore all of the theories and treatment recommendations they have read about or been given by well-meaning friends or neighbors, and instead follow a set of recommendations which sometimes "go against the grain" both in terms of the required expenditure of time and energy and in terms of their feelings about how they want to or should treat their pet. It can therefore be very helpful to owners at this stage if the counselor steps back

from the specific recommendations and tries to put the whole thing – the nature of the problem, the general type of treatment which is required, and the appropriateness and function of the specific instructions – into an easily understandable "package" for the client, one which sums up and reinforces everything which has been said up until this point.

Here too, the loop in the flowchart is a reminder that the counselor should assess how well the client understands each of these elements and be prepared to repeat, amplify, exemplify, etc. explanations whenever this seems to be helpful.

Phase V: Compliance maximization

When the point is reached where the client seems to understand everything, it is time for the counselor to ask him/herself the question of whether or not it is likely that the client will actually carry out the recommended treatment diligently. One never knows for sure. But there are signs that are useful to look for. For example, the client's facial expression when one is going through the recommendations for the last time. One sometimes gets the feeling here – perhaps the client winces slightly or glances somewhat evasively to the side – that says he/she is not really quite so sure about this one. Such a client reaction should not be ignored. One can simply ask clients outright whether they think that following this recommendation might be a problem. Clients generally have the tendency to quickly answer no. But if one is persistent and diplomatic, pointing out, for example, that many people find it extremely difficult to apply this recommendation because they don't think it's fair to the dog, clients can usually be persuaded to openly express their reservations.

Even when clients show none of these tell-tale signs, they still may not be entirely willing and able to follow every recommendation. Knowing this, it is often wise for the counselor to ask a few questions to probe this anticipated compliance area especially with recommendations like ignoring the dog's friendly behavior, which is difficult for anyone to do.

Is there likely to be some compliance problem? If not, it is time to end the interview. But if so, one must ask oneself whether the potential compliance problem is minor, and hence can be remedied by some additional explanation, or critical. If there are critical problems, they have usually been identified before this. But not always. Some clients deliberately keep their opinions to themselves and wait until the counselor has completely finished before they are prepared to reveal what *they* think about the treatment and whether they are willing or able to carry it out. And sometimes one learns at this very late stage that the approach recommended is just not feasible for one reason or another. Often, for example, clients reveal that another family member would not hear of such a thing, or the family schedule just doesn't allow for it. A more common scenario at this point is when one gets increasingly the feeling that carrying out the recommended treatment is probably just too much to expect from this particular client. For a client who lives for his dog and hangs on its every whim, asking him to make it move out of his way, keep it off the furniture, only pet it briefly, ignore it when it comes for its petting, and never give it what it wants when it begs may seem more and more unrealistic as the consultation goes on. But is there any realistic alternative? If there is, one might turn to it at this stage as is depicted by the loop in the flowchart in Figure 4.2 which takes one back to the "give recommendations" stage. But if not, as is usually the case, then one can do nothing other than to reemphasize what has been said previously and make it clear to the client in no uncertain terms that diligently following these recommendations is the only way of correcting the problem.

As a behavior problem counselor, one need not take this kind of client noncompliance personally or feel too discouraged by it. One is responsible for giving clients good, sound advice. But one is not responsible for solving clients' psychological problems. And people who are simply not capable of ignoring a dog's friendly approaches even though they understand this is required to keep themselves and other family members from being bitten again in future certainly have a problem.

Finally, one can add other recommendations or information at this very late stage in the consultation if one feels this might increase compliance. For example, one can ask the client to call the following Monday morning to give an initial report on how things are going, which sets up a kind of deadline situation to encourage clients to begin application of the recommendations immediately. Or one might discuss at this point how uncomfortable clients sometimes feel when they first start responding to the animal this way, but that this soon passes when they see that this doesn't seem to bother it at all. When one senses that the client remains somewhat skeptical, one can suggest that the treatment be tried only on a trial basis, as a kind of experiment. Some counselors also have clients keep a diary or record behaviors in some other way. These too are means to encourage clients to follow recommendations consistently. Finally, the counselor can point out that decades of experience treating this particular problem has shown that the recommended approach is the only way to solve it. This is an attempt to counteract the client's wishful thinking that there might be another approach which could be tried first before going as far as carrying out the rather extreme type of treatment being recommended.

Causes of noncompliance

Similar compliance problems are faced by veterinarians when, for example, recommending treatments like daily ear cleaning which both owner and dog find unpleasant. However, the noncompliance problem becomes especially serious with behavior problem treatments where recommendations may be elaborate, time-consuming, difficult to understand, require a great deal of client self-discipline, and run counter to what clients have always believed were the causes of the problem and how to treat it.

In doing one's best to encourage clients to comply with the recommended treatments, it is extremely helpful to be aware of the following kinds of factors which can lead to noncompliance, for it may then be possible to anticipate and counteract them.

Confidence in the counselor's expertise

This factor is especially critical for non-veterinary behavior counselors. In cases where referring family veterinarians have told clients that they attended one of my lectures or read several of my journal articles, clients assume from the start that I am the right person to give them the kind of help they need. If however the client has been given the phone number of a "dog psychiatrist" by a friend, the client's initial reaction may be more skeptical. Out of politeness, many clients do not openly ask about my background and educational qualifications until towards the end of the consultation when they do so seemingly just to make conversation. In other cases, however, clients' skepticism may be clear from the start, and one often feels sized up or tested by them early in the interview.

In general, these kinds of initial doubts do not represent a significant problem in knowledgeable and informed owners, for it is usually not long into the interview before they are convinced that they are talking to a genuine expert in the pet behavioral problem field. But with some relatively uneducated clients – or with clients who seem to have a particularly suspicious nature – there can be problems in this area. People who are totally ignorant of modern scientific views of animal behavior have no frame of reference which they can use to evaluate the counselor's level of expertise. For them, the counselor's opinion may seem like just one among many, essentially no better or worse than the opinions they have heard from others.

In general, it is best always to take the time to satisfy owners' curiosity or ease their suspicions by, for example, mentioning one's qualifications or briefly discussing the scientific basis of the pet problem field whenever owners indicate that they are interested or skeptical in this regard. Not only does satisfying clients' concerns and curiosity foster a productive co-operative atmosphere and maximize compliance, but clients are entitled to such information on ethical grounds.

Competition with the advice offered by others

As discussed previously, the pet behavior problem counselor is in the curious position of advising clients who are not only confronted with people offering advice on how to treat their pets wherever they turn, but at some level the clients too have always considered themselves to be fairly knowledgeable in this respect. If one were to ask a group of typical owners if they have ever given other owners advice on how to deal with pet behavior problems, many or most would answer yes, they have done so from time to time. The pet behavior counselor must always be conscious of this competitive dimension – that every explanation or treatment recommendation will be assessed by clients in terms of their own personal views, views they might have read in pet books, and views expressed by their friends, neighbors, relatives, etc. As a result, the pet behavior problem counselor must try harder than specialists in areas without such serious competitors/competing views to reassure clients that he/she is offering genuinely sound advice which is the result of decades of experience other qualified and experienced pet behavior counselors have had trying to help owners cope with similar kinds of problems.

Treatment is too much bother

Some clients seem to resent the idea that there has to be any kind of treatment at all. Intellectually they realize full well that the problem can only be resolved if they follow the counselor's recommendations, but emotionally they may be unwilling or only grudgingly willing to take the time and energy to carry them out. As clients, such people are relatively unappealing. They are dissatisfied with the recommendations. They may try repeatedly to get the counselor to recommend something simpler – some kind of drug perhaps. And when one points out, for example, that a dog is not getting enough exercise and needs to be taken out for at least a half and hour before going to work, they may reject this idea outright, explaining perhaps that their schedule just does not allow for it. Compared to most other clients, these owners often seem lazy, extremely self-centered, and whiny. Basically, clients like these sometimes give one the feeling that if they could snap their fingers and make the pet disappear, they would not hesitate. In fact, some have already essentially tried to do this. They might have taken the animal to the animal shelter and been told that the shelter does not accept problem animals. Or more commonly in the cases referred to behavior specialists, their family veterinarian has refused to put the animal to sleep on the grounds that it is healthy and the problem may be correctable. In a few cases, owners are obviously hoping that the specialist will conclude that putting the animal to sleep is a reasonable option.

Other than being firm in pointing out that there is no easier way to the solve the problem, and no grounds for recommending that the animal be put to sleep, there is nothing else the counselor can do here. These people just are not interested enough and do not feel responsible enough to do much about the problem. They simply want to get rid of the problem by getting rid of the pet, and in one way or another that's what they will probably eventually find a way to do.

However, not all clients who find the treatment too bothersome and time-consuming are as unlikable and hopeless as this. Some are sincerely interested in solving the problem, but they really are extremely busy, time-pressured, active people. To them, devoting a lot more time to the animal every day seems impossible. In theory, however, they are willing and seem sincere in this regard.

These time-pressured owners want fast, no-nonsense solutions. In the human behavior therapy area, this initial attitude or expectation is referred to the "drive-in syndrome" (Köhlke and Köhlke, 1994): essentially, solving the problem should be about as fast and effortless as buying a hamburger. While naturally disappointed to learn that things are not going to be nearly so easy, most owners successfully ad-

just to the realities of the situation and seem ready to give the recommended treatment a try. But whether or not they are motivated enough to carry out a genuinely demanding, long-term treatment is another matter. Probably the most likely prognosis here is for a partial solution. The owner will invest just enough time to bring the problem within tolerable limits and no more.

Treatment seems unnatural

Some owners cannot imagine, for example, ignoring a dog which comes to them to be petted, or giving it a command and then waiting until it performs the correct response before petting it. Particularly with some common dog problems like dominance aggression, owners may be asked to refrain from doing many things which they now do automatically with the animal like petting it or playing with it on demand, letting it go through doorways first, and walking around or stepping over it when it is lying in the way. Instead, the counselor is asking them to behave in a way which feels extremely *unnatural* to them such as never giving the dog what it wants when it begs, ordering it off the furniture, and making the sleeping animal get up and move out of the way whenever they want to pass by.

This element of unnaturalness, this idea that in the foreseeable future the owners will have to think about everything they are doing and inhibit their tendencies to do a lot of the things they have always done unthinkingly, represents a major problem for many owners. Some are pessimistic from the beginning. They know their own weaknesses and limitations, and they doubt whether they are self-disciplined enough to so drastically alter their behavior towards the animal. Others who are initially more optimistic find out quickly that it is not easy to remember to react correctly and exceedingly difficult to keep treating the animal like this day after day.

The fact that following some recommendations feels unnatural, requires a constant amount of effort, takes some time to learn to follow correctly, and takes more time before treating the animal this way becomes habitual must be dealt with at length during the consultation. One tries here to prepare owners for what to expect and encourage them to be persistent even if they find it is somewhat difficult initially. It can be emphasized to them that the fact that it feels so unnatural is precisely why carrying out the treatment is so difficult. Basically, they can't relax and just be themselves anymore but instead must continually playact, pretend that they don't see the dog sitting next to them apparently starved for affection, pretend they don't like him on the furniture, and so on.

Here again, the most likely outcome with many owners is that they will follow such recommendations only some of the time – or follow only some of the recommendations – and consequently achieve only part of the potential benefit this kind of treatment can achieve. Such an outcome is fully understandable given the existence of these competing motivations on the part of owners. On the one hand, they are highly motivated to follow the treatment recommendations that are necessary to correct a problem they can no longer live with. But on the other hand, they want to go on enjoying their pet the way they always have. Psychologically speaking, the resolution of such kinds of motivational conflict situations often involves finding a compromise solution which maximizes benefits and minimizes costs with regard to the competing motivational systems. And in this respect, one might expect that research into the compliance-versus-noncompliance phenomenon for problems such as dominance aggression would yield some interesting lawful relationships depending, for example, on *problem-related* aspects like how dangerous the dog is and how burdensome the problem is for family members on the one hand, and *human personality* characteristics like the degree to which owners enjoy treating or need to treat their dog like a human child on the other. My own observations certainly suggest that such relationships exist. For example, owners who have been severely bitten are naturally more inclined to diligently carry out extreme treatments than those who are only being growled at by their dogs. And compared to other owners, those whose attitudes towards their dogs reflect particularly high parental motivation are less likely to be able to inhibit anthropomorphic and spoiling tendencies to anything like the degree which the psychologically and emotionally demanding method for treating dominance aggression requires.

Treatment seems cruel

Try recommending to parents that they should ignore their small child every time it comes toddling up for attention. Even if parents might see a certain logic in doing so, they couldn't bear to go through with it. It would violate their deepest sense of what is right and fair to their child. And being parents to their animals, it is understandable why treating animals this way not only feels unnatural, but it feels cruel as well.

Thus, when one asks owners to completely ignore their dog when it comes for attention, it is therefore not surprising that their first reaction may be one of unease and discomfort. And such apprehensive feelings turn out to be fully justified: owners may indeed experience emotional difficulties when they try to consistently behave this way towards the dog. "We're the kind of people who like to treat our pets in a *friendly* way", explained the wife of a client couple in a recent case who admitted not following all of the recommendations during the week after my home visit. They were intelligent people who seemed to fully understand during the consultation why each of the recommendations was helpful and necessary. But when the time came to put my advice into practice, they just couldn't do it. It seemed and felt too extreme and cruel to them.

Reading well-known books and articles in the pet problem field, one sometimes gets the feeling that the authors don't really understand how far they are asking people to go when they prescribe "completely ignore the dog for a few days" as if this kind of pronouncement alone was enough to get owners to do something that goes against everything they feel and believe concerning how pets deserve to be treated. Basically, people need a lot of convincing in this regard if their reservations are to be overcome. One approach is to point out that to the dog, such reactions are much more understandable and far less cruel than it would be for a child – that underneath it all, the dog rather expects that its "pack leaders" won't react to its every gesture and bend over backwards to give it everything it wants. In short, that dog social groups don't function that way, and the dog will therefore not find it too surprising or disturbing when his human family becomes more like this as well.

Treatment requires people to make sacrifices

The main reason why most people keep pets, feel strongly attached to them, and feel so affectionate towards them is that pets are strong elicitors of self-rewarding physical contact, nurturance, and other social behavior. This in turn implies that one of the primary characteristics of owner-pet interactions is that it *feels good* to people to pet, talk to, play with, and take care of their pets. "What do I have him for if I can't pet him or hold him or play with him when I want?", one client told me challengingly after I had recommended a rather drastic treatment plan against the dog's dangerous dominance aggression. But another, more selfless client who was mainly concerned with bringing her dog's dominance aggression well enough under control to save it from being euthanized saw things differently: "I know I'll miss hugging him and cuddling him and petting him all the time, but it's something I just have to do. If it saves his life, it's worth it". For her it was. She followed the treatment advice to the letter and is now still enjoying her big shaggy friend, but in a somewhat more controlled, distant, and detached way than before.

The pet behavior counselor can put it this way to clients: "It feels good to pet our dogs and talk to them and play with them as much as we want – and anytime we feel like it. It's one of the pleasures of owning a dog. But you have the misfortune of having the kind of dog that does not react very well to this kind of treatment. Essentially, you will never be able to just relax and enjoy him the way other owners

can. Instead, you will have to give up doing a lot of things with your dog that you would often do and enjoy doing if there were no problems. Basically, correcting this problem requires a certain sacrifice on your part."

Pet problems may have "secondary gains"

This human psychology expression refers to the fact that people with psychological problems sometimes derive benefits from having the kind of problems they do and, hence, underneath it all, have a vested interest in making sure that the treatment fails. The classical example in human psychology is hysterical paralysis, where someone – most often a woman – would suddenly, inexplicably, but apparently quite genuinely loose the use or an arm or her legs. This disorder was fairly common until it was finally noticed that such patients always seem to somehow profit from their disorder (e.g. less work, more attention/sympathy) – an insight which drastically reduced the incidence of the condition practically overnight.

An amusing example of a similar phenomenon with pets is the common situation where the wife can't quite seem to handle the dog during walks and so this task is always left up to the bigger, stronger, more physically capable man to handle in his characteristically tough, masculine way – which makes some men beam with pride while their wives just quietly sit back and smile when the matter is being discussed. Although few people would consciously subvert the treatment for improving the dog's obedience and controllability during walks just to be able to stay out of the rain, one couldn't blame them too much if they didn't quite put as much effort into it as they otherwise might.

There may be more psychologically interesting secondary gains standing in the way of treatments in some cases. One often gets the feeling, for example, that clients rather like it that their dog is a tough, spunky, stubborn little customer even though this means that it is attacking every dog in sight and turning the family's neighbors into bitter enemies. In one of my cases, this went even farther. Two Welsh corgies had been viciously attacking a small dog which lived two doors away. In addition to the clients themselves, the owner of the victim dog was present for much of the consultation. But before she had come and after she had gone, the middle-aged couple who owned the problem corgies were not able to describe the various problem incidents without giggling. They basically could not have cared less about the attacks. But naturally they could not reveal this outwardly and had obviously called in a behavior specialist only as a kind of public demonstration to all in the neighborhood of their concern and sense of responsibility.

Effect of family dynamics on compliance

As Köhlke and Köhlke (1994) suggest, there are many ways in which the family dynamics interact with and can severely interfere with compliance. For example, there are often severe disagreements between family members concerning whether the animal should be kept, whether the problem is severe enough to require action, whether a pet behavior problem counselor should have been contacted, who and what is causing the problem, and what should be done about it. Many family situations which the counselor confronts are extremely sensitive in this regard. Husbands and wives may have been arguing over the pet for weeks already and their opinions on what should be done about its problem are severely polarized and highly emotionally charged. Also common, the parents want to have a problem pet euthanized and the children are prepared to fight to save its life. Such situations call for a great deal of diplomacy on the part of the counselor who, when facing a stern-faced panel of four or five family members of all ages, is in a curious position. He/she is a total stranger and yet is immediately given access to personal information (e.g. who sleeps where, who loves the animal more, what the death of the animal might mean to various family members) which quickly turns the brief counselor-family relationship into a surprisingly intimate one.

Also relevant to the matter of compliance is who in the family has the say when it comes to family decisions. Often some critical person in

the family is absent – either because of work or because they find the idea of consulting a pet behavior problem counselor foolish. And even when present, the person who ultimately will determine whether a certain treatment will be carried out may remain in the background and not exercise his/her ultimate authority until they have left the counselor's office or he/she has gone home. In many cases, the person with whom the counselor has dealt directly is highly cooperative and anxious to begin putting the recommendations into practice, but this doesn't happen because another family member doesn't cooperate. Sometimes the family member who must actually take care of the animal is the one who has the ultimate say in what is or is not to be done. And it is often the case that the family divides into two camps with this person on one side and the rest of the family on the other – particularly when the training required is particularly demanding or if the person who must deal most with the animal on a daily basis is the one who feels most threatened by and afraid of it.

In the last analysis, the fact that counselors must often deal with families rather than single individuals makes the factors which interfere with compliance much more complex and diverse than they might otherwise be.

Compliance is critical

The obvious potential importance of all of these compliance-related factors emphasizes once again that pet behavioral counseling is as much about changing *human behavior* as it is about changing the problem behaviors of pets. After the fact-finding phase of the consultation has been completed, it is generally clear to the counselor what sort of treatment method the clients must employ to improve their pet's problem behavior. But in the typical case, this phase may represent only half the length of the full interview. The rest is essentially focused on what, for the counselor, is the primary problem and real challenge of the pet behavioral problem field: saying things which will maximize the chances that *clients will in fact do what is necessary to solve their problem.*

Many skills and tactics are relevant here. Counselors must be good *teachers* of their clients. They must *understand* clients: their capabilities, attitudes, intellectual abilities, emotional tendencies, personal problems, and life situations. They must know how to effectively *influence* clients via explaining, demonstrating, emphasizing, warning, and pointing out positive and negative consequences. And to accomplish all of these things, they must first and foremost be *sincere*: they must like people, be able to relate easily to them, and be sincerely motivated to help them. For only then can they inspire the kind of confidence in their advice on which compliance depends.

References

Danneman, P.J., and Chodrow, R.E. (1982): History-taking and interviewing techniques. *Veterinary Clinics of North America: Small Animal Practice* **12**, 587–592

Köhlke, U., and Köhlke, K. (1994): Verhaltenstherapie bei Tieren: Besonderheiten und spezifische Problematik aus psychologischer Sicht. *Kleintierpraxis* **39**, 175–180.

5   Treating Dog and Cat Behavior Problems

The major causal factors which play a role in the development and maintenance of pet behavioral problems were briefly introduced in Chapter 3. In the present chapter, these factors will be considered in more detail with help of a descriptive model summarizing their relationship to the behavioral systems involved. As will be seen, most of the detailed features of the model represent potential focal points or "windows of opportunity" for treatment measures. Indeed, directly relating the various *causal factors* to the various types of *treatment possibilities* is the primary value of this simple scheme.

The model is shown in Figure 5.1. Briefly, the central vertical axis running from the problem situation box on top to the problem behavior box on the bottom represents what might be termed the *stimulus-response dimension*. Like other types of animal behavior, behavior problems are lawful reactions to detailed features of the surrounding environment. Something happens in the animal's environment, this is registered by the animal's sense organs, and information concerning the event is transmitted to and processed by its central nervous system which then in turn ultimately determines what the animal will do in this situation. The fact that individual animals may differ greatly in their reactions to identical situations implies that the basic parameters or operational characteristics of the underlying physiological mechanisms which generate their behavior differ in some way. The two side columns in the model list many types of preprogramming, physiological, interactional, and learning-mediated effects responsible for producing these kinds of inferred differences in the underlying physiological mechanisms. The central *animal's behavior system* component of the model is therefore analogous to the so-called "black box" of classical S-R or stimulus-response animal learning

theory. In effect, the model summarizes the various kinds of causal factors which can affect the behavior of animals without making any assumptions at all about what precisely is going on inside animals' nervous systems.

In the following sections, the nature and treatment-related implications of each of these three classes of causal factors (i.e. problem situation, system parameters, and environmental influences) will be considered in some detail. The general aim is to provide the reader with a comprehensive introduction to the full range of treatment measures which may be of potential benefit in controlling or eliminating dog and cat behavior problems.

Problem situation

For a few behavior problems like stereotypies, elimination in the home, or generalized nervousness/hyperactivity, obvious connections between immediate environmental events and the problem behavior are difficult or impossible to discern. However, with most aggression problems, fear problems, and many other types of behavior problems there is an obvious, precisely describable *problem situation*: a specific environmental context in which the problem always occurs and which, scientifically speaking, can be best described in terms of the various behavior-influencing effects some of the *stimuli* occurring in the situation have on the animal's problem behavior. These effects can be classified in the following way.

Arousing stimuli

The sound of a car door slamming outside, the sight of an owner becoming restless and peering out of the front window, or a strange odor

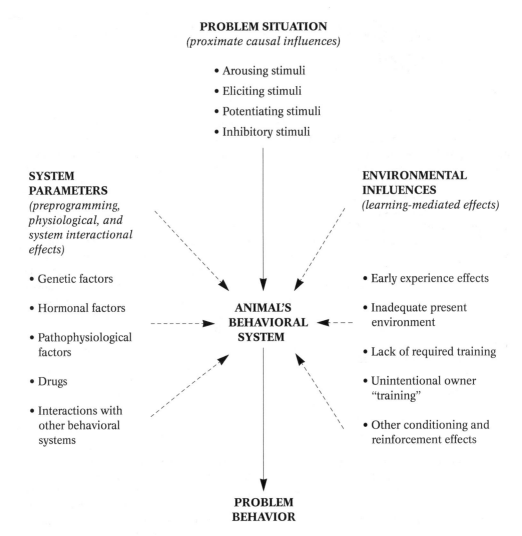

Figure 5.1: Etiology of pet behavior problems

which is suddenly perceived by the animal are examples of arousing stimuli which cause an animal to become more alert and active in a general, nonspecific way. The resting animal gets up, appears highly alert, tense perhaps; it searches, checks doors and windows, and carefully monitors the owner's behavior. While not directly responsible for eliciting or intensifying problem behaviors in the same way as the stimuli in the following two paragraphs, the probability and intensity of problem responses to

these other stimuli – and the owner's capability for preventing or counteracting such responses – may sometimes be greatly influenced by the animal's general state of arousal.

Eliciting stimuli

The doorbell rings and the territorially aggressive dog charges barking towards the front door. The first distant roll of thunder sends the dog with a thunderstorm phobia scurrying quickly to its owner's side for protection. The dominant aggressive dog bites when someone in the family tries to take a stolen sock away from it. These are types of stimuli which actually *elicit* the problem behavior. When questioned closely, owners of problem animals are generally able to describe them accurately.

Potentiating stimuli

Potentiating stimuli are environmental events which do not directly elicit a problem behavior, but act to increase its intensity or duration. A second dog may join in and cause a dog's barking at a stranger to increase. The stranger may stop, stiffen, perhaps cry out and turn and run away, stimulating a drastic increase in both dogs' aggressiveness. And the owner may feel threatened by the stranger and spur the dogs on, or his/her initial attempts to bring them under control by scolding them may be misinterpreted as support and thereby increase the intensity of the dogs' behavior as well.

Inhibitory stimuli

Pulling on a dog's leash more firmly, looking away when threatened by a dominant-aggressive dog, scolding a dog which has begun growling at a guest: these are inhibitory stimuli which can have the opposite effect on the problem behavior as eliciting or potentiating stimuli. They reduce its intensity or duration and perhaps bring it to an end.

Treatment "windows"

Treating pet behavior problems often involves advising owners to take or avoid specific actions which influence the effects of the various arousing, eliciting, potentiating, and inhibitory stimuli inherent in problem situations. With a dog which becomes anxious when alone, advising owners to behave in a calm and emotionally neutral way in the few minutes before they leave home is an attempt to *reduce arousing stimuli* emanating from their behavior. In general, owners tend to become aroused and nervous whenever any situation in which their dog often makes problems is anticipated like, for example, when they see that a stranger will soon enter the house or a thunderstorm is approaching. Such arousal and nervousness can have an adverse affect on animals, perhaps communicating to them that some sort of trouble is on the way. This in turn can make their initial reaction to the stimuli that actually elicit the problem behavior more intense than it might otherwise be.

The counselor's treatment advice often includes suggestions for the *avoidance of eliciting stimuli*. For example, avoid doing things which provoke aggression in dominant-aggressive dogs, don't expose the dog to intense fear-producing situations during treatment, deny the cat access to the room in which it is urine marking, or keep two cats which are aggressive to one another separated except during treatment sessions. Recommendations of this type are a major element in the treatment of many behavior problems. Indeed, owners tend naturally to try and cope with many behavior problems in this way. For example, the routine avoidance of aggression-eliciting stimuli by all family members sometimes makes it possible to live with a potentially dangerous dominant-aggressive dog indefinitely. Owners simply don't take food away from it, don't disturb it when it is sleeping, and stop doing whatever they are doing when the animal stiffens and gives them that sideways look which they know indicates that it is on the verge of attacking them.

Similarly, taking direct action to *reduce or avoid potentiating stimuli* (e.g. keeping a pair of dogs separated when introducing them to a stranger) or *apply or intensify inhibitory stimuli* (e.g. startling a marking cat, more severely scolding a barking dog) can exert extremely beneficial problem-reducing effects within the problem situation itself over and above their learning-mediated effects on the animal's future behavior.

System parameters

Animals differ greatly in their behavioral reactions to specific environmental situations.

While some dogs attack other dogs, chase bicycles, or react fearfully to thunderstorms, others never do. There are two possible reasons why. The first is that such differences are based on the operation of learning mechanisms in the sense that some problem animals have either learned to be that way or failed to learn to react with acceptable behavior in problem situations. The other possibility is that the behavior-generating physiological mechanisms of these animals differ in some other, more fundamental way: in effect, that the basic parameters or operational characteristics of the associated behavior systems differ in a way which is independent of the animals' past experience interacting with their environment.

Genetic factors

The behavioral systems themselves (e.g. dominance-related and self-defensive behavior in dogs; urine marking and territorial aggression in cats) are obviously inherited or *genetically preprogrammed*. Most behavior problems are basically inherited, species-typical behaviors that are problems for humans because, for example, they are elicited in inappropriate contexts (spraying in the home by cats), overly intense (territorial aggression in dogs), or directed towards inappropriate stimuli (dominance aggression towards human beings in dogs). The fact that strains of particularly fearful dogs have been selectively bred, illustrates the potential importance of genetic factors in determining fearful behavior tendencies to particular kinds of stimuli like noises or human beings (Dykman et. al, 1979). Similarly, the facts that some behavior problems may occur only in certain breeds (e.g. flank sucking in Doberman Pinschers) or run in families (e.g. the submissive urination case discussed in Chapter 17) indicate that genetic factors determining the basic characteristics of a behavioral system are sometimes involved. In general, a genetic basis is often strongly suspected in cases where no pathophysiological disorder can be identified, environmental factors (including early experience) do not appear to account for the development of the problem, and potentially effective training or environmental modification treatment approaches are of very limited benefit.

It is obvious to anyone who has had a great deal of experience with both problem and non-problem animals that there are often dramatic, largely inexplicable (based on prior history) differences between individual animals in the degree to which they are motivated to perform particular problem behaviors. Without extensive kinds of selective breeding or environmental manipulation experiments, there is no way to prove, for example, that some cats are especially highly motivated to mark for genetic reasons. However, it is often the only explanation which makes sense. Essentially, it is important to recognize the possibility that genetic preprogramming – rather than such things as mistakes by owners or inadequacies in a pet's environment – may be involved in some cases, particularly those in which animals have not favorably responded to treatments which are highly effective with other animals.

Hormonal factors

The dramatic differences between males and females in urine marking and dominance aggression in dogs, the beneficial effects of castrating males for behavior problems like intermale aggression, urine marking, and hypersexuality, and the beneficial effects of progestins on some of these behavior problems reveal the potential importance of hormones in affecting the behavioral systems underlying behavior problems.

Pathophysiologic factors

Most diseases have behavioral symptoms (e.g. lethargy, lack of appetite), and many behavior problems can be the result of some pathophysiologic disorder (Reisner, 1991). Especially common here are the sudden appearance of aggression in dogs which have never been aggressive before and the failure of cats to use the litter box after a history of always using it in the past. Such problems are often readily understandable responses to disease processes. In cats, a learned avoidance of the litter box due to painful experiences of eliminating there is often assumed to account for the shift to sites outside of the box. In dogs, uncharacteristic aggression often has a defensive character – keeping people and other animals away, or preventing them from touching it or manipulating it in certain ways.

Drugs

The facts that some drugs can have behavioral problem side effects or reduce the seriousness of behavior problems indicate the potential importance of drugs in directly affecting the behavioral systems underlying problem behaviors.

Interactions between behavioral systems

Certain behaviors like barking, scratching, digging, or eliminating which the animal exhibits in many kinds of environmental contexts may be symptoms of some behavior problem such as separation anxiety. Little is known of the physiological substrates of any of these kinds of specific behaviors or the separation anxiety problem itself. However, it is reasonable to assume that some sort of "linking" of the physiological systems underlying these specific behaviors on the one hand, and that underlying the animal's distressed reaction at being left alone on the other, is involved. Essentially, while vocalization may be the main symptom, it is the separation-related behavior system and not that controlling vocalization per se where the assumed origin of the problem lies. Another example is so-called fear aggression. While it is the aggression which represents the greatest problem for owners, it is mainly the fear which must be addressed by treatment measures.

Treatment "windows"

The question here is what kinds of possibilities exist for exerting beneficial effects on the undesirable behavior which do not directly depend on the operation of learning mechanisms. If there is major *genetic* component, an animal's unusually high motivation to perform the problem behavior in certain situations may be something that must somehow be coped with rather than eliminated. For example, the main treatment goal may be focused on response control (via muzzling, keeping the animal on the leash) rather reduction of undesirable behavioral tendencies by means of retraining measures.

Castration can be a very helpful treatment alternative in cases like intermale aggression, urine marking, roaming, and excessive sexual behavior in male dogs, and urine marking and intermale aggression in cats, where male hormones are playing an important role in the physiological mechanisms underlying the respective behavioral systems. Although most commonly beneficial in males, the alteration of hormone levels by means of castration can be indicated in females for problems which are directly connected with the estrous cycle.

When *pathophysiological factors* are interacting with the behavioral system, the treatment implications are obvious: it is the pathophysiological disorder which must be treated and not the problem behavior.

Of course, *drugs* represent a major "window of opportunity" for treating behavior problems if the possibility exists for directly producing beneficial changes in the physiological mechanisms underlying particular behavioral systems.

It is often reasonable to conceptualize behavior problems as involving more than one behavioral system. This is the case, for example, with fear aggression in both cats and dogs where the defensive aggression behavior system is being activated in fear-arousing problem situations. When such *interactions between behavioral systems* are involved, an additional window of opportunity for successful treatment may exist which is often the best or only means of solving the problem. As mentioned above, treating fear aggression, for example, often involves reducing an animal's fear in problem situations rather than trying to directly reduce the animal's aggression per se. However in practice, treatment may be focused on both behavior systems. In fear-related aggression towards human strangers in dogs, effective treatment may involve reducing the animal's fear of strangers on the one hand, and training it to respond less aggressively in fear-arousing situations on the other.

Environmental influences

Even if genetic and/or hormonal factors predispose an animal to show certain kinds of behavior problems, the development of such problems is still always the result of an interaction between the animal's behavioral systems and the characteristics of the environment in which it lives. Indeed, it is generally accepted that the development of most and perhaps all behavioral problems involve *learning* – a general concept subsuming all of the many ways in which an animal's behavior changes as a direct result of its experience interacting with its environment. The following sections summarize the nature of the various learning-mediated effects which are most commonly associated with dog and cat behavior problems.

Early experience effects

A particularly change-resistant form of learning occurs early in life in dogs and to some extent in cats as well. Here imprinting or an imprinting-like form of learning is involved: there is a critical time period during the first few weeks in life in which contact or lack of contact with certain environmental stimuli, conspecifics, and/or members of other species determines to a great extent the young animal's lifelong behavior towards them. Dogs that are taken away from their litter too early and deprived of contact with other dogs between the 3rd and 14th week of life often display abnormal social behavior towards other dogs later in life, essentially reacting to them almost as if they were members of an alien species. Similarly, lack of contact with humans during these first three months of life can also result in a permanent fear of human strangers. And finally, questioning the owners of noise phobic dogs often reveals that they spent the first few weeks of life in secluded kennel environments far removed from the hustle and bustle of the modern city environment.

Inadequate or otherwise problem-producing present environment

Some behavioral problems reflect inadequacies in the conditions under which animals are currently being kept. For example, dogs which are not given enough opportunities for physical exercise may become unruly and difficult to control under a variety of circumstances. Similarly, it is generally accepted that dogs and cats which exhibit stereotypies – odd, stereotyped, repetitive, and sometimes self-mutilating behaviors like tail biting, fly snapping, or licking, sucking, or chewing parts of the body – are often showing signs of stress, conflict, or frustration associated with a lack of contact with conspecifics, too little space, not enough opportunities for exercise, frequent exposure to aversive environmental stimuli, and so on.

Lack of required training

Aggression towards human visitors and house-soiling in dogs, for example, are often the obvious result of a *lack of training* which would have prevented the problems or kept them under control.

Unintentional owner "training"

A very common cause of the progressive worsening of behavior problems is *unintentional owner reinforcement* occurring, for example, when the owner attempts to quiet an aggressively excited animal or soothe a fearful animal by petting it, talking to it, distracting it with tidbits or playing. Such owner reactions tend to reward problem behaviors and thereby increase their future probability of occurrence and intensity. Similarly, owner reinforcement in the form of attention can maintain or strengthen stereotypies or be responsible for a variety of begging/pestering behavior problems in both cats and dogs. Sometimes *intentional reinforcement* is also involved as when puppies are rewarded with petting and praise for mild aggression towards human strangers that becomes increasingly a problem later in life. Finally, there are many other ways in which owners do things that act to *foster* or encourage problem behaviors – or what eventually develop into problem behaviors. Playing aggressive games with dogs may promote the development of play aggression problems or dominance aggression. Taking fearful dogs into environments in which they react particularly fearfully can lead to increased fear. Giving dogs various kinds of privileges like being allowed to sleep in human beds or jump up on other pieces of furniture may promote the development of dominance-aggression problems. And giving dogs what they want whenever they beg for something may make them extremely pushy and demanding.

Some of these types of owner behavior may have an indirect effect on behavior problems by promoting the development of an *owner-dog relationship problem*. This in turn makes a problem dog difficult for the owner to control and train in a variety of situations. For example, it is thought that allowing dogs on the furniture, allowing them to win all aggressive, test-of-strength games, and petting them whenever they come to be petted can help to create the kinds of dominance-related problems in dogs which severely restrict owners' abilities to control and train dogs exhibiting other behavior problems.

Other conditioning or reinforcement effects

Animals may become fearful after being exposed to some *traumatic event* (e.g. a traffic accident) or frequently subjected to some kind of *fear-arousing situation* (e.g. teasing by children, thunderstorms, owner temper tantrums). Many types of behavior problems may be affected by *other sources of positive reinforcement* besides those stemming from owners. Victims of aggressive threats by dogs may stop approaching and perhaps turn and walk or run away, which would reward a defensively aggressive dog's threatening behavior. Not coming immediately when called during walks may be rewarded every time the dog ignores its owner's calling to continue playing with another dog. Similarly, the dog which steals food and breaks out of a pen is rewarded in obvious ways. *Self-rewarding behavior* is also involved

in many problem cases. The aggressive barking of a socially deprived dog that is chained up outside alone all day may essentially be self-rewarding and, therefore, self-strengthening. The hunting of small animals like squirrels and cats seems to be highly rewarding for some dogs even though prey is never captured.

Treatment "windows"

The existence of these many types of causal connections between environmental characteristics and behavioral problems implies that there may be many approaches to treating problems by modifying the environmental conditions which are producing or maintaining them. Those which have proven useful in treating dog behavior problems are briefly introduced in the following paragraphs.

Like in the case of genetic factors determining various behavior system parameters, the effects of severe early experience deficits may be irreversible. But in milder cases where the deficiency was not so acute, there may be some potential for later change. *Care/maintenance condition changes* (e.g. taking a dog somewhere every day for extended contact with conspecifics or crowds of human strangers) can sometimes create conditions for gradually accustoming a dog to fear-eliciting stimuli. Theoretically, *systematic behavior therapy* to, for example, reduce fear of children or specific kinds of city noises might help in some cases.

If the animal's present environment is inadequate in some way, this may be remedied by *increasing owner understanding* (e.g. activity needs of animal must always be met, highly social animals need frequent contact with conspecifics), *specific environmental changes* (e.g. new type of litter for litter box, provide cat with toys, scratching post, etc.), *care/maintenance condition changes* (e.g. change dog's sleeping place, access to furniture, feeding times, etc.), or *systematic behavior therapy* (e.g. systematic desensitization and counter-conditioning to gradually reduce fear of specific type of feared stimulus).

In many dog cases, training or retraining is often required. Recommendations commonly given in this regard may take the form of encouraging *increased owner authority* (e.g. scold dog more energetically in problems situations), *conventional obedience training* (e.g. to increase owner control), *training in problem situations* (e.g. punish problem behavior while using rewards to strengthen acceptable behavior), and *systematic behavior therapy* (e.g. to train a dog which has never been alone to stay alone without becoming distressed).

If owners have been rewarding or in some other way fostering the development of behavior problems, it may be necessary to *correct owner misconceptions* (e.g. that fearful dog should be reassured by petting), *correct owner mistakes* (e.g. stop punishing more dominant dog for aggression directed towards more submissive dog in the household), *abandon ineffective treatment methods* (e.g. punishment long after the problem behavior occurred), or carry out *conventional obedience training*.

If other types of reinforcement above and beyond those administered by owners are involved in the maintenance of the problem, these too must obviously be stopped or counteracted. Using maximally rewarding food tidbits and making sure never to scold a dog even when it is slow to respond can help owners progressively strengthen the effect of their "come" command to the point where the rewarding effects of ignoring the owner's calling to keep playing with other dogs in the park can be overcome. Similarly, combining the application of effective punitive methods with the rewarding of acceptable behavior in problem situations can help to reduce behavior which is self-rewarding. Here again, therefore, *increasing owner understanding, correcting owner mistakes, carrying out conventional obedience training*, and the *cessation of ineffective training methods* can also be helpful problem-solving measures

Response control/prevention

Sometimes problems can be effectively coped with by using some kind of device such as a muzzle, head collar, cage, or simply keeping dogs on a leash to physically control or prevent the problem behavior in problem situations. These kinds of response control/prevention measures – which do not directly relate to any of the causal factors summarized in the model in Figure 5.1 – are often extremely helpful in many dog behavior problem cases.

Conclusion

The set of causal factors underlying many or most behavioral problems is a complex combination of several of the kinds of preprogramming, physiological, system interactional, and learning-mediated effects embodied in this chapter's descriptive model. As can be seen in the following Figure 5.2 which adds many details from this chapter's treatment-related discussion to the model of the pet behavior problem counseling process introduced in the last chapter, the treatment of behavior problems mirrors this complexity. Indeed, there are many different ways in which cat and dog behavioral problems can be influenced for the better. The treatment recommendations given to owners are always a combination of those which appear to the counselor to be optimal for the particular animal, problem, owner, and family situation.

References

Dykman, R.A., Murphree, O.D., and Reese, W.G. (1979): Familial anthropophobia in pointer dogs? *Archives Gen. Psychiatry* **36**, 988–993.

Reisner, I. (1991): The pathophysiologic basis of behavior problems. *Veterinary Clinics of North America: Small Animal Practice* **21**, 207–224.

CONSULTATION
(5-phase model)

- Fact-finding
- Problem explanation
- Recommendations
- Increase owner understanding
- Compliance maximization

**CHANGES IN OWNER
ATTITUDES/BEHAVIOR**

- Correct misconceptions
- Change attitudes
- Increase understanding
- Recommendations for modifying
  animal's environment
- Recommendations for modifying
  behavior towards animal
- Recommend contacting family
  veterinarian

**MODIFY ANIMAL'S
ENVIRONMENT**

- Specific environmental
  changes
- General care/maintenance
  condition changes

**CHANGE BEHAVIOR
TOWARDS ANIMAL**

- Correct owner mistakes
- Cessation of ineffective
  methods
- Avoid problem situations
- Conventional obedience
  training
- Training in problem situations
- Modify owner-animal
  interactional ground rules
- Systematic behavior
  therapy methods

**CONTACT FAMILY
VETERINARIAN**

- Medical examination
- Treat medical problem
- Castration
- Drug therapy

CHANGE IN ANIMAL'S BEHAVIOR

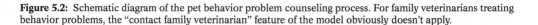

Figure 5.2: Schematic diagram of the pet behavior problem counseling process. For family veterinarians treating behavior problems, the "contact family veterinarian" feature of the model obviously doesn't apply.

6 Practice Organization

There are many organizational possibilities for carrying out pet behavior problem counseling. Counselors may make house calls, see clients in their office, or conduct extended interviews over the telephone. They may meet with clients only once for an extended consultation (with later contacts taking place via telephone), or they may meet with clients two, three, or even more times over a period of several weeks. Finally, although pet behavior problem counseling may be the only service the counselor offers, there is a large and steadily increasing number of small animal veterinarians who have added behavior problem counseling to the many other services they provide to pet owners.

The present chapter will use my own practice methods as an example in which to discuss the various elements and issues which are associated with all forms of pet behavior problem counseling. In doing so, I make no claim that this practice approach is best. To the contrary, meeting with clients only once is often an inadequate attempt to provide help to clients who are unwilling or unable to pay for the series of sessions required to maximize the chances for successful treatment. Then too, while the pet behavior problem counselor who sees clients in their homes has the considerable advantage of being able to observe the family and animal in their normal home environment, veterinary counselors who interview clients in their practices do not have to take the pains non-veterinary counselors who make house calls do to convince skeptical clients that they are in the hands of a qualified and competent specialist. Small animal veterinarians are therefore in an ideal position to function as pet behavior problem counselors on both counts: clients have no doubts as to their qualifications or competence, and clients are accustomed to

following their treatment recommendations and coming repeatedly to their practice when this is necessary or helpful. Family veterinarians also have the considerable advantage of knowing the clients, animal, and the nature of the problem before the consultation itself begins.

Practice elements

Consultation

As considered in Chapter 4, the pet behavior counselor must discuss the problem at length with the client in order to learn all of the necessary facts of the case and give, explain, and sometimes demonstrate recommendations. Not knowing anything about the case beforehand, my house calls tend to be quite long – often an hour or more for cat cases and 2-3 hours for dog cases. However, for the small animal veterinarian who is already familiar with clients, animal, and problem, half this time might be realistic – particularly if provision is made for one or two brief follow-up office visits to support the clients' treatment efforts during the following weeks.

Client information form

I use three special types of forms in my cases. The first is the *client information form* which I generally ask clients to fill out after the initial questioning has reached the point where I feel that I know most of what I need to know to understand the nature of the problem. Figures 6.1 and 6.2 present two versions of this form, one for dogs and one for cats. Readers should feel free to use or adapt these to suit their own counseling needs.

Having owners fill out this type of form offers the following advantages.

CLIENT INFORMATION FORM / DOG

Name of owner_____Telephone_____

Address_____

Name of dog_____ Breed_____Size/weight_____

Sex_____Age_____ Castrated?_____Age of acquisition_____

Source_____ Where is your home? city / suburbs / rural area

Size of home: approx._____m² How many persons in household?_____

Age(s) of child(ren):_____Occupation of head of household:_____

Number of walks/day:_____ How long (each):_____ On a leash? _____

How often does it play with other dogs during walks: Often / Sometimes / Never

Other animals in household:_____

Veterinarian (name)_____Date of last veterinary examination:_____

Please make a cross (**X**) in the appropriate column:

	YES	NO
– Obedience training at home?.............................	____	____
Using food tidbits?..................................	____	____
– Obedience training at obedience school?............	____	____
Using food tidbits?..................................	____	____
– The dog is: nervous..................................	____	____
underactive..............................	____	____
overactive...............................	____	____
pushy	____	____
stubborn...................................	____	____
affectionate..............................	____	____
playful......................................	____	____
obedient...................................	____	____

Does it sit on command? Always / Sometimes / Never

Does it lie down on command? Always / Sometimes / Never

Does it come when called? Always / Sometimes / Never

Please make a cross (**X**) in the appropriate column for the following behavior problems:

	OFTEN	OCCASIONALLY	NEVER
– Stealing food....................................	___	___	___
– Eating excrement	___	___	___
– Sexual behavior towards human beings	___	___	___
– Masturbation...................................	___	___	___
– Excessive fear reactions..................................	___	___	___
– Excessive licking or scratching of fur..............	___	___	___
– Disobedient....................................	___	___	___
– Difficult to control.............................	___	___	___
– Defending objects against family members......	___	___	___
– Excessive barking or growling at strangers......	___	___	___

	OFTEN	OCCASIONALLY	NEVER
– Biting strangers	——	——	——
– Aggressive to other dogs..............................	——	——	——
– Biting family members	——	——	——
– Growling at family members	——	——	——
– Aggressive when petted	——	——	——
– Aggressive when brushed	——	——	——
– Aggressive when touched	——	——	——
– Aggressive when pushed/shoved	——	——	——
– Aggressive when reached for.......................	——	——	——
– Aggressive when threatened	——	——	——
– Aggressive when punished	——	——	——
– Aggressive when disturbed while sleeping/resting	——	——	——
– Aggressive when eating...............................	——	——	——
– Urinating in home.......................................	——	——	——
– Defecating in home.....................................	——	——	——
– Destructive in home....................................	——	——	——
– Excessive whining, barking, howling, etc	——	——	——
– Roaming	——	——	——
– Destructive in the yard...............................	——	——	——

Please answer with "**YES**" or "**NO**":

– Do you consider your dog to be a member of the family? ....   ——
– Can it sleep in family members' beds?..   ——
– Is it allowed on the furniture?...   ——
– Do you take it with you on short errands?...   ——
– Do you take it with you on vacations? ....   ——
– Do you share food with it from the table?...   ——
– Do you share snacks with it? ....   ——
– Do you talk to it at least once a day? ....   ——
– Do you talk with it about important matters at least once a month?.......   ——
– Do you believe it is aware of your moods?...   ——
– Do you believe you are aware of its moods? ....   ——
– Do you have photographs of it? ....   ——
– Do you celebrate its birthday? ....   ——

Figure 6.1: Client information form for dogs (filled out by owner)

Collection of general client and animal information

It is a convenient method to collect information such as the client's name, address, telephone number, and family/home situation as well as the animal's breed, age, sex, size, and name, whether it is castrated, and where and when it was obtained.

Collection of information about conditions under which pet is kept, its general behavioral characteristics, and its other major and minor behavioral problems

Collection of such information helps round out the picture which has been formed up to this point in the consultation, and it sometimes brings new facts to light which, in turn, may open up new lines that need to be explored in further questioning. It also provides valuable data which can be useful for research purposes.

Collection of additional information about owner's attitudes and pet-keeping practices

The last set of questions on both forms were included purely for research purposes. They can be easily omitted without significant loss if the forms are adapted for use by the small animal practitioner. However, they do sometimes have the useful function of sensitizing owners to their own anthropomorphic attitudes and spoiling practices and thereby helping to lay the groundwork for changes in owner behaviors which may be required in cases, for example, like dominance aggression in dogs.

Important addition to case files

Clients often call months later when I cannot immediately recall anything about their case. When they do call, I ask them to hold the line for a minute while I get out their file which contains this *client information form*, a *case report form* (described below), a copy of the *treatment recommendation letter* sent to the client a few days after the consultation, and a copy of the *follow-up questionnaire* (described below) sent to the client several weeks

later. Glancing through all of this information, it takes only a couple of minutes to refresh one's memory about the particular case and its salient features.

Collection of statistical information concerning the various dog and cat behavioral problems

For example, a comparison of information collected with this form concerning the conditions under which the animal is kept (e.g. Are there other animals in home?), general behavioral characteristics (e.g. Is cat nervous?), and other behavioral problems (e.g. How often does cat show excessive fear reactions?) for spraying and non-spraying cats provided only limited support for the Hart and Hart (1985) contention that anxiety is the leading cause of urine marking problems in cats (see Chapter 20). Similarly, comparing the answers given by owners of problem and non-problem cats and dogs (see Chapter 3) indicated that the kinds of anthropomorphic attitudes and "spoiling" behavioral practices which are often cited in the popular pet press as being responsible for pet behavioral problems do not differ substantially between these various populations.

Essentially, information collected using forms of this kind can be profitably used for research purposes in a young field such as this one where there is a lack of reliable information relevant to many of the areas the forms address.

Case report form

The second major type of form is the *case report form* shown in Fig. 6.3. As soon as possible after the consultation, I go through this form and write down all relevant information. Not every question need be answered at this time, but in answering the main ones about the nature of the problem, eliciting situations, what people have done to try and combat the problem, and the existence of related problems, one can draw a fairly detailed portrait of the case for later reference in the space of perhaps 10 or 15 minutes. Unusual or unique features of each

CLIENT INFORMATION FORM / CAT

Name of owner_____Telephone_____
Address_____
Name of cat_____Breed_____Sex_____Age_____
Castrated?_____Age of acquisition_____Source_____
Where is your home?   city / suburbs / rural area   Size of home: approx._____m²
How many persons in household?_____ Age(s) of child(ren):_____
Occupation of head of household:_____Can the cat go outdoors?_____
On the balcony?_____ Other animals in household:_____
Veterinarian (name)_____Date of last veterinary examination:_____

Please make a cross (X) in the appropriate column:

		YES	NO
– The cat is:	nervous...........................	____	____
	underactive........................	____	____
	overactive..........................	____	____
	pushy .... ____		____
	affectionate.......................	____	____
	playful...............................	____	____
	independent.......................	____	____

Please make a cross (X) in the appropriate column for the following behavior problems:

	OFTEN	OCCASIONALLY	NEVER
– Aggressive to other cats....................................	____	____	____
– Playful scratching or biting of persons.............	____	____	____
– Aggressive scratching or biting of persons.......	____	____	____
– Excessive fear reactions...................................	____	____	____
– Excessive biting or licking of fur.	____	____	____
– Urination outside of litter box..........................	____	____	____
– Defecation outside of litter box........................	____	____	____
– Excessive begging (e.g. meowing).	____	____	____
– Scratching of furniture, carpets, etc.	____	____	____
– Aggressive to family members	____	____	____
– Aggressive to strangers	____	____	____
– Aggressive when petted	____	____	____
– Aggressive when touched.................................	____	____	____
– Aggressive when reached for............................	____	____	____
– Aggressive when punished	____	____	____
– Eating house plants	____	____	____
– Excessive running through the home..............	____	____	____
– Eating of non-food substances/objects............	____	____	____
– Lack of appetite	____	____	____
– Inadequate care of fur......................................	____	____	____
– Restlessness...	____	____	____

Please answer with "**YES**" or "**NO**":

– Do you consider your cat to be a member of the family?........................   _____
– Can it sleep in family members' beds? ....   _____
– Is it allowed on the furniture? ....   _____
– Do you take it with you on short errands? ....   _____
– Do you take it with you on vacations? ....   _____
– Do you share food with it from the table. ....   _____
– Do you share snacks with it?..   _____
– Do you talk to it at least once a day? ....   _____
– Do you talk with it about important matters at last once a month?.......   _____
– Do you believe it is aware of your moods?. ....   _____
– Do you believe you are aware of its moods?..   _____
– Do you have photographs of it?..   _____
– Do you celebrate its birthday?..   _____

Figure 6.2: Client information form for cats (filled out by owner)

case are also noted. Investing this additional time is the last thing one feels like doing after a long and tiring interview. However, when contacted by the client months later, or when it comes time to extract data from case files that is not provided by the client information form, this type of written record of the important, interesting, and unusual features of the case is invaluable.

Treatment recommendation letter

In addition to making recommendations during the consultation itself, I always send clients a letter a few days later containing a written summary of the most important recommendations. This is particularly helpful for clients when there are numerous recommendations or if family members other than those who participated in the consultation are to be involved in the treatment. A further advantage is that this approach allows the counselor to reflect on the case for a day or two after the consultation and alter the recommendations given or add new ones if this is necessary.

Of course, a copy of this letter is also an indispensable addition to clients' files, for one obviously needs to recall exactly what clients were instructed to do if they call several months later for additional advice.

Report to the referring veterinarian

Another necessary element in any referral practice is sending a report to the referring family veterinarian. The main functions of this type of letter are to inform veterinarians that a consultation took place, briefly describe the problem and general type of treatment recommended, encourage them to call if they would like to know more about the problem or treatment, and of course thank them for the referral.

Follow-up contacts with clients

Especially when one meets personally only once with clients, some provision for follow-up telephone contacts to support the treatment is indispensable. During the consultation, I encourage clients to call me if there is any problem, if the treatment does not work as well as expected, or if all has gone well and they would just simply like to report this. I also point out at this time that such follow-up calls are often necessary to modify the recommended treatment in some way, that most clients call often in the days and weeks following the consultation, and that they should feel free to call even months later if they have any kind of question. Even if clients do not in fact call later, it eases their mind during the days and weeks following the consultation to know that they will not be

CASE REPORT FORM

Owner (name, address)_____

_____ Animal _____

Date_____

NATURE OF THE PROBLEM
What is the main problem?

Are there other problems?

How frequently does each problem occur?

How serious is each problem?

BACKGROUND INFORMATION
How and when did the behavior problem(s) occur for the first time?

Were there other minor problems at that time or previously?

What illnesses has the animal had? (If relevant)

Description of other persons and animals in the household

Description of the living conditions
– inside the home:

– outside of the home:

SUMMARY OF RELEVANT INFORMATION
Main problem(s):

The methods the owners have applied to try to correct the problem. (What methods? How consistently? For how long? With what results?)

The circumstances in which the problem occurs:

Owners' opinions: about the animal, its problems, euthanasia, possible treatment measures, etc.

Relevant observations during the consultation:
– Behavior of animal:

– Reactions of the owners to the behavior of the animal:

Is there something else about the case which is important or unusual?

PROVISIONAL DIAGNOSIS

INSTRUCTIONS TO THE OWNERS

1.

2.

3.

4.

5.

Others:

PROGNOSIS (and relevant factors)

ADDITIONAL RELEVANT INFORMATION

Figure 6.3: Case report form (filled out by counselor)

left alone with the problem as before even if the treatment does not produce the expected results.

Follow-up questionnaire

It is helpful to collect follow-up information on cases for obvious reasons. In this connection, Figure 6.4 is a follow-up questionnaire which I sent to clients in a series of 161 consecutive cases including a few where the recommendation was to give the pet to someone else (most commonly, to find new homes without children for dogs that were aggressive to small children). The questionnaire was accompanied by a cover letter asking clients to cooperate and explaining to them how important such information is for helping counselors improve the advice given to clients. The survey was anonymous, but some owners nevertheless placed their return address on the envelope.

The results obtained for the 113 clients (approx. 70 %) who returned the form are presented below:

How helpful was the interview?

Very/quite helpful	59%
Somewhat helpful	37%
Not helpful	4%

The cost of the home visit was:

Much too high	4%
A little too high	21%
Reasonable	73%
Surprisingly low	2%

How many of the treatment recommendations were followed?

All of them	27%
Most of them	50%
Some/a few of them	20%
None of them	2%

How long were recommendations followed?

Few weeks or more	87%
One or two weeks	10%
Less than this	3%

How effective were the recommendations?

Very/quite effective	62%
Mildly effective	27%
Didn't help	11%

Extent to which recommended treatment improved the main problem?

Completely eliminated	18%
Greatly/considerably improved	47%
Mildly improved	23%
No improvement	12%
Problem got worse	0%

The following are some tentative conclusions which can be drawn from the answers to these survey questions:

- 96% of clients found the consultation helpful to some degree, and approx. 73% of clients found the cost of the home visit reasonable (approx. 140 and 110 dollars for dog and cat house calls respectively) with most of the remaining clients finding the cost a little too high rather than much too high or surprisingly low. These statistics indicate that in retrospect, almost all clients felt that they had received a useful service, and a substantial majority of them thought that it was worth the money they paid for it.
- According to clients' answers to the third and fourth questions, compliance with the recommended treatments was reasonably good: 77% stated that they followed most or all of the recommendations, and 87% indicated that they followed the recommendations for a few weeks or longer. However, only 27% of clients stated that they followed all of the recommendations – a fact which suggests that clients either found it impossible to follow some of the recommendations (e.g. for psychological or practical reasons) or that after the consultation, they felt free to pick and choose which they would follow and which not.
- In 65% of cases, clients found the recommended treatment quite effective in considerably or greatly improving the problem or eliminating it completely. In a further 23% of cases, the improvement was more modest. And in 12% of cases there was no im-

FOLLOW-UP QUESTIONNAIRE

1. The home visit was:

☐ Very/quite helpful   ☐ Somewhat helpful   ☐ Not helpful

2. The cost of the home visit was:

☐ Much too high   ☐ Reasonable
☐ A little too high   ☐ Surprisingly low

3. How many of the treatment recommendations did you consistently follow?

☐ All of them   ☐ Some of them   ☐ None of them
☐ Most of them   ☐ A few of them

4. For how long?

☐ Few weeks or more   ☐ One or two weeks   ☐ Less than this

5. How effective were these recommendations?

☐ Very effective   ☐ Mildly effective
☐ Quite effective   ☐ Didn't help

6. To what extent did the recommended treatment improve the main problem?

☐ Main problem **completely eliminated**
☐ Main problem **greatly improved**
☐ Main problem **considerably improved**
☐ Main problem **mildly improved**
☐ Main problem **did not improve**
☐ Main problem **got worse**

7. If the most serious problem did not improve after following my advice, did you find another method for eliminating or improving it?

☐ No   ☐ Yes. Please explain:_____

Comments on what has happened to the main probem(s) since my home visit

Figure 6.4: Follow-up questionnaire

provement at all. Although in a few of these cases (e.g. those in which finding a new home the dog was the primary or sole recommendation) no improvement was expected, in others clients may not have followed the most important recommendations, not followed them diligently enough, not applied them correctly, or the recommended treatment simply may not have been effective enough to cope with the problem. On balance, the overall improvement figure of 88% in the present survey is comparable with improvement figures ranging from 70% to 88% given by several other well-known pet behavior counselors (e.g. Houpt, 1983; Line and Voith, 1986; O'Farrell and Neville, 1994; Olm and Voith, 1988).

- While 88% of owners reported some degree of improvement, only 18% stated that the problem was completely eliminated. This means that realistically speaking, varying degrees of improvement but not complete elimination of the problem is the most likely outcome of single consultations. Studies reporting complete elimination (i.e. "cure") as opposed to improvement rates indicate that these vary greatly with the nature of the problem. For example, while Olm and Houpt (1988) reported a cure rate of approx. 30% in 43 cat housesoiling cases (with an overall improvement rate of 81%), Line and Voith (1886) reported the complete elimination of dominance in aggression in only 1 of 24 dogs (i.e. 4% cure rate with a high overall improvement rate of 88%).

General conclusions of the follow-up survey

Carrying out such a survey is extremely helpful for the pet behavior counselor. It provides needed feedback concerning retrospective client attitudes towards the counseling process, counselor, and costs of the counseling service. It also provides needed feedback concerning the effectiveness of the counseling process in solving client problems and thereby guards against complacency by providing the counselor with a realistic picture of the results of

his/her efforts. This in turn can have a major impact on future counseling effectiveness, for effective counseling implies providing clients with a realistic prognosis of whether and to what extent the problem can be improved or eliminated. If clients' initial expectations are too high, they may become quickly disappointed during the early stages of treatment, lose confidence in the counselor's advice, and therefore abandon the treatment method before major degrees of improvement can be achieved.

Naturally, knowing that only a small minority of problems are completely eliminated and something like one out of eight are not improved at all as a result of the consultation is sobering to the pet behavior problem counselor. Also disturbing is the realization that the 88% overall improvement figure may be somewhat inflated (particularly with regard to the "mildly improved" answer category). As Askew (1994) points out, given the facts that (1) there are spontaneous fluctuations in the severity of many behavior problems and (2) people often seek help only when problems are at their very worst, one might predict on purely statistical grounds an average improvement tendency in the days and weeks following the consultation even if the advice did not help at all. The behavior specialist often sees this effect in operation. People call. They are at their wits end. They can no longer cope with the problem. But when the time comes for the house call or office appointment a few days later, problems are rarely worse but sometimes have improved or normalized again.

The main point is, of course, that the quantitative results of such follow-up surveys should be interpreted with caution. For they lack the necessary control group which would allow one to determine the effectiveness of the counseling process as precisely as one would like. At best, they provide only a rough estimate of the effectiveness of the pet behavior problem counseling process.

Finally, it is also important to note that the results of follow-up surveys would be expected to vary greatly depending on the type of practice. In particular, the problem elimination and improvement figures for family veterinarians who combine behavior problem counseling with a normal small animal practice would be expected to be considerably higher simply because of having many more minor, easily-solvable problems among their cases. In contrast, in referral practices, problems tend to be unusually severe. For it is the more serious or difficult cases that have not responded favorably to the family veterinarian's treatment suggestions which are generally referred.

Professionalism

Although there are various ways in which a pet behavior problem referral practice or the behavior problem counseling activities of the small animal veterinarian can be organized, the following elements would seem to be the basic preconditions for responsible, professional, and ethical counseling in any setting.

Academic qualifications and a genuinely scientific approach

The importance of basic academic qualifications in a relevant area such as veterinary medicine, experimental psychology, human behavior therapy, or ethology cannot be overestimated. The main reason is not that one must be academically qualified to be skilled in dealing with people or training animals, but rather that professional training inclines and prepares one to base counseling activities on the relevant interdisciplinary and international *scientific literature*. A professional approach requires the application of the combined knowledge of the various types of specialists working in the field, and it requires some minimal knowledge of fields far removed from one's own (e.g. experimental psychology principles, knowledge concerning canine and feline ethology, knowledge of possible pathophysiological causes of behavior problems and possible side effects of commonly prescribed medicaments, etc.).

Many of the treatment measures that are now routinely recommended by today's academically qualified pet behavior problem counselors were first suggested by dog trainers and other poorly qualified or unqualified individuals. However, the time is past when the insights and simplistic, often dogmatic views of such individuals can play a useful role in the further development of the field. Competence in the pet behavior problem field of today requires that the counselor be knowledgeable in a number of scientific fields and intimately familiar with the large and still rapidly growing scientific literature in the pet behavior problem area itself. If there is one major difference between today's academically qualified veterinarian, psychologist, or biologist practitioners and the academically unqualified dog trainer who advertises his/her services as a "pet behavior therapist", "dog psychologist", or "canine behaviorist", it is the following: while academically qualified practitioners know that true competence can only be achieved by a combination of extensive counseling experience with a comprehensive knowledge of the interdisciplinary scientific literature, dog trainers are confident that they have learned everything they need to know about how to solve dog behavior problems in their obedience schools.

Responsible dealings with clients

Being responsible in one's dealings with clients means being sensitive to the human physical and psychological health-related aspects of pet keeping and pet behavior problems. It also means treating every client with respect and doing everything one can to provide a maximally effective service not only during the consultation, but also afterwards; for example, by giving the client written instructions and discussing aspects of the case as often as the client wishes over the telephone. In short, one should have a genuinely caring attitude and try one's best within the limits of the situation to help the client in any way one can.

Respecting the client's right to privacy is another crucial element. Cases can be discussed or summarized in written form at a later point, but names should never be mentioned and case details should not be so extensively discussed that the identity of the family would be recognized by acquaintances.

Keeping detailed records and files

Keeping detailed case records is extremely important for refreshing one's memory of the salient features of the case when clients call perhaps a month or two later to discuss some aspect of the problem or treatment. The possibility of some sort of future legal action either against the counselor or client involving the animal's problem behavior (e.g. animal has bitten a person or another animal, client is threatened with eviction because of an unsolved elimination or separation anxiety problem) is another reason for keeping detailed records. And finally, detailed case records are extremely useful for research purposes.

Carrying out basic field research

In the pet behavior problem field where the published research is minimal and there are too few university professors actively researching the area to remedy this situation in the near future, a special burden is placed on all practitioners to do what they can to advance the field in this regard. For one thing, records from a number of similar cases can be reviewed retrospectively to attempt to answer questions about specific types of problems which may arise like, for example, is aggression towards strangers more likely to develop in dogs which showed fear of strangers when young, or do spraying cats tend to be more nervous or fearful than other cats. Suggestive answers to such questions can sometimes be found simply by reading through all of the material collected on these types of cases.

A second research possibility is to administer to clients brief questionnaires such as the client information forms (Figures 6.1 and 6.2) during the consultation. Such questionnaires are not difficult to design, take no more than 5-10 minutes of the owner's time, and when coupled with information obtained by giving the same questionnaires to a control group of owners of non-problem animals, a wealth of extremely useful data can be obtained with a minimum investment of time and at practically no cost.

Specialist as advisor to animal shelters

Behavior counselors are sometimes asked to make visits to animal shelters to give advice on specific cases or to help make the decision of whether to euthanize particular animals. Generally, there is little to be done in the animal shelter itself about particular behavioral problems: the animal must be adopted into an appropriate home first and then the new owner helped to provide the kind of treatment required.

In discussing behavior problems with animal shelter personnel, the counselor should always stress the need for collecting detailed information about problems from the owners who are surrendering the animal. For only if such information is available is it possible to make decisions related to adoption vs. euthanasia and, if adoption is a realistic possibility, into what kind of family/setting and with what kind of treatment to counteract possible behavioral problems. Of course it is difficult in many cases for animal shelters to obtain this kind of information because those surrendering the animal are not prepared to cooperate or the shelter itself lacks the personnel to carry out this relatively time-consuming interviewing of owners on a routine basis.

In advising animal shelters concerning the kinds of information they must collect about, for example, aggressive dogs, it is often helpful to provide shelter personnel with a list of specific questions they should ask owners – perhaps with the help of a form they have drawn up for this purpose. While they may not always go this far, advising animal shelters in this way often helps considerably in the sense that when the counselor is called in later to give an opinion in specific cases, shelter personnel have taken pains in their interview of those surrendering the animal to obtain the kind of information he/she requires.

Ethical issues

Professionalism also implies ethical behavior. And the pet behavior consultation area is one in which several important ethical issues arise.

Giving human physical health and psychological well-being top priority

First and foremost, the veterinary or non-veterinary behavior counselor has been consulted to provide assistance to family members and not the animal. Usually the best interests of the two coincide: the correction of an aggression problem can make a dog or cat less dangerous for family members and ultimately save it from being euthanized. But when the choice must be made between the physical safety of family members and the welfare of the animal, it is human health which must be given top priority.

When the animal is exceedingly dangerous, this issue is straightforward and easy to resolve. But when it comes to problems where it is primarily people's psychological and emotional well-being which is involved, it can be a different story. Surrendering much-loved pets to animal shelters where they will face an uncertain future is the very last thing that most pet owners want to do. When things have gone so far that owners are seriously considering this option, it is usually a sign that owners simply cannot cope any longer with a problem situation that has been placing them under considerable stress for some time. Family members argue with one another, marriages are put to the test, and owners often break down and shed tears in the counselor's presence because of the problems they are having with their animals.

The primary lesson for the pet behavior problem counselor is that it is crucial to understand what a profound stress problem pets can represent for families. For this implies that the counselor should basically be supportive rather than critical of the client's view that life cannot and should not go on like this – that either the problem must be solved or the pet must go. It perhaps sounds harsh to put it this way, but the reality of life with an animal that is destroying your furniture, threatening your guests, or turning your neighbors into bitter enemies is also harsh. To encourage people to do everything in their power to correct behavior problems before considering surrendering the pet to an animal shelter is one thing. But it is quite another

to expect them to live with insoluble problems come what may, which would essentially amount to placing considerations of the animal's welfare above those of the members of its human family.

Animal protection aspects

Of course, pet behavior counselors also try to do what they can for the pets by, for example, correcting owner mistreatment when this is in evidence. In one of my recent cases, I tried everything short of shouting at a woman to convince her that either she must adjust her daily schedule to be able to give her dog the exercise it needs or she should give it to someone else who is willing and able to do this. Similarly, pet behavior counselors often advise owners to provide their dogs with more contacts with conspecifics, let them off the leash sometimes, or play with them more often during the day. Not necessarily because these things are crucial to solving some behavior problem, but simply because the counselor feels that the animal is not getting something important that it needs to live a normal and decent life. Essentially, looking at each case from the point of view of the pet's welfare as well – and making recommendations to improve it when they are called for – should also be recognized as one of the major aims of the pet behavior counseling process.

Protecting the general public

Responsible pet ownership means more than doing everything that is good for the pet. It also means protecting one's friends, neighbors, and other members of the community and their pets from, for example, one's aggressive dog. Here is another area in which pet behavior problem counselors are sometimes at odds with clients who can be surprisingly relaxed about such matters. "Well, if Rocky takes a dislike to someone once it a awhile, and bites him, that's his right, isn't it? I'm certainly no saint. So why shouldn't he be allowed to have his little faults too?"

When the pet behavior problem counselor feels that members of the general public or their pets are being clearly endangered by an owner's irresponsible attitude in this regard, it is sometimes necessary and appropriate to politely but firmly remind the owner of his/her responsibility towards others in the community. Accordingly, pet behavior counselors often strongly recommend that dangerous animals be muzzled and/or kept on a leash in potential problem situations. And particularly in the case of large dogs that are walked by not-so-large elderly people, it is often necessary to strongly emphasize to owners of potentially dangerous dogs that they must always be in a position of being able to physically control their animals even if this means using a special kind of collar which may attract attention and elicit criticism from passersby.

Use of medicaments

In my view, the routine prescription of progestins or other drugs for almost every serious behavioral problem case that walks in through the door which is practiced by some veterinarians – at least in Germany – should be questioned both on ethical and pragmatic grounds. As will be considered in the chapters throughout the remainder of the book, the available research evidence and combined experience of scores of behavior problem counselors indicate that drugs are effective only in certain types of cases. Taking all of the various dog and cat problems together, it is only in a small minority of cases that I recommend to the referring veterinarian that some drug be prescribed. This is not only because the animal doesn't really need them – which is the ethical side of the question – but also for the entirely practical reason that the prescription of a drug may act to reduce the chances that clients will comply with the behavior-oriented recommendations which are essential to coming to grips with the problem. Give people a set of demanding behavioral treatment recommendations and they might or might not carry out the treatment with the degree of consistency which is required. But give them the same recommendations and simultaneously prescribe a supposedly effective drug, and what might happen to compliance with the

recommended behavioral treatment then? Human nature being what it is, some owners will be lax as far as the time-consuming behavioral component of the treatment is concerned and instead tend to rely more heavily on the medicament than the counselor intended.

The problem is that it may be easier for people to give a dog a tablet every day or take it to their veterinarian now and again for an injection than it is to train it to stop threatening visitors. When clients come to their veterinarian's office because of some behavior problem, it is often this kind of quick and easy solution to their problem which they are hoping for. Thus prescribing some ineffective or mildly effective drug along with a behavior-oriented treatment tends naturally to strengthen the client's belief that there may indeed be an effective drug treatment against the problem. This in turn can lead to the half-hearted application or premature abandoning of behavioral recommendations that many clients will only diligently follow if they are convinced that this is their only hope for coping with the problem.

In Germany, where small animal practitioners are in severe competition with one another and with *Tierheilpraktiker*, non-medical specialists, veterinarians are under severe pressure to meet clients' drug-related expectations. This often results in prescribing homeopathic drugs whose producers claim are effective against behavioral problems. To the extent that such drugs are ineffective or so mild as to be practically ineffective against serious behavioral problems, only a kind of beneficial placebo effect which in some way parallels that often seen in human medicine could justify their use from the medical standpoint. However, in the case of serious behavior problems whose solution obviously requires major sorts of environmental modification or retraining efforts, it is difficult to imagine how such a placebo effect could result in the kind of change in the client's behavior towards the animal which would be genuinely effective in combating the animal's behavior problem.

Accustomed to viewing problems in medical terms and suspecting that behavior problems too may represent some kind of disorder of the normal functioning of the organism, it is not surprising that veterinarians without advanced training in behavior might be inclined to freely prescribe drugs which they have heard or read might be effective against such problems. In this connection, even excellent and balanced discussions such as that in Marder (1991), where the author has listed many drugs that are known to be, suspected to be, or might be effective for particular types of problems, have the unfortunate side effect of encouraging rather that counteracting this tendency by promoting a "try this, or try that" approach to solving problems which may be, in fact, inappropriately treated with drugs of any kind.

In the last analysis, the optimistic expectation voiced by some prominent American veterinary behavior specialists like Marder, Hart, and Voith that new and more effective drug treatments for pet behavioral problems are bound to be discovered in the coming years both reflects and acts to propagate the largely erroneous view that most behavior problems in pets directly parallel those severe behavior disorders in human beings for which drug treatment is appropriate and often highly effective. When one considers how and why behavior problems develop in companion animals from the behavioral science standpoint, it is clear that some kind of interaction between the species' normal learning processes with the individual animal's behavioral predispositions (both genetically preprogrammed and those directly resulting from the animal's past experience history) is at the heart of most behavior problems. It is seldom that some disease process or metabolic disorder is found to be the cause of the common behavioral problems considered in this book. In most cases, the behavioral tendencies that can eventually develop into serious behavior problems in a normal human family environment are statistically common enough and understandable enough from the behavioral science perspective to be considered as falling within the range of behavioral variation which is "normal" for the species. If this is indeed the case, then precisely what sort of effect are tomorrow's wonder drugs supposed to exert on animals' behavior systems? Are they to modify animals' nervous systems in some way? And if so, wouldn't this kind of chemical intervention in the internal physiological processes of an animal which is fully healthy be as ethically questionable as, for example, sedating an overactive dog whose only problem is its lack of opportunities for much-needed exercise?

Of course, sometimes every possible behavioral-oriented solution has been tried without success and, therefore, drug therapy with medicaments that are sometimes reported to be helpful in such cases is the only remaining means of trying to cope with the problem – and perhaps save the animal's life. But it is a different story in cases where there are potentially effective behavioral measures which clients seem to be simply too lazy, inconsistent, lacking in self-discipline, etc. to carry out. Should drug therapy be attempted in these cases? Often this is what happens. But perhaps such negative client attitudes and behavior should not be accepted as lightly and pessimistically as they often are. Even the laziest and normally most inconsistent clients can sometimes be persuaded to carry out demanding behavioral treatments providing that they are convinced that no drug solution to their problem exists. Obviously, it with these sorts of clients in particular where the prescription of an ineffective or only mildly effective drug can do the most harm.

References

Askew, H.R. (1994): Wie wissenschaftlich ist die Tierverhaltenstherapie? *Der praktische Tierarzt* **6**, 539–544.

Hart, B.L., and Hart, L.A. (1985): *Canine and Feline Behavioral Therapy*. Philadelphia: Lea & Febiger.

Houpt, K.A. (1983). Disruption of the Human-Companion Animal Bond: Aggressive Behavior in Dogs. In Katcher, A.H., and Beck, A.M. (eds): *New Perspectives on Our Lives with Companion Animals*. Philadelphia, University of Pennsylvania Press.

Line, S., and Voith, V.L. (1986): Dominance aggression of dogs towards people: Behavior profile and response to treatment. *Applied Animal Behaviour Science* **16**, 77–83.

Marder, A.R. (1991): Psychotropic drugs and behavioral therapy. *Veterinary Clinics of North America: Small Animal Practice* **21**, 329–342.

O'Farrell, V., and Neville, P. (1994): *Manual of Feline Behaviour.* Shurdington, Cheltenham, Glouce-

stershire, UK, British Small Animal Veterinary Association Publications.

Olm, D., and Houpt, K.A. (1988): Feline house soiling problems. *Applied Animal Behaviour Science* **20**, 335–345.

Part II

Treatment of Dog Behavior Problems

7 Understanding Dog Behavior

Clients contact a behavior problem counselor to obtain advice concerning exactly what they must do to solve the problem they are presently having with their pet. To help people solve or at least improve such problems, it is the effectiveness of the various recommendations the counselor gives along with his skill in convincing owners to consistently apply them which are most critical.

In the interest of maximizing the chances for compliance with treatment recommendations, owners must not only understand exactly *what* they must do, they must also understand to some extent *why* each of the various recommendations is important. While some clients are more curious about the behavior of their dog in the scientific sense than others, most are basically sensible, practically-minded people who are willing in theory to invest a great deal of time and energy retraining their animal if they are convinced that this is a reasonable and logical approach to the problem. Convincing them usually involves providing them with three types of information:

- Clients must understand the basic nature of the problem and how their dog's problem behaviors should be viewed within the context of what is normal and natural behavior for dogs – what might be termed canine ethology background information.
- Clients must understand how and why each of the various recommended treatment elements tend to produce behavioral changes in the desired direction – that is, the mode of action and expected effect of each treatment recommendation.
- Clients must be persuaded that such treatment methods have proven themselves to be effective means of coping with the type of problem involved – their demonstrated clinical effectiveness.

This chapter discusses the basic facts and related theoretical views that form the basis for the kind of canine ethology background information which the counselor must be able to explain to clients whenever this is helpful to their understanding of the problem, treatment goals, and treatment methods. The style of presentation will be brief: an attempt to summarize and integrate within the space of a few pages the most important features of an extensive literature whose detailed explication would require a book on its own. The views presented here will be those which most all behavioral scientists share, and specific references will therefore only be made at particular points in the text where there is some disagreement between authorities, where certain viewpoints have been expressed only by single individuals, or where some specific research project is being discussed. The list of references at the end of the chapter includes some titles not cited during the chapter as suggested sources for readers who would like to learn more about the various topics discussed.

Evolution and domestication

Archeological evidence indicates that the domestic dog, *Canis familiaris*, has existed as a separate species for at least 10,000 years. Experts now agree that the domestic dog evolved from the wolf, *Canis lupis*, perhaps with part of the great diversity between existing breeds of domestic dogs resulting from the domestication process having occurred independently with different wolf subspecies like the western Asiatic wolf, Chinese wolf, North American wolf, and Indian wolf.

The fossil record has little directly to say about the domestication process that gradually turned wolf into dog. One can only speculate here based on, for example, what is known about wolf behavior, the behavior of primitive human hunter-gatherers, the functions dogs perform in modern hunter-gatherer social groups, and the nature of interactions between modern pet owners and their dogs.

Biologically speaking, wolves are similar to human beings in being territorial, highly social predators which live in small, relatively stable social groups, engage in scavenging and cooperative group hunting, and establish temporary home base sites where some individuals remain behind (e.g. young offspring) and are supplied with food by returning group members. In addition, both wolves and human beings have a hierarchical group social structure based on dominance-submission relationships which function to avoid serious aggressive confrontations and thereby contribute to the cooperative character of group life. Both species are also extraordinarily adaptable and capable of adjusting group size, group behavior, and individual behavior to adapt to an extremely wide range of climates and environmental circumstances – something which can be inferred from the fact that subspecies or races of the two are as widely distributed throughout the world as they are.

Thought to be crucial to the beginnings of the domestication process when wolf pups were first brought into hunter-gatherer campsites is the fact that like many other complex animal species, wolves form bond relationships with parents and other members of their social group based on some variant of the process known as *imprinting* – basically where a very young animal develops a strong attachment to another individual or class of individuals during a relatively short period early in its life (between the 3rd and 14th week of life in dogs) which determines to a great extent the types of individuals (e.g. other wolves, dogs, or human beings) towards which it will direct its normal, species-typical social behavior later in life. This imprinting or imprinting-like effect would have resulted in the young wolf behaving towards its adoptive human group as if it were a wolf pack: following and approaching group members, re-

maining in close proximity to them under all circumstances, becoming distressed when separated from them, and being motivated to defend the band's home base area against intruders much the same as domestic dogs that were taken into human families as young puppies still do today.

The fact that an adopted young wolf would have consumed a portion of the band's food supply implies that it would only have been fed if it earned its keep in some way. Two of the most biologically significant ways in which tame wolves would have been useful to hunter-gatherer bands are providing assistance during hunting expeditions and guarding the band's home base area. Domestic dogs still perform such potentially useful tasks for human beings today. Not to be forgotten, however, is that a tame wolf which was fed and tolerated in campsites would also function as a kind of livestock food reserve for times of shortage. And it is also likely that it would have been killed and eaten as soon as it became useless (e.g. injury, old age) or displayed undesirable behavioral characteristics like attacking group members.

Once adopted wolves began to breed in this new hunter-gatherer band context, powerful new selection pressures associated with the preferences of their human hosts were applied which were ultimately responsible for the evolution of a new species, *Canis familiaris*. It is probably reasonable to assume that these selection pressures were applied unintentionally in the sense that young wolves which appealed to band members (e.g. because they were useful in some way and easy to manage) were fed, rather than killed and eaten, without the conscious motivation to progressively develop certain morphological or behavioral traits which characterizes modern selective breeding.

The early stages of this process of domestication must have favored general behavioral characteristics like docility, tameness, reduced aggressiveness, reduced fearfulness, and ease of handling. Individuals which were dangerous to humans or difficult to manage would not have lived long. Those which remained more calm, allowed humans to approach, submissively allowed themselves to be handled and manipulated without becoming aggressive or extremely fearful, and were more flexible and able to adapt to diverse or unnatural (for wolves) physical and social environmental conditions would have been allowed to stay around long enough to breed and pass on the genetic basis of these traits to their offspring. Later at various places and times during the long domestication process, additional selection pressures favoring more specific behavioral characteristics related to working tasks like hunting (sight hounds, scent hounds, dogs which pursued prey underground), war, and agriculture (guarding livestock/crops, herding) began operating which ultimately produced many of the major behavioral differences seen between types of dog breeds today.

Comparison of wolf and dog behavior

Most dog behavioral problems involve social behavior. Characterizing what is normal and natural dog social behavior is, however, complicated by the fact that most modern dogs live as members of human family social groups rather than packs composed only of conspecifics. The approach taken by many authors is therefore to take the social behavior of the dog's immediate progenitor, the wolf, as a starting point, and then characterize the various evolutionary modifications of wolf social behavior that occurred during the domestication process based on (1) observations of the social behavior of feral dogs (abandoned or stray dogs and their offspring living in human city or rural environments) and (2) direct comparisons of the behavior of groups of captive wolves and dogs living under similar conditions. This approach will be followed throughout the remainder of the chapter.

Social behavior of wolves

Wolves live in packs which are small, cohesive, highly organized and stable social groups composed mainly of individuals which are genetically related to one another. A pack may consist of as many as 20 or 30 wolves under some

conditions (e.g. where the survival of the group depends on killing particularly large prey like moose). However, the usual size of packs is between 4 and 7 individuals. In the typical pack, these would be the breeding pair along with varying numbers of subordinate mature adults, juveniles less than 2 years of age, and pups. Pack size tends to be dependent on the available food supply. But it may also reflect the influence of human killing and the fact that generally only dominant members of the pack are allowed to breed. When food is abundant, subdominant wolves may leave the pack and establish packs of their own. The main advantages of pack living are protection against large predators such as bears, the ability to defend (against other wolf packs) and exploit a territory large enough to provide a continuous supply of food, and the ability to employ group hunting strategies to kill very large prey animals.

Reproduction in a wolf pack is usually confined to a single breeding pair consisting of the male and female which occupy the highest positions in the dominance hierarchies which can be separately discerned for males and females. Exceptions to this rule sometimes occur, however, in groups which produce two litters or where another male besides the alpha animal succeeds in copulating and reproducing. Apparently, female mate preferences based on factors other than dominance can also sometimes be involved. Although one may wonder why adult individuals would continue to live in a pack even when they are entirely prevented from breeding, pack living helps these individuals survive and remain healthy while waiting for the opportunity to mate. And even if this never happens, playing their role in helping the group survive and prosper is still doing justice to the genes they carry. For most pack members are genetically related to one another and, in effect, assisting one's blood relatives is, like reproduction itself, a way of ensuring that the portion of one's own genes are passed on to the next generation.

Wolves breed once a year during a particular few-week period which varies, depending on the latitude, between January and April. Immediately prior to and during this time, the level of dominance-related fighting between males and between females increases, reflecting the great importance of individuals' positions in the group's dominance hierarchies to their chances of successfully reproducing. Females first come into estrus at 2 years of age. Litter size is often five or six pups with only about half of the offspring surviving the first two years of life.

Dominance-submission relationships between pack members are therefore a distinctive and critically important feature of pack social organization. Although the male and female dominance hierarchies are commonly thought of as being linear – that is, the alpha individual above all others, the beta individual above all others except the alpha individual, and so on – the situation is far more complex than this. Indeed, the hierarchy obtained by systematically observing a pack can vary greatly depending on how (e.g. aggressive behavior initiated versus submissive displays received) and when (i.e. time versus type of group behavior) dominance is measured. The simple linear peck order seen, for example, in chickens therefore turns out to be a relatively poor model of dominance-related interactions between wolf pack members. In general, dominance between major classes of group members is more predictable: dominance tends to be positively correlated with body weight, sex, and age. Thus, larger animals, males, or adults tend to be dominant over smaller animals, females, and juveniles respectively.

The formation and maintenance of dominance hierarchies within complex animal social groups is basically a way of dealing with the survival- and reproduction-related competition over resources like food, mates, and secure resting places. It eliminates the need for frequent fighting by establishing stable *relationships* between individuals that essentially determine which individual gets potentially contested resources without having to actually fight for them. Fighting may be involved in establishing dominance-submission relationships between individuals that are fairly evenly matched in terms of size and strength. However, these relationships are then maintained by social interactions involving various kinds of communicative postures and gestures that function to confirm which is the dominant and which the submissive member of the pair without fighting and usually without threatening. In wolves, dominance signals include body postures and behavioral gestures like standing in a tall posture with head held up and ears and tail erect while directly staring at the other individual. The dominant animal may also "stand over" the submissive animal by placing its forepaws or chin on the other animal's back. When threatening, the dominant individual may show vertical retraction of the lips, bared teeth, and piloerection of the fur on the back. Submissive postures and gestures are to some extent the opposite of dominance signals with the body held lower, ears laid back close to the head, tail held low, head held lower than the body, and breaking eye contact first and looking away from the dominant animal when stared at. The subordinate individual may also nose, nip, or lick the muzzle of the dominant individual – a behavior which commonly occurs when the submissive individual greets a returning dominant individual. These so-called active submissive behaviors are often contrasted with passive submissive behaviors which may be elicited when the individual is threatened by a more dominant wolf. Here, the submissive wolf rolls over onto its side or back with its ears laid back and tail tucked up between its legs.

The fact that dominance-submission relationships are found in such a wide variety of complex animal species (including human beings) is a measure of how useful this form of social organization is in helping to maintain cohesive, cooperative, largely peaceable social groups composed of basically "selfish" individuals which are genetically preprogrammed to do everything they can to further their own chances for survival and ultimate reproductive success. The cohesive, cooperative character of the wolf social group is in evidence in hunting, territorial defense, caring for young, and indeed in most all of the pack's movements and activities. It has been suggested that one of the major functions of many distinctive wolf behaviors like urine marking of the same sites, group howling, muzzle-to-muzzle greeting behavior, and mutual investigation of ano-genital regions may be to somehow reinforce this group cohesion.

In general, the group's most dominant individuals tend to act as leaders by instigating important pack activities like group defense, hunting, and territorial urine marking. On the level of dominance-submission relationships between pairs of individuals, it has been suggested that dominance is associated with leadership here too in the sense that the dominant member of the pair tends to initiate the most social interactions while responding to the fewest.

Displays signaling dominance and submission are just one example of the extraordinarily complex and refined ways in which wolves use body postures and behavioral movements to communicate with one another. Facial expressions are also extremely important, with the position of the lips, degree of opening of the eyes, and positioning of the ears combining to communicate to others in group that an animal is excited, playful, nervous, curious, frightened, attentive, etc.

Olfactory communication via feces, urine, and glandular secretions is also an important aspect of wolf behavior. Packs often deposit feces and urine at trail junctions and along the edges of territories presumably to inform possible wolf intruders that this territory is occupied. This in turn usually elicits avoidance by lone wolves, for example, which may otherwise be killed by the resident pack. The observation that urine marking frequency increases if foreign scent marks are encountered is also consistent with this view. Urine marking is not, however, only territory-related. It is also thought to play a role in communicating reproductive status (e.g. estrus) and in pair formation and courtship.

Social behavior of feral dogs

To what extent do domestic dogs still exhibit social behavior comparable to that of their not-too-distant and not-too-dissimilar wolf ancestors? One approach to answering this question is to examine the behavior of feral dogs which live our city and rural environments.

In the city, the majority of the dogs wandering about are owned dogs which are allowed to roam. Others are however genuinely feral in that they have no human home and must fend for their own food. In contrast to what might expect judging by the eagerness with which most family dogs look forward to opportunities to socialize with other dogs in the neighborhood during walks, feral dogs are not particularly sociable. Most individuals sighted are solitary and relatively few groups of more than two dogs are encountered. The dogs seen together are usually dogs which are well-acquainted with each other in the sense that their home ranges (i.e. areas in which they are observed at least 95% of the time) overlap and the core areas within these home ranges in which they are sighted at least half the time are no more than 50 m apart.

In cities, both feral and owned, free-roaming dogs seem to be territorial in the sense of having home ranges, an identifiable core area within these, and an identifiable home site within the core area: the dog's most frequently used shelter – which naturally would be an owned dog's family home. However, there is little evidence that these home ranges and core areas are territories in the normal animal behavior sense of being areas which are defended against intruders. Indeed, dogs which are new to a neighborhood seem to move about at will with resident dogs making little or no effort to expel them unless they come too close to the residents' normal resting places – perhaps a vestige of the wolf pattern of more intensely defending the den or home site area of the pack's territory.

Overall, aggressive confrontations are infrequently observed between feral dogs. When aggression does occur, however, it is usually between unfamiliar dogs indicating perhaps that the familiarity dimension rather than some territorial element per se is primary. In wolves too, this familiarity dimension is assumed to be important. Some of the species' social behavioral patterns like urine marking within sight of other animals, investigating of the urine marks, and mutual investigating ano-genital regions of fellow groups members are thought to function as ways of confirming that other group members are familiar, known individuals rather than strangers.

Familiarity may also be a crucial factor in determining mating success. Daniels (1983b) reported that when large numbers of feral or free-roaming owned male dogs have congregated around an estrous female, unfamiliar males were attacked more often than familiar males by males familiar with the female, remained part of the group for a shorter time, and were never observed to successfully mate. Female selection seems to play a major role in determining mating success on such occasions, and females do not mate indiscriminately but rather select mates from among those she is already familiar with. This represents if not a "vestige of monogamous ancestors with long-term pair-bonds" as Daniels suggests, at least of vestige of wolf pattern of mating only with individuals from one's own pack. Wolf-like too is the observation of increased aggression and dominance-submission relationship formation around the estrous female – presumably a vestige of the increased aggression that occurs among male wolves during the breeding season.

Congregations and hence the temporary formation of groups of more than two individuals are also sometimes seen around other resources like food sources or desirable sheltering locations. The rarity with which groups larger than two individuals are sighted in the urban environment is probably related to the facts that scavenging is more efficient when dogs are alone than when in a group, shelters for larger groups are scarce, and larger groups tend to quickly come to the attention of city dogcatchers.

One long-term observational field study of the behavior of a group of three feral dogs (Fox et al., 1975) observed few of the ritualized dominance-submission display dialogues between group members commonly seen among the members of a wolf pack. However, consistent leadership was observed with one individual tending to more frequently initiate activities and determine the direction of group movement after resting, eating, and ranging in the park. The observers also found no indications that urine marks had any kind of territorial function in this group. Although feral city dogs live from food scavenged from what humans throw away or put out for them, these dogs were also observed to hunt in the sense of frequently chasing squirrels in the park within their home range (without success: the 61 recorded chases did not yield a single squirrel). And finally, more aggression towards other dogs was seen in this study than in the other studies discussed above. Of the 33 interactions with other dogs observed, six were classified as "neutral" (dog was ignored), eight were "friendly" (reciprocal tail-wagging), and 19 were "aggressive or offensive" (dogs either intimidated or chased a strange dog away).

In rural environments, larger packs with a consistent leadership hierarchy determining pack movements sometimes form. These appear to be stable packs with a constant membership which maintain territories and repel neighboring groups. While dependent on human scraps and handouts, such packs may also feed on dead livestock and kill wild animals such as rabbits for food. In effect, social organization and behavior which is much more similar to the wolf-like pattern seems to develop in the rural environment.

Direct comparisons of the behavior of wolves and dogs under similar environmental conditions

The most productive research strategy for comparing the behavior of wolves and domestic dogs is to observe groups of both under highly similar environmental conditions. For example, Zimen (1988) discussed the results of this kind of research project which he and his wife carried out 20 years previously. Briefly described, the couple spent three years observing and recording the behaviors occurring both in a wolf pack kept in a large enclosure and in a large group of poodles which had free use of the rest of the property outside of the enclosure. Poodles were an ideal choice for this project, for they were largely bred to be family dogs rather than to perform certain specialized tasks (e.g. hunting, guarding, herding, transport, etc.) as is the case with most other breeds.

The goal of this project was to obtain a detailed *ethogram* or catalogue of each species' characteristic types of behavior for comparison purposes. For the wolf, the end result was a list of 362 individual behaviors organized into several major functional categories like play, sexual behavior, movement behavior, care of young, etc. Overall, the observers found 231 (i.e. 64%) of these individual behaviors to be identical or very similar in the poodles. Only 46 (13%) of the wolf behaviors were no longer present in the dogs – mainly communicative behaviors in wolves which poodles cannot display because of their floppy ears. For the 85 (23%) behaviors which were obviously derived from their wolf ancestors but are now shown in poodles in considerably or greatly changed form, the following general types of changes were noted:

- Many poodle behaviors are performed less skillfully or intensely than corresponding behaviors in the wolf.
- Although many interrelated behavioral sequences in the wolf are displayed in uncoordinated and incomplete form in the poodle, the poodle also shows some new behavioral combinations.
- Some poodle behaviors occur only in a playful form lacking the dimension of "seriousness" seen in the corresponding wolf pattern. In this respect, the poodle behaviors are comparable with those of young wolves.
- A few poodle behaviors occur in a more complex form than in the wolf.
- Changes in or the disappearance of specific behaviors has occurred to a much greater degree in some functional categories than in others.

The following is a brief account based on that presented in Zimen (1988) of the nature of the changes or lack of changes in the various functional categories.

General forms of movement

Approx. 30% (8 out of 27) of the wolf behaviors in this functional category have changed – mostly movements which require great strength, physical skill, and coordination like various forms of jumping. For trotting and galloping as well, the poodles' gait appears stiff and clumsy compared to the smooth, elegant, energy-economizing gait of adult wolves.

Orientation behaviors

Many of these behaviors have changed (41 %). These mainly involve the distinct body posture and movement of particular parts of the body (unlike poodles, wolves use changes in ear positions to help assess incoming auditory stimuli) when orienting towards distant stimuli, and the comparatively greater restlessness or agitation of wolves in response to minor disturbances.

Protection and defense

Many changes were seen here too (46%), with passive forms of defense like fleeing remaining similar while the active, attacking defensive behaviors having become clearly less intense. Poodles no longer display the great strength, leaping capability, and speed of reaction seen in defensive wolves. Related expressive behaviors like growling and baring the teeth are much less pronounced in poodles. Finally, the urination, defecation, and trembling shown by very fearful wolves occur in much weaker form in poodles, if at all.

Hunting behavior

Three-quarters of these behaviors have changed. Poodles don't and cannot successfully hunt large prey, and their hunting of small prey is much less skillful, quick, concentrated, and persistent. Instead, their hunting behavior resembles the chasing after moving objects shown by young wolves. Poodles too chase everything that moves like rabbits, crows, falling leaves, or bicyclists without catching them. In contrast, wolves quickly learn to recognize genuine prey and know what can be successfully chased. Their behavior is purposeful and goal-oriented whereas that of poodles is an end in itself which appears to be self-reinforcing.

Eating and elimination

With 22% and 16% changed respectively, specific behaviors in the eating and elimination categories are fairly similar in poodles and wolves. However, poodles tend to eat in a much more "civilized" manner compared to the wolves' rapid devouring of large quantities of food. And poodle bitches rarely if ever lift their legs to urinate the way female wolves do.

Transport and storage of food

Many changes (47%) were observed in this category, mainly behaviors related to providing for the future and caring for young. The systematic, coordinated behavioral sequence used to bury food seen in wolves is no longer present in poodles. Here too, the remnants of this wolf behavior seem playful and lacking in seriousness in poodles. Poodle mothers may carry food to their puppies, but they seldom regurgitate food for them. Poodle fathers and other group members do not share in supplying food to young as is common in wolf packs.

Care of the body surface and comfort behavior

Few changes (8%) were observed here. Basically wolves and poodles stretch, scratch and lick themselves, yawn, sneeze, pant, etc. in precisely the same way.

Expressive behaviors

Expressive behaviors involved in *visual* communication between animals have changed to the greatest extent (67%). Facial expressions, gestures, and body postures are the most important forms of expressive social behavior in wolves. In poodles, many of these postures and movements of particular parts of the body like the tail, legs, head, ears, and face are seen only in reduced form, or have disappeared. In comparison to wolves, poodle expressive behavior seems much less complex and pronounced – a crudely stereotyped and greatly simplified version of what it once was. One implication of this evolutionary development is that while the human observer knows precisely what sort of mood or intention a wolf is communicating, in poodles it is often more difficult to discriminate between an aggressive, friendly, playful, or fearful mood on the basis of these visual expressive postures and movements alone. In general, poodles can only convey comparatively crude signals with the few elementary expressive behaviors they possess to the full extent (e.g. lowering of the tail or tucking it between the legs when fearful or submissive, wagging the tail to show positive excitement).

In contrast, poodles exhibit much more complex *vocal* expressive behavior than wolves. As Zimen puts it, what dogs can't express with their gestures, facial expressions, and body postures, they "say" with their barking. And there are many situations in which this is the main or exclusive form of expressive behavior exhibited. It also occurs in new combinations with other types of behavior. Wolves, for example, hunt soundlessly whereas dogs bark when following a trail and even more so when prey is sighted. The same is true of play: unlike dogs, wolves usually play without making sounds. While barking has become the most important vehicle of communication when warning or during defense in dogs, visual communicative behavior like agitated restlessness, staring, and baring the teeth are predominantly exhibited by wolves in this context. Finally, wolves exhibit more snarling and growling in aggressive and defensive situations, and they more frequently howl – presumably to coordinate and synchronize pack mood and behavior as well as serving as a method of long-distance communication.

Other types of social behavior

Changes in many other social behavior patterns have taken place (37%). Here too, only the simplest and most elementary types of wolf behavior are still seen in poodles. More complex and differentiated types of behavior are present only in cruder forms or have completely disappeared. For example, although neither species shows much in the way of expressive behavior at this time, serious fighting between poodles has little in common with the powerful and uninhibited fighting of wolves. For play behavior (35% of behaviors changed), simple play fighting and more solitary forms of play involving few expressive behaviors have remained quite similar whereas those involving much expressive behavior like play elicitation, play movements, and running games have changed greatly. When playing, poodles no longer show the rich mixture of social behaviors from other functional contexts seen in wolves.

Sexual behavior

The behaviors associated with mating itself have been faithfully preserved: no changes in the form of sexual behaviors during estrus were observed. However, reproduction in dogs differs enormously in other ways from that of wolves. Female dogs become sexually mature within the first year whereas wolves require a year longer. Similarly, female dogs come into their relatively shorter estrous period twice a year rather than just once. During this time, the insistent, somewhat frantic, and highly vocal attempts of every male in the vicinity to mate with the bitch in dogs contrasts sharply with the more subdued character of wolf behavior under these circumstances. Also no longer in evidence in the dog are the restriction of mating to the highest-ranking pack female and incest taboos between mother and son, littermates, and father and daughter.

Parturition, rearing young, infantile behavior

Poodle bitches do not dig a den and hide food there in preparation for birth. And poodle males do not participate in caring for the young. But otherwise, no differences between wolves and poodles were observed in these areas. The behavior of poodle and wolf pups during the first two or three weeks is identical.

In discussing the results of this illuminating research project, Zimen poses the question of why poodles eat, defecate, scratch, lick, and mate like their wolf ancestors and yet defend themselves and communicate with each other is such very different ways. His answer: dog behavior represents a biologically understandable

evolutionary adaptation of wolf behavior to the new human-dominated social and physical environment. Basically, the fact that even changes such as those in which vitally important behavior patterns in the wolf have become cruder, functionless, or disappeared in the dog should be viewed positively rather than regarded as a kind of degeneration.

Domestication as evolutionary adaptation

That a new species, the domestic dog, evolved within the space of only a few thousand years is a measure of how powerful the impact of the change in natural environment from that in which wolf packs live to life in our human-dominated modern societies has turned out to be. Such rapid and far-reaching evolutionary development implies two sorts of major changes in the selection pressures operating on populations of the evolving species: many of the *evolutionary constraints* characteristic of the former environment no longer apply, and the new environment brings with it a host of *new selection pressures* which progressively shape and mold the species in new directions.

Being provided with food implied that the wolf's natural hunting behaviors were no longer needed except to the extent that these were useful to their new hosts. There was no longer a need to be territorial in the wolf sense of the pack defending an area large enough to feed itself. Food no longer needed to be cached in holes dug for this purpose. The number of litters no longer needed to be limited to that which the pack could successfully raise. And the protection against predators afforded by life in the human social group meant that the wolf's great strength, speed, agility, and wariness of anything novel were no longer critical to survival. Essentially, many of the wolf's behaviors had lost their importance for the survival and well-being of species members – including many of those expressive behaviors which are so critical to maintaining the wolf's social organization and abilities for cooperative hunting and territorial defense. As Zimen emphasizes, the loss of such now-superfluous, energy-wasting behaviors was advantageous and not disadvantageous, for it helped the developing new species to take full advantage of the opportunities provided by its new alien world.

Other behaviors were not only no longer useful, they were disadvantageous and therefore strongly selected against such as aggression towards fellow group members and extreme fearfulness of minor novel changes in the environment. And finally, the new selection pressures favored the species' development of earlier breeding, promiscuous breeding, a complex repertoire of vocal behavior to communicate with its highly vocal human hosts, extreme submissiveness towards humans of all ages, and what might be termed general behavioral flexibility in the sense of readily learning to perform various behavioral sequences which were fostered by its hosts while quickly reducing those which were discouraged.

With its many inappropriate, unnecessary, or potentially dangerous behavior patterns, even a tame wolf which has been born and raised in this alien human environment remains a misfit which is strangely out of place. In contrast, it is only in such an environment in which the domestic dog is genuinely at home. For *Canis familiaris* is the end result of evolutionary processes which have taken the basic wolf stock and molded and shaped it to fit the demands of a new natural environment – the human interspecies family group living in harmony with the seemingly endless sea of human and dog strangers which surrounds it.

References

Borchelt, P.L., and Voith V.L. (1986): Dominance aggression in dogs. *Compendium on Continuing Education for the Practicing Veterinarian* 8, 36–45.

Daniels, T.J. (1983a): The social organization of free-ranging urban dogs: I. Non-estrous social behavior. *Applied Animal Ethology* 10, 341–363.

Daniels, T.J. (1983b): The social organization of free-ranging urban dogs: II. Estrous groups and the mating system. *Applied Animal Ethology* 10, 365–373.

Fox, M.W. (1963): *Canine Behavior*. Springfield, Illinois, Charles C. Thomas.

Fox, M.W., Beck, A.M., and Blackman, E. (1975): Behavior and ecology of a small group of urban dogs (*Canis familiaris*). *Applied Animal Ethology* 1, 119–137.

Fox, M.W., and Bekoff, M. (1975): The behaviour of dogs. In Hafez, E.S.E. (ed) *The Behaviour of Domestic Animals*. London, Bailliere Tindall.

Klinghammer, E. (ed) (1979): *The Behavior and Ecology of Wolves*. New York, Garland STPM Press.

Mech, L.D. (1970): *The Wolf: The Ecology and Behavior of an Endangered Species*. New York, The Natural History Press.

O'Farrell, V. (1992): *Manual of Canine Behaviour*, 2nd Edition. Shurdington, Cheltenham, Gloucestershire, UK, British Small Animal Veterinary Association Publications.

Thorne, C. (ed) (1992): *The Waltham Book of Dog and Cat Behaviour*. Oxford, Pergamon Press.

Zimen, E. (1988): *Der Hund*. München, C. Bertelsmann Verlag.

8   General Treatment Principles

Briefly summarizing the treatment-related discussion presented in Chapter 5, treating dog behavior problems such as aggression, separation anxiety, and elimination problems often involves a combination of several measures of one or more of the three following types:

- *Taking or avoiding direct actions in problem situations* to reduce arousing stimuli, avoid eliciting stimuli, reduce or avoid potentiating stimuli, or apply or intensify inhibitory stimuli that are exerting, or have the potential for exerting, a proximate causal influence on the problem behavior.
- *Influencing underlying behavior system parameters* by means of castration, correction of possible pathophysiological conditions, administering drugs, or by affecting interactions between behavioral systems.
- *Altering environmental influences on the underlying behavioral system* via the operation of learning processes that are directly or indirectly affected by changing general care/maintenance conditions, altering human-dog interactive ground rules, making specific environmental changes, applying systematic behavior therapy methods, carrying out conventional obedience training and/or training in specific problem situations, abandoning ineffective training or behavior control methods, increasing owner authority, correcting owner misconceptions, correcting owner mistakes, and producing changes in owner attitudes. All of these measures can drastically alter either the owner's behavior towards the animal or some other portion of the animal's environment which, in turn, can cause it to learn to behave differently in problems situations.

Successful resolution of behavior problems requires not only recommending the right training, behavior therapy, environmental change,

etc. measures, but also confronting and modifying owners' basic attitudes towards their animal and how it should be treated. Thus, working through the owner to change the pet's problem behavior implies much more than just feeding the appropriate training or behavior therapy recommendations into the owner as if he/she were a passive piece of equipment which automatically responds as programmed. Indeed it is the fact that the pet behavior counselor can only successfully treat many pet behavior problems by being skillful in changing owners' cognitive beliefs and attitudes, and dealing with owners' emotional reactions, which makes pet behavior counseling so challenging on the one hand, and so diverse and interesting on the other.

Changing owner beliefs and attitudes concerning the dog and its problem behavior

Establishing an appropriate general perspective

Encouraging owners to view the problem correctly means putting it in an appropriate general perspective by explaining the specific nature of the problem behavior, its relationship to normal canine behavior, and the reasons for its development. Discussing a certain amount of canine ethology is always helpful in this connection. It is also important to explain to owners the general reasons for the development of problems such as those they are having with their dog. Most often it is a case of a dog that has always displayed certain problem tendencies eventually developing serious behavior problems when it is treated "normally" – that is, like most other owners treat their dogs. To put the blame for the development of the problem solely on owner foolishness, ignorance, or mistakes is seldom appropriate or accurate even though most owners suspect that this is the case and are therefore quite prepared from the start to believe it.

Identifying and correcting counterproductive owner beliefs and attitudes

Many owners believe, for example, that all dogs aggressively defend bones against family members, certain breeds of dogs must necessarily be a problem in some respects, dogs will feel miserable if ignored (as children would), animals feel guilty about their problem behaviors, one must always be polite to animals, and treating animals well means always trying to do what they want. These kinds of erroneous beliefs are often associated with general treatment practices which have helped create the problem. And if not corrected, these beliefs may interfere with compliance with the recommended treatment measures.

Concerned here are often clients' most strongly held beliefs about their animals, themselves, and how animals should be treated by human beings. This has two major implications. Firstly, by calling owners' beliefs about such important and sensitive topics into question, one may be running the risk of alienating them or making them defensive. Obviously, the pet behavior counselor must be diplomatic in this regard. It is often better, for example, to say something like "people often wrongly think that ....." rather than "No. You're wrong there" when one is about to set owners straight on some point. When owners remain stubborn in their conviction, the counselor can be just as stubborn – but tactfully: "I know you feel strongly about this, but let's look at it this way ..... Don't you think that might be possible too?"

The second and most important implication of the fact that attitudes and beliefs which stand in the way of successful resolution of the problem may be strongly held is of course that they can be extremely resistant to change. During the consultation, owners may tentatively accept the counselor's argument that it would

be better if they always supported the larger, more aggressive of their two male dogs even though it is the one that is apparently causing all the trouble. However, so firmly convincing them to view the victim's behavior as being the true source of the difficulty that they will go against all of their democratic and parental instincts and side with the aggressor later is not easy. And as we have considered in Chapter 2, convincing some owners that they must stop treating their dominant-aggressive dogs like small children – in effect, that their most strongly held beliefs about what are fair, appropriate, cruel, etc. ways of treating pets must be drastically revised – can sometimes be next to impossible.

But nevertheless, the attempt must be made to do just this. For without changes in those beliefs and attitudes which represent obstacles to owners changing their behavior towards their pet, even the most highly effective treatment will fail because of lack of compliance – or only half-hearted compliance – with the counselor's recommendations.

Changing the ground rules of owners' normal interactions with their dog

In many or most dog cases, owners are given a few basic rules of how to behave towards their animals outside of the particular situations in which the problem behavior occurs. The following are some examples: don't allow the dog on the furniture, don't feed it just before family meals, don't let it sleep in the family bedrooms, never reward begging or pushy behavior of any kind, take the dog to a place where it can play with other dogs every day, always make it follow a command before you give it what it wants, ignore it when it comes to you for attention or petting, etc. The following sections discuss various principles that are relevant when recommending such important interactive ground rules to owners.

Reason for recommendation

It may not be necessary to explain in detail the reason behind every single recommendation.

But it is best to give owners at least a brief rationale for most of them. Not only do owners have a right to know why they are being asked to follow these in part unappealing recommendations, but such understanding fosters compliance for obvious reasons. Recommendations such as these generally require a major change in owner behavior where owners must essentially be persuaded to do something other than what they have always done. Therefore, the counselor must be aware that such recommendations always carry with them the message that something the owners have always been doing, and always thought was right or acceptable, is indeed wrong – a mistake, at least for their particular animal. Under these circumstances, the chances of being able to successfully alter human behavior are increased if owners understand *why* changing their behavior in these ways will help solve their problem.

In general, counselors must be sensitive to the client's reactions and frame of mind at all times, and when they see that uncertain, questioning look on the client's face, they must be prepared to take as much time as is necessary to explain the logic behind the recommendation involved in terms the client can understand and accept.

Difference between "mistakes" and practices that are inappropriate for the particular problem or animal

Having admitted to themselves that they are not capable of solving the problem on their own, and having contacted a behavior counselor for advice, most clients are ready to accept and comply with the treatment recommendations. Often, however, clients go too far by essentially holding themselves entirely responsible for a problem which is only partially their fault. While it might foster compliance to let clients go on thinking this way, doing so would seem questionable on ethical grounds. Out of a sense of fairness to clients, their misconceptions concerning their role in the development of the problem should also be corrected; in this case, by pointing out that there is a difference between mistakes in some general, for-all-dogs

sense and treatment practices which are inappropriate for dogs displaying certain types of problems. Essentially, that it's not so much that they have been making mistakes which most owners don't make, but rather with the inherently somewhat difficult animal they have, they must be far more careful about what they do or don't do than the average pet owner.

Erroneous views posing obstacles to compliance must be identified and corrected

As considered above, convincing owners to change their behavior towards their animals often involves changing their underlying attitudes and beliefs. The causal connection between such cognitive phenomena and overt behavior need not be a one-way street – owners may be reacting "instinctively" and then justifying their behavior in cognitive terms later. However, the fact remains that one stands a much greater chance of successfully changing owners' behavior towards their animals if one can change the various kinds of cognitive views which are somehow associated with it. Here again, the problem of intermale aggression between two dogs in the same home is a good example. Owners commonly make the mistake of scolding the aggressor whenever there is trouble between the family's two dogs. They do so "instinctively" as the human parent would to protect a smaller or weaker child from an older sibling. When asked why they react in this way, owners usually justify their behavior either by pointing to the practical, problem-suppressing effect of punishing undesirable aggression or by bringing in the concept of fairness. While there are indeed cases of aggression between dogs in the same home in which it might be appropriate to recommend scolding the aggressor to directly suppress aggression, the notion that it would be "unfair" to scold an apparently innocent victim must be counteracted. For example, one can explain to owners that fighting is a sign that a stable dominance-submission relationship which will eventually prevent fighting has not yet developed, and that they should foster this desirable development process by always preferring and siding with the more dominant of the two dogs regardless of which one has apparently started the trouble. Fortunately, most owners accept this new explanation readily and are then in a position to view the aggression between the two dogs in a new light – one which facilitates making the kind of change in their behavior towards the two dogs that promotes rather than counteracts the formation of a stable dominance-submission relationship.

Resistance must be overcome

Many owners are not at all pleased when the counselor recommends that the dog should not be allowed on the furniture or that it should be ignored every time it comes for attention. In general, people like treating their pets the way they do, and they sometimes require a lot of convincing before they are prepared to give up what is for them one of the pleasures of owning a pet.

Of course such feelings and associated resistance to acceptance of treatment recommendations must be overcome. Often, it is best to deal with these possible sources of resistance or noncompliance directly as soon as they are sensed by asking owners whether, for example, they think it will be difficult for them to follow this particular recommendation. Some owners are quite open here and go right to the heart of the problem: "But I *like* it when he puts his head in my lap" or "I couldn't possibly ignore him when he's just trying to be friendly!" But many owners are not so candid. They reply, albeit rather more distantly or guardedly than before, that of course they can do that if it is necessary. However, in spite of their statements to the contrary, one often senses at this point that they really can't see themselves doing something so extreme or unappealing.

Pet behavior problem counselors are not human psychologists. But they must nevertheless try to deal with such feelings during the consultation and not simply ignore or gloss over them. The best approach is first try to encourage owners to speak openly about their reservations concerning the recommendations. After making it clear that these are perfectly understandable and normal feelings that all owners have, one can then go on to explain how using these feelings as a guide to how to treat a pet can lead to problems like those they are now having. When it comes to giving up some of the pleasures of pet ownership, one can try to deal with this directly as well by making it clear to owners that there is in effect no other choice: "If you go on treating your dog the way you do now, you are bound to get bitten again – perhaps even more severely. Most other dog owners can treat their dogs any way they like. But unfortunately with the kind of dog you have, you can't do that."

Exact description of required owner behavior

Although one might assume that anyone would understand exactly what is meant by ignoring an animal or scolding it, this isn't the case. Sometimes, for example, people think that following the recommendation to ignore a dog when it comes to be petted means only that they shouldn't pet it, and not – as intended – that they should also refrain from talking to it or even looking at it by essentially pretending that it wasn't there. And to a few owners, scolding a dog means calmly explaining to it that it really shouldn't have done what it just did.

If there is any question in the counselor's mind that owners may not quite understand precisely how they should behave, this must be remedied: "When I say ignore the dog, I mean that when it comes to you, you shouldn't talk to it or look at it or react to it in any way. Basically, you should do your best to pretend that you don't even know its there".

Establish realistic expectations

Here as with other types of recommendations, it is important to give owners an idea of how the dog will react to this change in interactive ground rules and how far this will go towards solving the various specific problems which they are having with it. With the drastic change in owner-dog interactive ground rules which is recommended for dominant-aggressive dogs (see Chapter 10), owners are cautioned that the dog may act shocked, somewhat confused, and otherwise not like its usual self for 2 or 3 days. Furthermore, it is explained that this change in general treatment practices usually produces an improvement in some of the problem symptoms fairly quickly (e.g. dog quicker to follow commands) but not in others (e.g. still can't safely take food away from it).

In general, giving the owner a realistic picture of what to expect is not only fair, it also acts to maximize compliance by eliminating unrealistic expectations which could be a source of disappointment and lead to premature abandoning of the treatment method.

Consistency is critical

This must always be stressed to owners not only because human nature is what it is, but also because a lack of consistency can create new conditions which may worsen the problem. If, for example, excessive barking to beg for or demand something is to be treated by never giving the dog what it wants, following this recommendation with 100% consistency will correct the problem within a few days. However, following it with only 90% consistency probably won't work. The dog will simply adjust to the fact that begging is only rewarded sometimes and therefore continue barking whenever it wants something. And not only will the problem behavior continue as before, but when the time comes to stop rewarding the begging entirely in the future, the dog won't learn to stop begging nearly as quickly as it otherwise would have. In general, learned behaviors which are maintained on an intermittent, rewarded-only-sometimes schedule continue for much longer periods of time after all sources of rewards are eliminated than behaviors which have been rewarded in the past every single time they were performed. Here is a case where inconsistent treatment does more harm than no treatment at all.

In general, it is also always worth strongly emphasizing to owners the connection between consistency and efficiency of treatment. An inconsistent treatment might help bring the problem under control, but it probably will not provide as satisfactory a solution and it will have to be applied for a much longer period of time than otherwise need be the case.

Human feelings critical

The fact that people are attached to their pets, love them, regard them as family members, and feel inclined to be as kind and polite to them as they are to their own children helps explain why people choose to allow their pets on the furniture, reward begging, are not too strict with them, give them food from the table, and walk around them when they are sleeping so as not to disturb them. In advising clients to change the basic ground rules of how they interact with their pet, the matter of how they feel about their animals must therefore play a prominent role in the discussion between owners and counselor. In general, there are three guidelines to keep in mind when dealing with matters involving very strong feelings on the part of owners: (1) owners feelings should always be recognized and respected, (2) ways in which the new recommended treatment practices are as compatible with such feelings as former practices should be stressed, and (3) where owners feelings may pose an obstacle to their carrying out the recommended treatment, it must be clearly explained to them that their feelings are not the best guide as to how they should behave towards their pets.

If the counselor suspects that owners are going to have difficulty complying with recommended treatment for psychological or emotional reasons, the situation addressed in the last of the three guidelines is normally involved: owners don't *want* to give up petting their dog on demand or stop letting it sleep in bed with them. They want their present relationship with the dog and their behavior towards it to remain just the same. They *like* treating the dog this way and might even feel that they *need* it or that it would be cruel or unfair to their dog if they did otherwise. And they feel all of these feelings very strongly – so much so that some owners get upset to the point of shedding tears when they are told that a drastic change in their behavior in these areas will be necessary to solve the problem. Obviously, there is little counselors can do to change such feelings. But they can remain firm and unyielding in their opinion concerning changes in owner behavior that are required to modify the animal's problem behaviors on the one hand, while at the same time remaining sensitive and respectful to the owners' feelings in this regard on the other. Empathy on the part of the counselor demonstrates genuine concern and gives clients the feeling that he/she is on their side. This in turn encourages them to call later, honestly report failures as well as successes, and try as best they can to follow even the most difficult recommendations. In short, sensitivity to and respect for owners' feelings is critical not only to the relationship between client and counselor, but also in terms of maximizing compliance with the treatment recommendations.

Obedience training

The owners of many problem dogs complain that their dog is disobedient in the sense that it doesn't reliably come when it is called outdoors, or that it is difficult or impossible to control in problem situations like when it is threatening a person or fighting with another dog. Accordingly, increasing the dog's responsiveness to commands and, therefore, the degree to which owners have this kind of control over its behavior is a major element in the treatment approach recommended for many dog behavior problems.

Above and beyond the fact that part of the solution to many dog problems requires that the dogs be trained to respond more quickly and reliably to owners' commands, there is another, more general rationale for including obedience training as a major treatment element. In universities, it is common that experimental psychology students must take a course in which groups of 2 or 3 students are assigned their own rat or pigeon which they must train to press a lever (rats) or peck a lighted plastic disc (pigeons) to obtain food rewards which the student can administer by pressing a button. After the bar-pressing or disc-pecking res-

ponse has been well-learned, students must then demonstrate numerous animal learning principles by recording changes in rates of bar-pressing or disc-pecking which occur as a result of, for example, giving rewards intermittently, stopping all rewards for awhile, rewarding the animal only when a light is on, etc. Even for students who know beforehand exactly what will happen, the experience of actually interacting with the animal in this way is illuminating and provides a much deeper insight into how animal's learn than the students could ever get through books and lectures alone. Understanding something also in part means "having a feel for it", and for many activities in life this can only be acquired through direct, hands-on experience. Thus, when counselors recommend teaching dogs a few simple commands, demonstrate how to do this, and then supervise the owners' initial attempts to continue the training process themselves, they are always conscious of the fact that carrying out such training may be beneficial to owners' future capabilities of managing and training their animals in ways which go far beyond merely achieving the immediate goal of training their dogs to sit down, lie down, come, etc.

The following adaptation of obedience training methods recommended by Campbell (1992) and Voith (1982b, 1982c) is an approach the present author has successfully employed over the course of several years.

Using food rewards

Food tidbits which the dog really loves should be used as rewards. Initially, some owners say that their dog doesn't particularly like tidbits. But when questioned further, owners admit that although the dog doesn't care all that much for the kind of food rewards they usually buy, there are other foods like cheese, sausage, or chocolate that it would walk through fire for. The owner is then asked to prepare a plate of one of these cut in 30 or so very small, pea-sized pieces.

Use very small, pea-sized pieces of food which the dog loves as rewards

There are two reasons for using very small pieces of food as rewards. Firstly, it has been well-established in animal learning experiments comparing food rewards of various sizes that the size of the reward is not critical to learning. While animals will run faster down a long runway to obtain a larger reward, they learn to perform new behaviors just as quickly with very small rewards as with much larger ones. Secondly, many small rewards can be given to the animal within a short period of time without reducing its motivation to earn more tidbits or wasting the extra time it takes the dog to consume large tidbits.

Many owners have quite a different approach to giving food rewards than the behavior counselor. Food rewards are something big and substantial which may be given to the dog once every day, for example, after the mid-afternoon walk. And when tidbits are given for good behavior, it is usually long after the fact. Following a walk in which the dog has been especially well-behaved, the owner may "reward" it for its good behavior, verbally explaining this to it as the dried beef stick or whatever is handed over. For these owners, simply watching the counselor giving two dozen small tidbits in rapid succession, practically simultaneously with the desired response, as a means of quickly training the animal to sit or lie down is illuminating. This in itself may be a great help to them later when it comes to training their dog to come more reliably during walks or sit down and stay at their side rather than chase after joggers.

Teaching the "sit", "stay", "down", and "come" commands

Using the following method, it is possible for the counselor to teach any dog which does not fear or behave aggressively towards him/her the basics of all four commands in a maximum of 5 to 10 minutes. With this method, one never touches the dog or physically manipulates its postures by, for example, pushing its rump down to get it to sit. Instead, one takes advantages of the dog's natural tendencies by essentially luring or enticing it into body postures in

which it is natural for the dog to sit or lie down of its own accord while waiting for something.

First, call the dog and give it a food reward for coming. If the dog doesn't come when called, hold up the tidbit and gesture with your hand that it should come. When it finally does come, give it the tidbit *immediately*. One simply holds out one's hand to the dog, opens it, and allows the dog to take the tidbit gently out of the palm or from between the thumb and forefingers. If the dog has a tendency to snap, it is easily trained to take rewards more gently by snapping your hand closed in front of its nose every time the dog lunges forward towards the reward and then opening it again and keeping it open if and only if the dog slowly leans forward to take the tidbit more gingerly. Owners learn another lesson by watching their dog rapidly learn to be more restrained when it takes the reward: if the trainer has a good clear idea of the target behavior, and if he/she is 100% consistent in refusing to reward anything else, learning of the desired response proceeds rapidly.

> Rewards must be given immediately – less than one second after the dog has performed the desired behavior

Giving the food reward immediately – if possible, just as the dog is in the process of performing the desired behavior – is exceedingly important. Laboratory experiments indicate that the optimal time interval between response and reward for producing new learning is less than a second. Accordingly, owners must understand that the key to any reward-based training procedure is this extremely close temporal connection between the response and reward. Essentially, to be maximally effective, rewards must be given *practically at the same instant the desired behavior is performed*. Even 2 or 3 seconds later is much too late.

At the end of the counselor's obedience training demonstration when it is time to pass the plate of rewards to owners and ask them to take over, the owners' timing of giving rewards is one of the main things the counselor must pay attention to. If owners are a little too slow, it must be pointed out to them that they must plan ahead and get ready with the reward so that their hand opens practically at the same instant the dog begins performing the desired response. Basically, owners must understand a concept which is fundamental to using either rewards or punishments to train animals: one must think in terms of rewarding or punishing not *the animal* – as owners tend to view the situation – but rather of rewarding or punishing *specific behaviors*. Giving the dog a reward several seconds after coming in response to being called rewards something. However, it is certainly not the act of coming, but rather something like staring up at the owner, standing quietly, looking around, or whatever else the dog was doing at the moment the hand that dispenses the tidbits opened.

> One doesn't reward the animal, one rewards a *behavior*

To teach the dog to sit when it is standing in front of you and gazing hopefully up at you, open your hand far enough to show it the tidbit, move your hand slowly closer to its nose until it is concentrating fully on it, then move your hand upwards towards a point above the top of its head so slowly and smoothly that its gaze follows the tidbit and it must tilt its head backwards to keep tracking it. If it stops watching your hand and looks back at you, bring the tidbit back down and get its attention focused on it again before you again try to lure its gaze upwards and its head backwards in this way. When the dog is looking up with its head tilted back, you only need to wait – it will sit down on its own within a few seconds, probably because this is a more comfortable, energy-saving waiting posture which doesn't involve craning its neck back so far. If however it doesn't sit down quickly, slowly moving your hand even farther behind his head so that it has to crane its neck backwards even more to follow it will surely cause it to sit down.

As soon as the dog sits and is rewarded practically the instant its hindquarters hit the floor, take a few steps away from it, give it a tidbit when it comes when called, and then repeat

the sit-eliciting process – always saying the word "sit" so that eventually it will learn to sit in response to the word alone. In the beginning, it is only the sight of the tidbit, your hand movements, your body language, and perhaps the tone of your voice which the dog is responding to. Another basic animal training principle is involved here: the first step in training any new behavior is to get the dog to perform the desired response – or some close approximation to it – by any means whatsoever. In effect, one can worry later about training the dog to sit in response to a quietly uttered command not accompanied by the bribe of a food reward, elaborate hand movements, or emphatic body language support. But initially, one is facing a type of communication problem. The dog is eager to earn the food reward by doing whatever it must to get it, but it simply doesn't understand what to do. Like the traditional dog trainer's approach of pushing the dog's hindquarters down to more or less force it to sit the first few times, the present method of using hand movements and food rewards to entice the dog into sitting of its own accord is an effective way of getting it to perform the desired behavior so that it can be immediately rewarded – which in turn "tells" the dog what it must do to earn more food rewards.

> To train the dog to do something new, the first step is always to give it all the help that you can (hand gestures, showing reward, kneeling down, physically maneuvering the dog, etc.) to get it to perform the desired response. Later on in the training process, all of the special "prompting" aids initially used to encourage the dog make the desired response the first few times can be gradually phased out or "faded".

After the dog is reliably coming and sitting on command, it can be taught to lie down in a similar way. First call it and reward it for coming, and then tell it to sit and reward it for sitting. Then show the dog the next tidbit, hold it only partly visible in your hand directly in front of its nose, and then move your hand very slowly away from its nose and down to the floor a foot or so in front of its forepaws. Move the tidbit so gradually and slowly that the dog has a tendency to follow it with its nose almost right down to the floor. The distance away from its feet should be such that it has to stretch its neck and body somewhat forward to stay close to it. Now try waiting a few moments. Some dogs lie down immediately – presumably because this a more comfortable waiting position than remaining stretched forward. Other dogs simply try and get at tidbit by mouthing the hand (which is now lying on the floor) or scratching it with their forepaws. It is not necessary to scold these unwanted behaviors. Just keep your hand closed on the floor so that the dog can't get at the tidbit no matter what it does. The dog will abandon these vain attempts to get the tidbit by mouthing or scratching as soon as it has tried them a few times without success.

Unwanted behaviors which the dog tries to use during training to get the reward (mouthing or scratching the trainer's hand, jumping up, snapping, barking, etc.) need not be scolded – just ignored with 100 % consistency. The dog will quickly stop doing such things if there is no payoff.

If the dog is stretching far forwards but gets tired of waiting and gives up and goes back into a normal sitting posture, hold the tidbit in front of its nose and try again to entice it into stretching its body and neck forwards to follow the tidbit back down to the floor with its nose – perhaps not so far away from its feet this time so it doesn't have to stretch quite as far. Another thing the dog might do is simply remain awkwardly stretched out without doing anything else. If it does, slowly move the tidbit a little farther away from it – to get it to stretch just a little farther.

This strategy will get perhaps 90% of dogs to lie down within 1 or 2 min. However, if the dog is one of those which doesn't have a strong natural tendency to lie down when straining forwards with its head close to the floor, one need not wait longer. One can simply reward the first step in the lying-down process – that of sliding

its forepaws farther forwards along the floor. At this stage, one can simply move the hand holding the reward very slowly away from the dog's nose – trying to do so in a way which makes it stretch to follow it as before – and, at the same time, watch its forepaws. The instant it moves one noticeably forwards, the hand immediately opens. After a few rewards for stretching its body and neck forwards and downwards and then sliding or moving its forepaws forwards, the ground rules are changed so that doing this is no longer enough to get a reward, and the dog will soon lie down.

If getting the dog to perform the desired response for the first time takes too long or is too difficult, reward some more easily-elicited "first approximation" of it (e.g. sliding the forepaws forwards along the floor as a first approximation to lying down). When the behavior to be trained is complex and not part of the animal's normal behavioral repertoire (like jumping through a raised hoop), the necessary training process may involve the rewarding of a long series of successively closer and closer approximations to the target behavior like, for example, approaching the hoop, walking through it when it held on the ground, stepping through it when it is held 1 inch above the ground, then 2 inches, 4 inches, etc.

After the dog is reliably and quickly lying down under these circumstances, the "stay" command is added to the other three. Say "sit", reward the dog for sitting, then say "stay", take a step or two backwards away from the dog, and then say something like "good" while quickly going back and giving it a reward before it has had a chance to get up. If the dog is faster than you are and gets up to come after you, call it back to the original spot, say "sit" again – without rewarding it this time – take only one step backwards, and don't wait nearly as long as you did previously before you say "good" and quickly move back and give the dog its reward.

Now repeat the whole sequence. Take a few steps backwards, call the dog, reward it for coming, say "sit", reward it for sitting, then say "stay", take a step or two backwards, and say "good" just as you start to go back to reward it. After many repetitions, your saying "good" will eventually come to signal the dog from a distance that it has indeed performed the correct response and a reward is on the way. Technically speaking, this kind of stimulus becomes what is referred to as a *secondary reward* (or secondary reinforcement), which means that it takes on behavior-rewarding properties as a result of its reliable association with the food (or *primary reward)* which follows. Such secondary rewards are extremely useful for training animals, for they provide a means of bridging the delay between the time the desired response is performed and the time the food is delivered. In effect, one can still reward the behavior immediately even though the distance between animal and trainer might be several yards or more.

As soon as the animal is reliably performing all four behaviors, clients are asked to take over and continue rewarding the dog for following the commands for an additional few minutes. This allows the counselor to correct owners' mistakes or reassure them that they are indeed carrying out the training correctly

In general, this kind of obedience training demonstration is extremely important with owners who have had little or no experience training their dog. In the first place, it demonstrates both the power of rewards and specifically how to administer them so as to produce desired behavior in the animal. Secondly, it demonstrates the importance of being firm and unyielding and never giving a reward to the animal when it hasn't performed correctly. Thirdly, it demonstrates to the owner the importance of setting specific goals of exactly what behaviors are to be rewarded at every stage in training. And finally, it demonstrates the behavior-changing power of a calm, firm, systematic approach – which contrasts sharply with the kind of macho, bullying approach espoused by many dog trainers.

In the beginning, clients who have never trained an animal tend to be very awkward and uncertain about exactly what to do and when

to do it. Of course, this is to be expected given that being an effective animal trainer requires not only possessing an intellectual understanding, but also a good "feel" for the process – that is, a kind of instinctive knowing of when exactly to give each reward, what to reward next, and so on. Given that the perceptions and skills which underlie this kind of "feel" for the training process can only come through first-hand training experience, it is therefore important to get clients involved in training their animals themselves right from the start. Not only does this result in a more obedient and controllable animal, but the experience gained by the owner may transfer to other situations in which the dog must be trained to behave in more acceptable ways.

Using petting, praise, and play as rewards

Dogs can also be trained without using food rewards, and many dog trainers teach owners to only use petting or praise as rewards. However, dogs which are petted and otherwise doted upon from morning to night are generally not nearly as highly motivated to work for such rewards as for tidbits – especially if owners are instructed to withhold all tidbits at other times so that the only opportunity the dog has of obtaining tidbits is by earning them during training sessions. Basically, dogs like petting and praise, but most will do anything and everything short of walking through fire to get those choice morsels of cheese, sausage, or cookies which are usually denied them.

This does not mean, however, that petting and praise rewards need not or should not be used as well. To the contrary, owners are also instructed to pet and praise their dogs when they are giving food rewards. Essentially, food rewards are mainly used as a temporary obedience training aid to maximize the efficiency of the initial training process. Later, once the behavior has been well-learned, it is suggested that the owner gradually phase out food rewards in favor of a progressively more exclusive reliance on petting and praise alone to maintain or strengthen the new sequences of behavior (i.e. the animal is petted and praised every time but only given food rewards on average every second time they perform correctly, then every third or fourth time, and then increasingly less frequently until the animal is only occasionally rewarded with food).

Play can also be a powerful reward for most dogs. Many owners seem to understand this instinctively when they refrain from immediately throwing a ball or stick but instead make the dog sit or stay first. Although play rewards do not lend themselves to use within the initial basic obedience training sessions discussed in this section, they are ideal for use in some of the other contexts discussed later in the chapter such as when training a dog to stop chasing after joggers or bicyclists.

Generalizing obedience training to everyday situations

Once the dog is reliably following the four basic commands of "come", "sit", "down", and "stay" during the special daily training sessions in the home, owners are instructed to *generalize* this training by carrying it out in other situations like during walks and during the course of normal interactions between owner and pet in the home.

"Nothing in life is free"

A very useful approach owners can use to incorporate continued obedience training into the normal daily family routine is to institute a new family-dog interactive ground rule which Voith (1982a) refers to as "nothing in life is free". Basically, the animal must follow one of the four basic sit, come, down, and stay commands in order to earn everything it wants – not only food rewards, but also its dinner, being allowed to go through the door to go outside or come back inside after a walk, having its leash put on before walks, having a ball or stick thrown during play, being petted when it is waiting to be petted, etc. The owner is instructed to never give the dog what it wants immediately, but rather to give it a command first and then insist that the dog perform the required re-

sponse before it gets whatever rewarding object, privilege, or owner behavior it is waiting for.

Primarily known as one of the standard recommendations for the treatment of dominance aggression (Chapter 10), this interactive ground rule can also be profitably employed in any type of case in which there is a need to increase the dog's tendency to follow owner commands under any and all circumstances. It can be, however, a difficult strategy for owners to implement properly. Essentially, they must think every time they interact with the dog and resist their tendency to, for example, automatically reach down and pet the dog as soon as it comes to them for attention. And for owners this can therefore be a somewhat unpleasant change in the relaxed, spontaneous relationship they have always had with their dog.

Nevertheless, consistently implementing the "nothing in life is free" policy can be extremely beneficial and well worth the effort it might take for the counselor to convince a skeptical owner to implement it. To overcome owner resistance, one can stress how easy it is with this method to strengthen the dog's general habit of obeying commands. It also strengthens the dog's submissive, cooperative, "follower" behavioral tendencies, which can greatly improve the behavior of stubborn, pushy, strong-willed, "leader type" dogs. The counselor can also stress that although it is psychologically somewhat difficult to implement, in the long run it is the most efficient way to improve obedience from the point of view of time and energy; no obedience school, no special training sessions every day. Instead, just make sure that the dog must earn everything it wants by following commands.

Strengthening obedience during walks

Many problem dogs are often disobedient during walks. Either they don't come when called or they come only reluctantly and never when there is something more interesting to do. Often this problem is associated with what might be loosely described as a "lack of respect" for the owner which is almost always in evidence when there is a dominance problem between owner and dog. When this is the case, it is the basic nature of the relationship between the two and not merely the dog's behavior during walks which needs improving. Even in this case, however, some additional obedience training during walks often helps.

There are two approaches. The first is a straightforward extension of basic obedience training. The owner is instructed to always take a bag of 30 or so tidbits on walks and use these to strengthen particularly the "come" command, the main focus of outdoor obedience training. The training procedure is simply to call the animal and then give it a food reward immediately after it comes. If the animal takes its good time to come, it still gets its reward and associated praise and petting. Basically, the animal is always rewarded no matter how long it takes to come, and it is never scolded either for coming late or for something it did when it was far away from the owner. Getting angry at an animal for not coming when it is called and then scolding it for not coming when it finally does come is the critical mistake which owners must avoid making. For this essentially punishes the dog for coming and therefore sets up a situation where the dog can delay punishment by staying away when called. Owners should be reminded in this context too that their tendency to think in terms of rewarding or punishing *the animal* for something it did a little while ago is counterproductive: it is *behavior* which is rewarded or punished, and therefore it is what the animal is in the process of doing at the time a reward or punishment is administered which will be affected.

In connection with the application of this simple training method, several other basic animal training principles are explained or re-emphasized to owners:

- Rewards must be given *immediately,* which means the owner should have the reward ready in his/her hand to give to the dog the moment it arrives.
- The dog should not be rewarded when it comes on its own, only when it comes after it is called. This sets up optimal conditions for the command to become a *discrimina-*

tive stimulus or sign to the animal that the behavior of going to the owner will now be rewarded.

- Food rewards should always be accompanied by petting and praise. This accustoms the owner to rewarding desirable behavior in this way. It may also strengthen the rewarding properties of petting and praise themselves by means of their close temporal association with food rewards.
- Over the course of time, the use of food rewards can either be phased out entirely or cut down to a minimal level. Owners are instructed to reward the dog with food every single time it comes on command for the first few days. Once it has learned to come quickly when called and is doing so reliably, the number of tidbits given can be gradually reduced while continuing to always reward the dog with petting and praise.
- During this process of gradual reduction of the frequency of rewards when the desired behavior is first rewarded every time, then every second time, every third time, etc., these are average rates and not literal descriptions of when the rewards are given. For example, every third time means every third time *on average*, and the animal is therefore sometimes rewarded twice in a row and sometimes not for 4 or 5 times. Basically these types of intermittent reward schedules should always be *variable* so that the rewards are given on an irregular and unpredictable basis. Under such conditions, animals never know in advance if the behavior is going to pay off or not. And they therefore remain highly motivated to keep performing the learned behavior even when it is only occasionally rewarded.
- If in spite of using the dog's favorite food rewards, it still ignores the owner's call when it has better things to do like play with another dog, responding correctly to the come command should be initially practiced either at times during walks when there are no distractions of this sort or at times when the owner sees that the dog has played enough and is just about ready to come anyway.

A second method for teaching a dog to come is for owners to call it only once and if it doesn't start coming within a few seconds, turn and walk away until it comes after them. With dogs that do not like to be too far away from their owners (i.e. most dogs), the consistent application of this simple rule can be a highly effective approach to the problem. Essentially, the dog soon learns that the command signals the owner's departure, an important elicitor of following in dogs that become uneasy when left on their own. When the dog catches up to the owner, it can be immediately rewarded with petting, praise, a food reward, and the owner's continuing the walk in some other direction than towards home, which signals to the dog that the walk is not over after all. (See Chapter 18 for a more detailed discussion of this latter method and sample recommendations related to both methods which can be given to owners).

Training in problem situations

By adding a *punishment* dimension to the principles on which the previous discussion of using food rewards, petting, and praise to improve obedience is based, one is equipped with a powerful behavioral training strategy. The general nature of this dual strategy is for the owner to consistently react in problem situations or potential problem situations so as to both *punish* the problem behavior and *reward* any acceptable alternative behavior which the animal performs instead. From the list of the principles of effective punishment which follows, it is clear why this approach is often an extremely effective way to eliminate or reduce the severity of many dog behavior problems.

Principles for the effective use of punishment measures

- In experimental psychology, punishment is defined in terms of the suppressive effect particular stimuli have on an animal's future behavior: an aversive stimulus which lowers the future probability of performance of a behavior which it regularly follows – and is therefore contingent upon – is by definition

a punishing stimulus. Pain, for example, is a punishing stimulus for animals since it tends to reduce the future probability of behaviors which it consistently follows. But for a masochistic human being, it can function as a reward or positive reinforcement which increases the frequency or intensity of behaviors. Similarly, while mild scolding is punishing for most dogs, it may be rewarding for a socially deprived animal which is kept outside alone in a kennel most of the time. In short, it is the effect on behavior and not how aversive the stimulus might appear to the observer that counts.

In correcting pet behavior problems, the most commonly recommended punishments are scolding, leash correction, and startling noises. Hitting animals is not recommended by most counselors. It is not necessary to go that far to effectively punish animals, and hitting may have various undesirable side effects (e.g. increases fear of owner, possible elicitation of fear- or pain-elicited aggression) which can be avoided by using something like a startling noise.

- Laboratory experiments and everyday experience indicate that the most likely effect of punishment is to produce only a *temporary suppression* of behavior. Behaviors which have been apparently eliminated with punishment methods alone tend to recur again and again in the future. The never-ending-battle character of owners' attempts to rely solely on punishment to counteract problem behaviors like barking at strangers during walks or jumping up on visitors is an example of this effect. Punishment is effective in the sense of immediately stopping the behavior and suppressing it for awhile, but its effects are short-lived. In most cases, the problem can never be completely eliminated with this method alone. Under special circumstances, punishment can sometimes be successful in producing long-term suppression of problem behaviors. But here the punishment must be of traumatic or near-traumatic intensity, which makes it undesirable on both ethical and practical (i.e. side effects) grounds.

- The most effective way to use the punishment procedure to suppress a problem behavior is to combine it with rewarding an alternative, acceptable behavior in problem situations. Technically, this other behavior is referred to by behavioral scientists as a *competing behavior* in the sense that physically speaking, the animal can do one thing or the other but not both simultaneously (e.g. jumping up on a visitor and lying down when a visitor enters the house are competing behaviors). The method of eliminating unacceptable problem behaviors by using reward-based training procedures to elicit and strengthen acceptable competing behaviors in problem situations is called *counterconditioning*, and it is widely applied in many training and behavior therapy procedures.

- A punishing stimulus should be intense enough to stop the punished behavior *immediately* and *every time* it is administered, but it should not be so intense that it produces highly fearful behavior. Essentially, when an animal is often able to ignore an owner's scolding to simply keep on performing the punished behavior even when scolded, the scolding is not punishing enough – and either the owner must increase the amount of authority behind it or turn to another punishing stimulus. Alternatively, if the animal cowers in fear and runs away and hides for a few minutes, the stimulus is far more intense than it need or should be.

- Unlike rewards which are best administered intermittently to maintain a behavior which was originally learned under a continuous reinforcement schedule (i.e. the behavior was initially rewarded every time it occurred but is later only rewarded sometimes), laboratory experiments indicate that the punishment method is most effective when a behavior is always punished every single time it occurs. In effect, a point is never reached where a behavior should be punished every second time, every third time, etc. as is the case with food rewards.

- Laboratory experiments and practical exper-

ience indicate that effective punishment works almost immediately, mostly within just a few applications of the punishing stimulus. Therefore a basic rule of thumb is that when an owner must keep punishing an animal again and again for performing some problem behavior, something is fundamentally wrong with the training method. It could be that the punishing stimulus is simply not intense enough to suppress the behavior for long or, more commonly, punishment alone cannot do more than temporarily suppress a behavior which the dog is highly motivated to perform. In the latter case, the punishment method is effective as far as it goes, but the use of rewards to train and strengthen some competing behavior in problem situations is indispensable if a satisfactory and permanent solution to the problem is to be achieved.

- Punishment can have the side effect of eliciting aggressive behavior if it is painful, elicits fear in a fear-aggressive dog, or is seen as a status-threatening challenge by a dominant aggressive dog. For many dogs, it is therefore contraindicated for reasons of owner safety.

Early or pre-problem intervention method

For many problems like aggression towards human strangers on the street, a third element can be an extremely helpful addition to the dual strategy of punishing the problem behavior while rewarding acceptable competing behaviors in problem situations. Here the owner is instructed to attract the animal's attention and get it involved in some sort of rewarding activity *just before it begins to show the problem behavior* when the stimuli that normally elicit the behavior first appear or occur. For a dog which is aggressive to joggers, for example, the owner might call the dog and reward it with tidbits for following commands as soon as both owner and dog first notice that a jogger is approaching but still too far away to elicit aggressive behavior from the dog. This short obedience training session – which dogs that are not given food rewards at any other time enjoy immensely – is simply continued until the jogger has passed by and is out of range. Instead of rewarding commands, owners could also use play at this time by taking the dog's favorite toy out of their pocket and throwing it to get the dog involved in a chase-and-fetch game while the jogger passes by. Campbell (1992) often recommends a similar approach which he refers to as the "jolly routine". Here, owners are instructed to start acting particularly happy and do whatever usually gets the dog's tail wagging as soon as a potential problem situation starts developing.

This early intervention approach is often referred to as a "distraction" method. However, one must be careful not to give owners the wrong impression that any kind of distraction is to be recommended. Distraction is involved to the extent that the dog's attention is diverted to something other than the jogger, but this approach is quite different than distracting the dog with something like tidbits or playing *after* it has already started being aggressive – which rewards the problem behavior and is therefore strictly contraindicated. Basically, one must emphasize to owners that this early intervention type of "distraction" is only appropriately applied *before* the problem behavior is exhibited. However, if the dog has already begun to be aggressive, it is too late: the problem behavior must be suppressed by punishing the animal rather than rewarding it with tidbits or playing.

Cessation of rewards for problem behaviors

The behavior problem counselor often sees cases in which unintentional rewards from the owner have caused a problem to develop, are maintaining it, or are steadily making it worse. For example, some dogs are difficult for owners to walk because they refuse to go in certain directions, take five minutes of persuading before they are ready to cross a street, or stop every 20 or 30 yards and wait for the owner to pet or talk to them before they consent to continue onwards. Similarly, some dogs pester for playing, attention, or food in the home in such a demanding and persistent way that the owner must comply or be driven crazy.

In such cases, punishment is rarely necessary. Usually, it is enough simply to have owners fully ignore the behavior and not give the dog what it wants at this time. Behavioral scientists refer to this behavior modification procedure involving the cessation of all positive reinforcements which are maintaining an undesirable behavior as *extinction*. One simply ignores the dog when it tries to stop on the street during walks and instead walks normally onwards without talking to or even looking at it no matter what it does. And in the case of pestering for petting, playing or food in the home, one makes it a hard and fast family rule that the dog *never* gets what it wants at such times.

The extinction procedure is an extremely effective approach to eliminating problem behaviors that are being entirely maintained by external sources of reinforcement (e.g. from the owner) which the owner can control. However, this approach is only effective if three conditions are met: (1) owners must be completely convinced that this is what they must do, (2) they must have enough self-discipline or be stubborn enough to apply it with 100% consistency, and (3) they must be fully prepared by the counselor for what will happen when they first stop rewarding a problem behavior – namely, that the problem will temporarily worsen before it finally improves.

Laboratory experiments clearly show that at the very beginning of the extinction process when the rewards that are maintaining the behavior are first completely discontinued, both the frequency and intensity of the response increase greatly before they start a long, gradual, extremely uneven and irregular decline which precedes permanent abandonment. Also sometimes observed at this time are aggressive responses – apparently a natural response of animals to the situation where rewards which an animal is accustomed to receiving do not materialize. Watch someone operating a soft drink machine which doesn't work (i.e. the learned behavior of putting money in the slot doesn't bring its usual reward) and both effects can be seen: money is put in repeatedly if the machine doesn't accept it; buttons or levers are repeatedly operated with increased speed and vigor, and finally a few bangs with the fist and a last sound kick with the foot express more than the person's desire to coax the machine back into working order. Basically, human beings too don't just passively accept the failure of a learned response to produce its usual reward on the first attempt and turn and walk meekly away. Owners must be forewarned about other distinctive features of the extinction process as well like, for example, that each new day will bring a renewed tendency to try the behavior that seemed to have been completely abandoned the day before (called *spontaneous recovery*) and the actual course of the extinction process is highly uneven, with increasingly widely-spaced bursts of rapid responding rather than a smooth and continuous decline in frequency seen in a graph of the extinction process averaged over a group of animals. In other words, the animal will give up for an hour, try hard again, give up for another hour or two, try it more often the next day, give up for a day or so, try hard again for a few minutes perhaps four or five times the next day, etc.

Behavior therapy methods

The expression *animal behavior therapy* is commonly used in two senses. The more general meaning subsumes both the pet behavior counselor's efforts in providing assistance to problem owners as well as all of the various kinds of treatment measures recommended such as training, modifying environments, castration, drugs, counterconditioning, systematic desensitization, etc. In this sense, the term animal behavior therapy is synonymous with that of pet behavioral counseling.

Throughout the discussions in this book, the use of the term will be restricted however to its second, more specific meaning. Namely, systematic and often somewhat elaborate retraining procedures which are either directly derived from or based on the same principles as procedures used in human behavior therapy. An example is *systematic desensitization* for the treatment of phobic fear reactions. Here, animals are so gradually and carefully exposed to a progressive sequence of situations more and

more closely resembling that in which fear was previously elicited that the animals never become fearful – a standard procedure for treating phobias in human behavior therapy.

However, just as there are few direct parallels between behavior problems in pets and human beings, so too are the parallels between pet and human behavior therapies strictly limited. It is more in the application of principles which form the basis of the common procedural approaches (e.g. gradual exposure, habituation, counterconditioning, extinction, etc.), and their use in specially designed, systematic, and often elaborate procedures to train animals to behave differently in specific problem situations, where the resemblance lies. Some specific examples of behavior therapy approaches commonly recommended to pet owners are the following:

- Gradually training a dog to ride in a car without becoming afraid by using food rewards for following sit, down, stay, etc. commands without showing signs of fear when near a car, in a parked car with the motor off, then with the motor on, for a short trip of 5 meters, and then for increasingly longer trips.
- Using food rewards to gradually train a dog not to growl when being brushed by rewarding it for not growling when touched with the brush on its head, then on its neck, back, then when given one light brush stroke on its back, then several, and then for tolerating brushing with gradually increasing pressure and for increasingly longer periods of time over the course of several days.
- Training dogs which become agitated and bark, are destructive, or eliminate in the home when left alone (i.e. separation anxiety) to better tolerate these lonely times by at first leaving them only briefly alone (e.g. for a minute or so) before returning and rewarding them for quietly waiting, and then very gradually increasing the length of time one is absent over the course of several days and weeks.

Non-training measures

Pet behavior problems are also often treated with measures other than behavioral training or environmental modification such as castration, drug therapy, and the use of physical response prevention or response control aids like muzzles or head collars. As will be discussed often in later chapters, these too have their own principles in terms of how they should be used and when they are indicated. In the present discussion of various kinds of training measures, they should not however be completely forgotten. For sometimes they can be a fully acceptable alternative to behavioral training as, for example, where intermale aggression is completely eliminated by castration. Most commonly, however, castration, drug therapy, and response control measures are recommended as auxiliary methods which are applied along with behavior-related training measures.

Drug therapy

The following lengthy quote from Marder (1991) provides an excellent and balanced summary of factors which the veterinarian must keep in mind when considering or prescribing drugs, particularly psychotropic drugs, for the treatment of behavior problems:

"There are few good controlled studies of the effectiveness of drug therapy for the treatment of specific behavior problems in dogs and cats. Although animals have been used in experimental studies of some of the psychoactive drugs, most of these studies have involved unnatural circumstances or brain lesions and are not applicable to pet behavior in a home environment. Furthermore, there are no documented animal analogues of human psychiatric diagnoses, so it is extremely difficult to extrapolate from the human literature when deciding which drug to use for a certain problem. For example, there are no known animal psychotics or schizophrenics. Although some behaviors clearly are not adaptive (e.g. flank sucking and other stereotypies), most of the behavior problems seen by animal behaviorists are normal species-typical behaviors (e.g. aggression) that clash with the human lifestyle. Very little is know about effective dosages and therapeutic blood levels of specific drugs for dogs and cats. Drug dosages have been based
on human recommendations, which may be inaccurate and, sometimes, dangerous.

When prescribing drug therapy to help change the behavior of a pet, the veterinarian should be thoroughly familiar with dosages, possible side effects, and contraindications of the specific drug. A recent and complete physical examination should always precede the use of any psychotropic drug; this also applies to prescribing a drug on the advice of a dog trainer or nonveterinary behavior consultant. Because the veterinarian prescribes the drug, the veterinarian is responsible if complications occur. Furthermore, the owner must be informed that behavioral drug therapy still is experimental. One should consider having the owner sign a legal release form, as most of the psychotropic drugs are not approved for use in animals. Because there are both species and individual variability in response to each drug, the pet should be observed closely for any serious side effects for its entire duration the first time the drug is given.

Until more is learned, drug therapy should not be relied upon as the sole treatment for a behavior problem. Psychotropic drugs can be helpful adjuvants to a behavior modification program, but unfortunately, they rarely are curative alone. Quite frequently, a drug has little or no effect on the problem behavior; when it does, the effects seen while the animal is taking the drug do not transfer to the nondrugged state". (pp. 329–330)

The matter of side effects should not be taken lightly. The following is a list of the possible side effects discussed by authors such as Marder (1991), Overall and Beebe (1994), Burghardt (1991), and Voith (1989) for most of the drugs commonly prescribed for the treatment of behavior problems:

Progestins (e.g. megestrol acetate, medroxyprogesterone acetate): increased appetite, lethargy, depression, mammary gland hyperplasia and tumors, diabetes mellitus, hyperglycemia, adrenocortical suppression or atrophy, temperament changes.

Benzodiazepines (e.g. diazepam, clorazepate dipotassium): increased aggression in fear-aggressive dogs, ataxia, lethargy, increased appetite, paradoxical excitement or increased activity, hepatic side effects.

Tricyclics and other antidepressants (e.g. amitriptyline HCl, imipramine, doxepin, clomipramine): mydriasis, cardiac arrhythmia, dry mouth, constipation, urinary retention, marked sedation, hypotension, decreased seizure threshold, skin reactions.

Phenothiazines (e.g. acetylpromazine, promazine, chlorpromazine): lowered seizure threshold, hypotension, paradoxical excitation.

Buspirone: renal and hepatic side effects

Narcotic antagonists (e.g. naloxone, naltrexone, hydrocodone): lethargy, wakefulness, activity changes, anorexia.

Fortunately given the considerable uncertainties related to appropriateness, dosages, and possible serious side effects inherent in the prescription of these various experimental drugs, medicaments are only potentially helpful in a minority of cat and dog behavior problem cases, and there are very few cases (e.g. where behavioral measures alone have failed to resolve urine marking problems in cats or stereotypies in dogs and cats) where drug therapy is really essential.

Cautionary note: In providing drug and dosage information throughout this book, I am essentially only reporting what is recommended by well-known veterinary behavior specialists like Voith, Marder, Hart, Burghardt, Overall, and others. As an experimental psychologist, I am not qualified or competent to prescribe drugs or provide drug-related or associated medical information to any greater extent than this. When including such information at various places, I have been careful to provide the reference or references from which the recommendation was taken. I would strongly urge the veterinarian who is contemplating the prescribing drug therapy not to rely solely on the information provided in this book, but rather to first consult the accompanying references as well as those referred to in the previous few paragraphs which extensively discuss a variety of drugs, side effects, and associated issues related to the use of drugs to treat pet behavior problems.

Constraints on the treatment of dog behavioral problems

It is not always possible to completely eliminate or considerably reduce the seriousness of dog behavior problems by modifying owner attitudes, changing interactive ground rules, obedience training animals, training them to behave more acceptably in specific problem situations, castrating them, administering drugs, or carrying out some kind of systematic behavior therapy procedure. There are several major reasons why.

Genetic constraints

Some dogs are unusually highly motivated – compared to the average dog – to kill cats, fight with other dogs, or direct dominance-related aggressive behavior towards human family members. Rather than simply having learned to be that way, it is likely in many cases that such undesirable behavioral tendencies at least partly reflect the individual's genetic makeup, which is unalterable. When this is the case and a dog's problem behavioral tendencies must essentially be accepted as if they were an immutable feature of its "personality", the possibilities for solution are often limited. Here, the goal of treatment may not be to completely solve the problem in the sense of eliminating the dog's problem behavior, but rather to minimize its impact by avoiding or changing the nature of problem situations, by training the dog to be more obedient and hence more controllable in all situations, and/or by using physical aids such as muzzles or head collars.

Of course, one can never be entirely sure that such severe genetic constraints are involved. But if the behavior is unusually intense, unusually easily elicited, and has long existed and survived in the face of changes in owners, environments, and the application of measures which are normally effective with such problems, then it is likely that this is the case. However, this rarely means that the case is hopeless. Rather that solution possibilities are limited and may be of a different character than with an animal whose behavior problem has developed as result, for example, of unintentional owner reinforcement or substandard living conditions.

Practical constraints

The owner's schedule may not permit training sessions at several times during the day, it may not be possible for the owner who has no car to take the dog somewhere where it can play with other animals, thin walls between apartments may make using a loud noise to startle an animal unfeasible, or there may be other practical reasons why it is impossible for the owner to carry out the required treatment in the form in which it is usually recommended. Normally, such practical constraints are not so insurmountable as to preclude effective treatment, but they are a feature of many cases. Indeed having to tailor the specific treatment recommendations so that they are compatible with whatever practical constraints are associated with, for example, the physical environment inside and outside of the home, who in the family is charged with looking after and training the dog, and family members' schedules and lifestyles is one of the reasons why problem cases are as individual as they are.

The human factor

As discussed in previous chapters, for the treatment of problems like dominance aggression where success requires that the manner in which family members interact with the dog be drastically altered in a way which does not come naturally to them, one sometimes has the feeling that the treatment is doomed to failure from the start because these particular people with their particular attitudes, needs, and personalities are simply not psychologically or emotionally capable of changing their behavior in the way required. Another type of human factor constraint is related to particular kinds of cost-benefit calculations on the part of owners – that is, between the amount of time and effort they must devote to correcting the problem on the one hand, and the benefits which will result if they do this on the other. Some owners are not willing to go as far as an optimal treatment plan

might require because they are simply not willing to pay the kind of time or effort price doing so entails. For them, only easy-to-apply methods come under consideration. If there is no easy way to solve the problem, they will just keep on living with it as they have been doing, give the animal away, or have it put to sleep.

Essentially, there are as many kinds of human factors as there are idiosyncratic owner personalities and life situations. Indeed these human factors which determine what kinds of treatments are recommended and how well recommended treatments will be complied with are in some ways the most critical and interesting "problems" which the pet behavior problem counselor faces. For although the training methods introduced in this chapter are effective means of coping with almost all dog behavior problems, whether problems are actually solved or improved depends entirely on owner's willingness and capability to diligently carry out the recommended treatment measures. Given that it is probably in the area of owner compliance where most treatments fail, it is learning to deal more effectively with the human factors affecting compliance, and not designing new and more effective treatments per se, which is the greatest challenge faced by the pet behavior problem field.

References

Burghardt, W. F. (1991): Using drugs to control behavior problems in pets. *Veterinary Medicine* **November,** 1066–1075.

Campbell, W. E. (1992): *Behavior Problems in Dogs. Second Edition.* Goleta, California, American Veterinary Publications, Inc.

Marder, A. R. (1991): Psychotropic drugs and behavioral therapy. *Veterinary Clinics of North America: Small Animal Practice* **21**, 329–342.

Overall, K., and Beebe, A. (1994): *VHUP Behavior Clinic Newsletter* **Summer.**

Voith, V.L. (1982a): Treatment of dominance aggression of dogs towards people. *Modern Veterinary Practice* **63**, 149–152.

Voith, V.L. (1982b): Teaching sit-stay. *Modern Veterinary Practice* **63**, 317–320.

Voith, V.L. (1982c): Teaching the down-stay. *Modern Veterinary Practice* **63**, 425.

Voith, V.L. (1989): Behavioral disorders. In Ettinger, S. (ed): *Textbook of Veterinary Internal Medicine*. Philadelphia, WB Saunders.

9   Introduction to Aggression Problems

As Figure 9.1 indicates, roughly two-thirds of the dog problem cases seen by the non-veterinary pet behavior problem specialist involve one or more forms of aggression towards humans or other dogs.

From the beginning, it was clear to early workers in the pet behavior problem field that aggression in dogs was best considered not as a single problem but as a group of problems which differed from each other in major ways. For example, Table 9.1 summarizes some of the information presented in Borchelt and Voith's (1982) aggression problem summary table in a way which emphasizes features of the various problems that are most relevant to the present discussion.

This is basically an empirical classification system, a simple unordered, descriptive listing of the various types of aggression problems which emerges from the counselor's years of case experience. The basis of the categorization is the nature of the target or victim of the aggression and the nature of the specific kinds of eliciting situations in which the aggression occurs.

Two features of this system are worth noticing. Firstly, it has no overall structure which helps either to place the various aggression problems within some biologically meaningful

context or to relate the problems to one another. Secondly, the concepts used to label the various problems are either *functional* (possessive, protective, predatory), *descriptive* without any functional implications (intermale, interfemale, maternal), *eliciting situation*-related (pain-elicited, punishment-elicited), or *motivation*-related (fear, redirected, dominance) – scientifically speaking, an indefensible mixture of different levels or classes of concepts. The fact that various versions of this empirical classification system still predominate in the field today is a measure of how little progress has been made on the theoretical front since the formal establishment of the field more than two decades ago.

As Borchelt and Voith (1982) point out by presenting an alternative classification system for behavior problems based on etiology, in theory there are many different ways to classify behavior and behavior problems. Table 9.2 presents a classification system of the nature of the most common dog aggression problems that attempts to go somewhat beyond the mere listing and describing of problems. While this system too simply lists problems which are commonly observed within the three major categories of *intraspecific-intragroup*, *intraspecific-extragroup*, and *interspecific* aggression, the de-

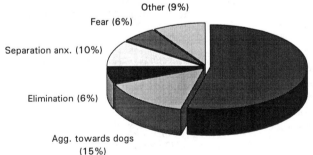

Other (9%)

Fear (6%)

Separation anx. (10%)

Elimination (6%)

Agg. towards dogs (15%)

Agg. towards humans (54%)

Figure 9.1: Relative frequency of general classes of behavior problems in dogs (n=267 major problems in 147 dogs)

Table 9.1: Classical dog aggression problem classification system adapted from Borchelt and Voith (1982)

Problem	Target	Eliciting situation
Dominance aggression	Family members	Response to dominant gestures by owner (e.g. petting, scolding); competitive situations over resting place, food, etc.
Possessive aggression	Person/animal	Target approaches dog when it is in possession of food, toys, objects.
Protective aggression	Person/animal	Target approaches area (home), owners, other animals.
Predatory aggression	Animal/human	Stalking, etc.
Fear aggression	Human	Dog approached, reached for, threatened, punished.
Intermale aggression	Other male	Target seen at distance, approaches.
Interfemale aggression	Other female	Usually competitive situations between two females in same home.
Pain-elicited aggression	Person	Target tries to groom, medicate, manipulate painful area.
Punishment-elicited aggression	Person	Dog exposed to aversive/painful punishment.
Maternal aggression	Person	Target approaches puppies, puppy surrogates, nest area.
Redirected aggression	Person	Target interferes when dog threatened or fighting.

scription of most of the aggression problems in proximate, function-related terms (i.e. "self-protective" rather than "fear aggression"), the placement of some forms of aggression (e.g. self-protective, group-defensive) in more than one major category, and the emphasis on the sociobiologically critical dimensions of *group member vs. outsider* and *conspecific vs. member of another species* are useful features. For they focus attention on several important theoretical questions which arise in connection with these types of problems.

Intraspecific vs. interspecific aggression

From the biological viewpoint, it is natural to distinguish between *intraspecific* behavior which is directed towards the members of one's own species – true social behavior – and *interspecific* behavior which is directed towards the members of other species. Both can be highly complex and involve behavior ranging from cooperative and non-aggressive to competitive and aggressive. There are times when dogs play together and hunt cooperatively, and there are other times when the same dogs may fight with and bite one another. Similarly, interspecific behavior too can range from mutually beneficial (mutualism) to exploitive (parasitism, predation) to competitive (interspecific competition), which in this latter case can sometimes involve aggressive behavioral interactions between members of the two species as, for example, when scavengers from two different species fight over a carcass.

Technically speaking, the aggression of dogs towards human beings is interspecific behavior. However, it makes little sense to try to understand and account for such behavior in terms of the various concepts and principles that are commonly used by animal behaviorists to understand and account for interspecific relationships in the animal world. For the form and

Table 9.2: Functional classification system of the nature of the most common dog aggression problems towards human beings and other dogs

Intraspecific aggression *(dog responding to human being/dog as conspecific)*		Interspecific aggression *(human being/dog responded to as member of alien species)*
Intragroup aggression *(between fellow group members)*	**Extragroup aggression** *(towards human beings/dogs outside of the family)*	
Competitive aggression *(dominance-related or possessive)*	Competitive aggression *(dominance-related or possessive)*	Competitive aggression *(interspecific competition)*
Self-protective aggression	Self-protective aggression	Self-protective aggression
Defense of young	Group-defensive aggression	Group-defensive aggression
Playful aggression		Predatory behavior

eliciting context characteristic of many of the types of aggression dogs display towards human beings clearly indicate that the basic nature of such aggression is *intraspecific*. To understand why dominant-aggressive dogs attack human family members in the particular types of situations they do, for example, it helps to assume that the dogs are responding to human beings as if they were fellow dog pack members by (1) reacting aggressively towards human behaviors which resemble dominant behaviors among dogs or (2) by behaving aggressively in the kinds of competitive situations over food, resting places, etc. in which dominance-related threatening and fighting commonly occurs in dog packs.

Rather than implying that the *inter-* versus *intraspecific* dimension is not as relevant to the phenomenon of dog aggression towards human beings as it is to other types of animal behavior, the fact that this basic distinction which is so easily drawn for other animal behavior phenomena seems somewhat difficult to directly apply to the human-dog relationship should be welcomed. For it forces one to squarely confront the issue of the biological nature of dogs' aggressive behavior towards human beings. Like the similar issue of the biological nature of the behavior of pet owners towards their pets discussed in Chapter 2, it is a difficult and complex problem which is nevertheless crucial to understanding dog behavior problems.

Several key assumptions underlie the classification scheme presented in Table 9.2. The first is that the nature of dog aggressive behavior directed towards human beings may be either *interspecific* or *intraspecific*. In interspecific aggression, the dog is indeed behaving towards a human being as it might towards the member of any other potentially dangerous or competitor species. Fundamentally speaking, this form of aggression can be either (1) *defensive* (e.g. defending oneself or helping to defend one's group against some large predator – *self-protective* and *group-defensive* aggression respectively), (2) a form of *interspecific competition* as when members of another species are aggressively driven away because they too are predators competing with a pack of dogs for available game, or (3) *predatory* behavior directed towards chickens, other livestock, and in rare cases human children or frail adults. Animal behavioral scientists do not consider predatory behavior to be a form of aggression – which always consists of species-typical threat displays and fighting behaviors quite dramatically different than those exhibited during predatory attacks on prey animals. However, given that the present discussion is focused on the wide range of dog behavior problems that involve some sort of physical threat or danger to human beings or others animals, it makes sense to include predatory attacks in the classification scheme even though these are, biologically speaking, more appropriately regarded as a form of feeding or ingestive behavior.

Another key assumption made by the present scheme is that it can be applied equally appropriately to the most common problems involving aggression towards humans and other dogs. In effect, just as it is appropriate to consider some attacks on human beings as involving *intraspecific* aggression, so too is it appropriate to consider some attacks on other dogs as involving *interspecific* aggression. As discussed in Chapter 15, there are dogs which attack all other dogs on sight and essentially do not seem capable of responding to other dogs as conspecifics. In such cases, it is tempting to assume that the dogs do not in fact recognize other dogs as conspecifics and are therefore behaving towards them as if they were members of another animal species.

How could it be possible that an animal like a human being which is physically and behaviorally so different from a dog could nevertheless elicit behavior in dogs which in the wild would only be directed towards other dogs? Three possible complementary hypotheses can be offered. Firstly, dogs display a pronounced imprinting or imprinting-like effect where early experiences with other dogs, for example, are critical determinants of the dog's social behavior towards dogs later in life. Most authors assume that the degree of flexibility here is great enough for some type of imprinting-like process to affect the dog's basic orientation and later social behavior towards human beings as well: in effect, dogs which have spent their first few months in close contact with human beings are predisposed to behave towards them and perhaps perceive them as fellow conspeci-

fics. Secondly, there are strong resemblances between the human family and dog pack social structure and group dynamics which might also predispose a dog which interacts almost exclusively with human beings to respond to and view human group members as conspecifics. Finally, living almost exclusively in the company of human beings, it may be fair to regard the normal family dog as being somewhat socially deprived as far as the possibilities for interacting with real conspecifics are concerned. As ethological research with a variety of species clearly indicates, social deprivation circumstances may to lead minimally adequate or sometimes normally completely inadequate stimuli eliciting social behavior in the absence of biologically normal eliciting stimuli. In short, the social dynamics within the human family group are close enough to those of the dog pack to elicit the intraspecific social behavior which the somewhat socially deprived, human-imprinted dog is highly motivated to and in a certain sense therefore "needs" to perform.

Intragroup vs. extragroup aggression

The second biologically important distinction embodied in the classification scheme presented in Table 9.2 is that between *intragroup* and *extragroup* aggression problems. *Intragroup* aggression is seen when dogs are aggressive towards human family members or other dogs in the family whereas *extragroup* aggression involves aggression either towards strange dogs or humans or towards humans or dogs outside of the family with whom the dog has had contact before and therefore recognizes as individuals.

In thinking about these various types of relationships, it may be helpful to recall what is known about wolves and rural feral dogs (see Chapter 7) and imagine the pattern of social interactions which might develop between dogs and dog packs if they were reintroduced into the wild to live away from all contact with human beings much the same as their wolf ancestors still live today. In the absence of abundant, human-provided food sources, packs would be small, stable groups, mostly composed of individuals that are in some way genetically related to one another. A pack would have a hunting/scavenging territory which it defends against outsiders. The various packs inhabiting a given geographical area would have their own, largely non-overlapping territories with relatively stable border areas between neighboring packs. Basically, the relations between neighboring packs in such a natural setting would be predominantly antagonistic in the sense that defense of territory and the food and other survival resources it contains would be directed towards one's immediate neighbors.

However, our domestic dogs live under a vastly different and more complex set of spatial and social conditions. The human family has no territory which it defends, and even the core home base area is rarely defended by human beings. Strangers come to the door, enter the home, conduct their business, and go with perhaps only the hint of an initial suspicious, sizing-up inspection by the human resident at the time of first face-to-face contact. Similarly, on their walks, dogs and owners move through a world full of indifferent human strangers, friendly human acquaintances, strange dogs of all types and sizes, known enemy dogs which are waiting for the day's bout of mutual threatening, and known perpetually juvenile friends that are always ready and eager to play. Like the new demands placed on human beings by the process of civilization which replaced the small, simple, well-ordered world of the primitive hunter-gatherer with the diverse, dynamic, and exceedingly complex modern society world in which we live today, the process of domestication has made similar demands on our dogs. For them, the simple world involving only the natural and unambiguous distinctions between a group's hunting territory and everything outside of it, fellow group members and outsiders, and conspecifics and the members of other species no long exists. And they, like we, must do the best they can to cope with this often stressful and sometimes confusingly complex new physical and social environment with behavioral systems which although modified somewhat during the domestication process, are still

not so different in terms of fundamentals from those of their wolf ancestors.

Considering the degree to which our complex modern society environment differs from that in which the dog's (i.e. wolf's) basic behavioral system equipment evolved, the great diversity among dogs in how they react to "outsiders" – to strange and known humans and dogs which they encounter on the street, walk by the yard, or visit family homes – should not be too surprising. Some dogs are extremely friendly to strange humans and/or strange dogs under all circumstances while others are always extremely wary and aggressive. Some dogs are only aggressive to strange humans and not to strange dogs, while others are the opposite. Some dogs are aggressive to strange humans and/or dogs within the home but not outside of it. Finally, the special friendly or agonistic relationships dogs form with dog and human "acquaintances" which it occasionally encounters in the home or while wandering on the streets represents a third element which considerably complicates the simple intragroup vs. extragroup picture which could be drawn if the species still lived in the kind of natural environment in which its wolf ancestors evolved.

While sometimes difficult to directly or simply apply, the *intra-* vs. *extragroup* dimension is nevertheless of both theoretical and practical importance to the pet behavior problem counselor. When questioning owners of aggressive dogs, it is crucial to view and attempt to understand aggression towards family members and aggression towards human strangers as if they were two quite separate phenomena in which the dog is motivated differently and perceives the target of its aggression in a quite distinctly different way. Dominance aggression towards human beings, for example, is almost exclusively an intragroup problem – one in which the relationship between fellow group members must be examined and in some way modified. So-called intermale aggression towards other dogs on the other hand, takes somewhat different intragroup and extragroup forms that not only require different types of treatment measures, but which also give rise to somewhat different kinds of questions concerning why particular animals are a problem in this regard. Similarly, so-called "fear aggression" can be elicited by human or dog family members, strangers, or non-family members with whom the dog occasionally interacts. However, the nature of problem situations, causes, and treatments differ enormously depending on such things, for example, as whether the problem is a reflection of past owner punishment or fights between dogs in the same home (common in intragroup self-protective aggression), inadequate early experiences (e.g. extragroup self-protective aggression towards all dogs or all human strangers), or past aversive experiences with particular known human or dog individuals or particular types of non-family members (e.g. children). In short, it is just as important for understanding and treating dog aggression problems to question owners in detail concerning whether the dog is being aggressive to human or animal members of its family group, complete strangers, or familiar outsiders or types of outsiders as it is to ask oneself the question of whether the dog is behaving towards the victim as if it were a conspecific or member of another species. Both facilitate understanding the basic nature and detailed form of the problem, and both are crucial for determining the nature of the treatment which will be required to reduce or eliminate it.

Having introduced the general nature of the classification scheme presented in Table 9.2, the remaining sections will be devoted to briefly describing the various common types of dog behavior problems and how they fit into it.

Intragroup aggression

When interacting with members of its human family, the behavior shown by dogs can only be understood if it is assumed that they are basically treating family members as conspecifics – in effect, as albeit somewhat strange-acting and strange-looking dogs. This applies to aggressive behavior as well. When directed towards human beings, it seems reasonable to assume that all of the types of aggression problems discussed in the following section are examples of

fundamentally *intraspecific* behavior which closely resembles both in terms of causal factors and form aggression shown towards other dogs in the family.

Competitive aggression

Competitive aggression between dogs in the same home

Two family dogs may threaten each other and fight in a wide variety of contexts because each is basically trying to establish and maintain a dominant position in relation to the other. In effect, so called intermale and interfemale aggression between two dogs in the same home are forms of *competitive* or *dominance-related aggression*.

With regard to problems between two family dogs which are always fighting over the possession of some object like food, toys, etc. – what Borchelt and Voith (1982) call possessive aggression – there are two possibilities. The first is that this too may be a form of dominance-related competitive aggression where the animals are basically fighting over the "right of possession" of objects (i.e. when there is only one bone, one toy, etc.). The second is that while the aggression is obviously competitive, it may not in fact be dominance-related. Even the most stable dominance-submission relationship may not be able to prevent all aggression in competitive contexts like, for example, if the dominant animal tries to take food practically out of a subdominant animal's mouth. In this connection, it has been observed that normally subordinate wolves can often successfully defend meat or bones which they are in possession of by growling and snapping at a dominant animal which approaches (Mech, 1970).

Competitive aggression towards human beings

Perhaps the most common serious dog behavior problem, dominance aggression, involves growling at and biting human family members in situations which either have a directly competitive element (e.g. owner tries to take something away from the dog or pushes it off the bed) or where the owner shows one of several kinds of behaviors or gestures towards the dog like touching it in certain ways, bending over it, scolding it, or punishing it which are thought to provoke aggression because they resemble dominant dog behavior towards a subordinate dog.

In most cases of so-called "redirected aggression" (Borchelt and Voith, 1982) when owners are bitten when they interfere in their dog's threatening of or fighting with another dog, there is usually some kind of dominance-related relationship problem between owner and dog. Here it is possible that from the dog's point of view, the subordinate owner does not have the right to interfere in this crucial situation and a bite is a fully appropriate way to teach a fellow group member a lesson it obviously needs to be taught.

Although dominance-related competitive aggression towards human beings is normally a form of intragroup aggression which has little or nothing to do with the dog's behavior towards humans outside of the family, there are a few dogs which direct dominance-related behavior (e.g. putting paws on visitors' shoulders) towards strange humans, particularly when they are visitors in the dog's home. However, too little is known about this rather uncommon form of behavior to know whether it should be regarded as the kind of dominance-related extragroup behavior shown towards strange male dogs or, alternatively, a special form of intragroup dominance-related behavior towards a person who perhaps appears (from the dog's viewpoint) to have joined the family group.

Self-protective aggression

Although dominance aggression towards human beings too almost always has a defensive character (i.e. the dog reacts aggressively towards someone who disturbs it while sleeping or tries to take its bone away), the dog is presumably defending its rank and associated "rights". In intragroup *self-protective* aggression, however, the dog is defending itself in a more direct and obvious way. Several of Borchelt and Voith's (1982) types of aggression fall

into this category when directed towards family members. In pain-elicited aggression (e.g. the dog reacts aggressively when a family member examines an injured limb or applies medication to a wound), the dog is reacting to defend itself from what it may perceive as an immediate threat to its physical well-being. As many experiments have demonstrated, pain is one of the most powerful elicitors of self-protective aggression in all complex animal species. So-called redirected aggression in situations where a dog which is in pain lashes out at the nearest family member who is present or restraining it can be understood similarly. Punishment-elicited aggression towards family members differs in that it may be more the anticipation or threat of pain caused by the punishment rather than pain itself which explains why the situation is aversive enough for animals to evoke aggression. Finally, in so-called fear aggression towards family members, animals which have been punished too severely or badly frightened by a family member in the past may show aggression when too closely approached or reached for by the person it has learned to fear. Of course, the feared group member may just as easily be another dog which is growled and snapped at whenever it approaches too closely – usually a legacy of past fighting between the two.

Defense of young

While usually referred to as maternal aggression, males too can show this kind of defensive reaction when a person or another animal in the family approaches puppies or a nest area. This is one of the more understandable and least complicated behavior problems which small animal veterinarians usually deal with themselves rather than referring clients to a behavior problem specialist.

Playful aggression

The aggressive play of young dogs can be a problem for some types of owners. Particularly young children and frail elderly people are sometimes put a risk by overly frisky and aggressively playful animals. Owners and veterinarians sometimes suspect that some more dangerous form of aggression is involved here, which is usually the reason why such cases are referred to behavior specialists.

Extragroup aggression

The biological function of extragroup aggression is to safeguard and protect oneself, other group members, or critical resources needed for the group's survival against members of *other groups of conspecifics* – which may include both dogs and human beings for dogs which have had adequate early experience with other dogs and lived from several weeks of age onwards within a human family.

Group-defensive aggression

Biologically speaking, a territory is by definition a defended area. Wolves are highly territorial in the sense that they hunt and scavenge within the confines of a group territory which is defended against incursions by neighboring packs. By in large, it is clear however that domestic dogs which live in human families in the city environment are not territorial in the basic biological sense of defending a relatively large geographical area against outsiders. Like wolves, feral dog packs which live in a rural environment seem also to defend group territories against incursions by other packs. However, feral dogs living in the city streets behave more like family dogs in this regard, and it is generally only the core resting and shelter areas within the much larger home ranges which are normally defended against other dogs.

Within the group territory in wolves, particularly during the breeding season, there is often a core area containing several dens which the group defends much more intensely than the remainder of the territory. It is probably the defense of this kind of core area which is involved when feral city dogs defend their primary shelter areas and family dogs defend yard and home against outsiders. Basically then, what is normally described as "territorial aggression" in

dogs in the literature (e.g. Hart and Hart, 1985) appears to be comparable not with wolf territorial aggression per se, but rather with the wolf's tendency to defend the group itself by defending its home base area and the sheltering areas, cached food, and mother with pups which it may contain.

Interestingly, Borchelt and Voith (1982) do not define a separate territorial aggression category but rather combine cases of aggression "when person or animal approaches area (home, room, yard), owners, or other animals" under the general heading of protective aggression. The present classification does something similar and essentially makes the same assumption that the dog barking at passersby from its yard and that barking at approaching pedestrians during walks are displaying the same general type of aggression problem.

In the present scheme, the term *group-defensive* is used as a descriptive label for this category of aggression problem for two reasons. Firstly, it allows a relatively clear-cut distinction to be drawn with the *self-protective* aggression problem category defined below. Boldly threatening and attacking – instead of remaining quiet and perhaps heading in the opposite direction, surely the safer strategy – indicates that the function of the behavior is to defend not only the individual itself but the group and its members as well. Secondly, it is consistent with the fact that such bold threatening and attacking behavior may often form the basis of cooperative, coordinated *group defensive behavior*. This can be clearly seen in the pronounced social facilitation effect which can take place in this situation when more than one animal from the family is present. If one family dog barks at a passerby or passing dog, the other family dog is likely to join in even if it would never do this on its own and never starts barking at strange individuals first. Whether it is a case of dogs kept together in the yard or dogs which are walked together – or roam together – on the streets, this form of aggression towards human beings and other dogs is highly infectious: one dog's aggression stimulates the other and causes it too to orient towards the target and join in with the initiator's threats and attacks. It can be assumed therefore that if the dog were a member of a pack, this social facilitation effect might well trigger off a group aggressive display by both alerting and recruiting the assistance of fellow group members.

Self-protective aggression

Some dogs do not go out of their way to bark and growl at or attack strange dogs or humans, but rather prefer to quietly avoid them and only become aggressive "in self-defense", when approached too closely or threatened or attacked by a stranger.

It is natural for any dog to defend itself when attacked by a strange dog or human being under certain conditions, but not when it is simply approached by a dog or human which is clearly displaying friendly or otherwise non-aggressive intentions. A problem therefore exists when the dog perceives certain types of individuals as threatening or dangerous which the normal dog would not perceive this way. Thus, exploring the reasons why dogs tend to find certain individuals or types of individuals threatening is the key to understanding the dog's aggressive behavior in specific cases. Some sort of partial early experience deficit may be involved where, for example, dogs which had no experience with young children during their first few months of life remain always suspicious and uneasy around them throughout their lives. More conventional learning processes play a major role in most cases with past negative experiences with particular individuals or types of individuals determining the dog's present reactions when encountering similar dogs or humans. As with most behavior problems, genetic factors may be important as well – perhaps partially determining, for example, the dog's general tendency to become fearful in a variety of circumstances, how aversive it finds particular stimuli (e.g. high-pitched sounds like the crying and screaming of very young children), how submissively it tends to react to assertive or aggressive behavior on part of others, or how low is its threshold for self-protective aggression.

It is interesting to consider at this point whether these two major types of group-defensive and self-protective aggression problems have something in common in the sense that dogs which show the group-defensive pattern of aggression towards other dogs or human strangers on the street or in the home may also be reacting this way "out of fear" in spite of appearances to the contrary. In many of cases, owners of dogs which are quite offensively and boldly aggressive to human or dog visitors in the home report that the dogs were noticeably fearful of other dogs or strange humans when they were very young. In effect, this often seems to owners to be the original source of the dog's strongly negative orientation towards or perception of them. It is possible, therefore, that group-defensive aggression problems too are a form of "fear aggression" in the sense that they too involve the keeping away or driving away of what is basically a feared individual or at least a type of individual which is perceived by the dog as being threatening or potentially dangerous for some reason. Some survey data bearing on this hypothesis will be presented in Chapter 12.

Competitive aggression

Some male dogs are aggressive to many or most other strange males which they encounter during walks. When the dog meets a strange male, it assumes body postures (e.g. head and tail held high) and engages in behaviors (e.g. standing over) which serve as displays communicating high rank in a group dominance hierarchy. In this situation, the other dog must behave submissively or at least accept such dominant behavior without protest or else a fight will ensue.

Those writing in pet behavior problem field commonly suggest two possibilities for accounting for this intermale aggression scenario. First, that it is basically a form of group-defensive aggression whose aim is to communicate to an intruder that the resident of this territory is a tough customer to whom the dog is wise to pay its respects and then do its best to avoid in future. In effect, that the primary function of the behavior involved is to pass territory-related information from one dog to another and settle what amounts to a kind of potential territorial dispute relatively peaceably without the need for overt fighting.

The second possibility is that such behavior can be profitably viewed as a form of true dominance aggression which has little or nothing to do with territoriality – i.e. that the behavior is aimed at quickly settling the dominance question so that future aggressive competition between two individuals which are now in the process of establishing some kind of new social relationship with one another will be avoided. Indeed, the initial sequence of aggressive behavior interactions described above can turn out to be a prelude to more positive behavioral interactions between the two animals. For example, if the less aggressive dog reacts submissively to the other's dominant behavior, the tone of the social interactions may change dramatically and the two may soon end up playing together. In effect, although the two individuals may be strangers to one another, the function of such behavior would not be to encourage the submissive animal to depart and keep out of this territory in the future, but rather to form or confirm a certain kind of relationship between individuals which allows them to engage in more peaceful forms of social behavior.

Essentially this view postulates that for our domestic dogs, the distinction between intragroup and extragroup behavior is not always as clear as it would be if the dogs were living wild in packs which establish group territories and regularly keep or drive intruders away. More specifically, it is being suggested here that this type of extragroup competitive aggression might lead naturally and quickly to intragroup behavior – that perhaps it is the first step in the *group formation* process which must occur when, for example, strays which eventually band together to form a stable social group initially encounter one another or when a new individual is allowed to join an existing group.

Basically then, this type of intermale aggression along with play between strange dogs and indeed the tendency for most family-owned dogs to be strongly drawn to one another other during walks may be another indication of how highly our pet dogs are motivated to form groups with real conspecifics in spite of our belief that we are providing them with all that they need. Essentially, the degree of partial social deprivation inherent in the domestics dog's life isolated from true conspecifics for all but a small proportion of every day may be in evidence here as well.

Interspecific aggression

True interspecific aggression towards human beings or other dogs is probably relatively rare. Growing up as they do in a human family surrounded by an environment which is populated mostly by human beings, the vast majority of dogs behave towards human beings to a certain extent as if they were other dogs. And most dogs have had enough contact with other dogs throughout their lives to establish and maintain normal species identification. In some cases, however, dogs may either lack the normal kind of early socialization experience with humans or other dogs, or a normal family dog may temporarily come under the influence of the "group psychology" of the dog pack and thus be induced to treat a particular human being (e.g. frightened young child) as if it were a member of an alien species.

Self-protective and group-defensive aggression

Dogs which have had no experience with humans during the first three months of life tend to remain extremely fearful of them for the rest of their lives (e.g. Scott and Fuller, 1965). In some dogs, this fear of strangers is extraordinarily intense and gives one the feeling that the dog may indeed view human beings as a totally alien, potentially dangerous species rather than as a potential social partner.

Dogs with this syndrome do not make good pets for obvious reasons. Therefore most of the family dogs which have problems resulting from inadequate early experience show only milder symptoms in this regard. They accept

and are friendly to some human beings like family members, relatives, and neighbors they
know well, but are fearful and potentially aggressive to all others. In these cases, it is impossible to say whether interspecific aggression
is involved. Even though the dog may respond
fearfully and aggressively to strangers, the fact
that it interacts normally with human family
members and other known individuals seems
to argue against lack of species' identification
as being the sole explanation for its negative reactions.

However, some dogs threaten and are ready
to attack *all* other dogs which approach them
regardless of size, sex, signaled behavioral intention (e.g. friendly tail-wagging, play-bow),
familiarity with them, etc. These dog-aggressive
dogs act as if they simply do not "like" other
dogs and respond to them as enemies to be feared and fought against or at best, entirely ignored. Here, the interpretation of the behavior
seems more straightforward: the early experience with other dogs which is necessary for them
to be perceived and later responded to as conspecifics is lacking, and the dog therefore
seems to be reacting to them as if they were
members of some alien species.

Interspecific competition

The competition between the members of different species over survival-related resources like
food, nesting sites, protective cover, etc. can be
indirect as in *exploitation competition*, where
both simply exploit the same resources but do
not interact, or *interference competition*,
where members of the two species interact directly with one another and may display territorial behavior and/or aggression (Grier and
Burk, 1992). Examples of this latter type of
competition are the fighting between large
mammalian and avian predators/scavengers
over a carcass and the aggressive confrontations between birds and squirrels around win-
ter bird feeders.

One possible type of problem aggression in
dogs involving interspecific competition is the
cat-killing behavior shown by dogs which
chase, catch, and coolly dispatch cats as a mat-

ter of course. Given that both species are mammalian predators which may compete for some
small prey animals – or for the choicest human
table scraps in city garbage cans – it is possible
that such behavior may be interpretable from
an evolutionary viewpoint not as predatory behavior, as is conventional in the literature, but
as a reflection of potential competition between the two species over the same food resources. One might also speculate that this aggressive form of interspecific competition might
also help to account for why some dog-aggressive dogs are ruthless killers of other dogs –
particularly those much smaller than themselves. Perhaps this too is an indication that the
victim dogs are seen not as conspecifics, but as
members of a competitor species.

Human interspecific competition aggression
directed towards feral dogs, coyotes, wolves,
etc. is common. When marauding packs begin
essentially competing (*exploitation competition*) with farmers for the livestock by killing
sheep and chickens, the farmer's "aggressive"
response (*interference competition*), or that of
community agencies acting on his/her behalf,
is usually immediate and intense. In many parts
of the world, wolves have been hunted to extinction for interspecific competition reasons.
Interestingly, however, one is hard pressed to
find an example of similar interference competition aggression of dogs towards human beings
(the aggression of a dog towards a person who
tries to take a bone away is presumably intraspecific with the person essentially being treated like the dog would treat a fellow dog member of its pack). Perhaps remnants of the relationship   between   wolves   and   human
hunter-gatherers which evolved over millions
of years are involved here: dogs which perceive
humans as an alien species simply avoid
contact with them and defer to them without a
struggle in situations potentially involving direct, aggressive competition over food or other
resources.

Predation

Although the behavior patterns used for hunting, capturing, and killing prey are quite diffe-

rent in a number of respects from those normally involved in threatening and fighting of any sort, it is conventional in the pet behavior problem literature to consider predatory behavioral problems along with aggression problems because of the element of danger involved for the members of other species and, in rare cases, human beings.

In rural areas, the predatory killing of chickens or sheep by packs of feral dogs or stray family dogs can sometimes be a problem. Typically, dogs which are highly motivated to engage in such behavior – and have done so successfully a few times in the past – are difficult to reform presumably because of the powerful self-rewarding properties of engaging in predatory behavior itself and the rewarding effects associated with having caught and killed prey in the past.

In cases of predatory behavior towards human beings which have been reported (e.g. Borchelt et al., 1983), the behavior was elicited in a group of dogs in relatively unusual situations where the child or elderly person victim reacted in a way (e.g. trying to run away, screaming, etc.) which in some way stimulated an escalation of the hunting pack "psychology" of an otherwise not particularly dangerous group of animals. As will be discussed in Chapter 13, one theory to account for sudden, sometimes fatal attacks on human newborns by family dogs is that it is a form of predatory behavior where the dog simply does not recognize the infant as a human being and therefore basically predatory behavior is involved (Voith 1984).

Concluding remarks

As will be considered in the following several chapters, the biological classification system presented here can sometimes be difficult to apply with any degree of certainty in specific cases. Is a dog that reacts aggressively to a human stranger on the street showing fundamentally interspecific or intraspecific behavior from the point of view of the underlying behavioral systems which are involved? This may not always be clear. Perhaps some dogs are "con-

fused" about this matter themselves – or more scientifically, perhaps under certain conditions, human beings are only weak or inconsistent elicitors of intraspecific behavior. Likewise, classifying dogs' reactions to other dogs they meet during walks can sometimes be equally problematic. Is a dog displaying intragroup or extragroup behavior when it plays with another dog it knows well in the neighborhood? While one often suspects that intragroup behavior is being elicited here, the situation may not be so clear when such behavioral interactions are aggressive. Also not entirely clear are cases where dogs which are complete strangers to one another immediately begin playing like they were juvenile members of the same pack. Perhaps being more or less continuously deprived of opportunities for various kinds of positive and aggressive social behavior because human family members are by no means optimal elicitors of highly motivated intraspecific behavior creates conditions favoring its easy elicitation by canine strangers.

Is it clear that this kind of biological categorization system raises more questions than it answers. But perhaps that is a measure of its potential utility. Certainly one of the major conclusions which can be drawn from this chapter is that the area of dog aggression problems is highly complex and is badly in need of scientific study. Different problem animals need to be observed in the same kind of careful and systematic way in which modern ethologists observe wild animals in their natural environment. And the behaviors involved need to be carefully recorded, analyzed, classified in terms of both form and eliciting context and then compared with those of animals which do not exhibit serious behavior problems. Basically, it is time to go beyond the rather crude descriptive level which, for example, simply lumps all forms of fear-related aggression under a single general rubric and all but ignores the kinds of interesting and theoretically important issues which this chapter's classification system raises. And it is with the goal in mind of developing a more biologically meaningful conceptual framework which may help to stimulate thinking and suggest future lines of research in this area that the present approach is offered.

References

Borchelt, P.L., Lockwood, R., Beck, A.M., and Voith, V.L. (1983): Attacks by packs of dogs involving predation on human beings. *Public Health Reports* **98**, 59–68.

Borchelt, P.L., and Voith, V.L. (1982): Classification of animal behavior problems. *Veterinary Clinics of North America: Small Animal Practice* **12**, 571–585.

Grier, J.W., and Burk, T. (1992): *Biology of Animal Behavior.* 2nd edition. St. Louis, Missouri, Mosby – Year Book, Inc.

Hart, B. L., and Hart, L.A. (1985): *Canine and Feline Behavior Therapy.* Philadelphia, Lea & Febiger.

Mech, L.D. (1970): *The Wolf: The Ecology and Behavior of an Endangered Species.* New York, The Natural History Press.

Scott, J.P., and Fuller, J.L. (1965):*Genetics and Social Behavior of the Dog.* Chicago, Chicago University Press.

Voith, V.L. (1984): Procedures for introducing a baby to a dog. *Mod. Vet. Pract.* **65**, 539–541.

10   Dominance Aggression Towards Human Family Members

As Figure 10.1 indicates, more than half of the problems involving serious aggression towards human beings in 147 dog cases involved aggression towards family members (i.e. intragroup aggression). And as Figure 10.2 shows, approximately 72% of these involved dominance-related *competitive aggression* or so-called *dominance aggression*. Overall, 56 of the 147 dogs (i.e. approx. 38%) showed this form of aggression to a degree ranging from moderate to severe – a substantially higher percentage than the 23.3 and 19.6% figures quoted by Borchelt and Voith (1986). Fifty-one of these dogs were males (i.e. approx. 91%, which closely agrees with Borchelt and Voith's figures).

Dominance aggression towards family members always occurs in one or both of the following situations:

> Dog and family member are competing over something

- When a family member tries to take food or other objects (e.g. bones, toys, napkins) away from the dog – or approaches it when it is in possession of one of these.
- When a family member approaches or touches the dog's "favorite person" or another dog (e.g. a bitch in estrus).
- When a family member approaches the dog when it is in its bed or disturbs in at any time when it is resting or sleeping (i.e. widely assumed in the literature to involve competition over resting/sleeping locations).
- When a family member walks into a room occupied by a dog or meets it coming the other way in a narrow hall or doorway.

> Owner behaves in dominant manner towards the dog

- Petting, hugging, grooming, bathing, medicating, or towel-drying the dog; touching its feet or face; lifting, pushing, or pulling it; putting on its collar; pulling it with its leash; jerking on its leash; staring at it or threatening, scolding, commanding, hitting, or yelling at it; reaching for or bending over it. Although many of these owner behaviors would not be considered "dominant" in human terms, they are assumed to be common elicitors of dominance aggression because they resemble dominant dog behavior towards another dog.

Other common features of dominance aggression cases:

- Owners often describe the attacks as completely unprovoked, and they often describe the dog as "moody" or unpredictable in the

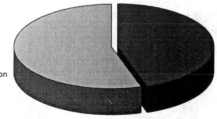

Intragroup aggression
(55%)

Extragroup aggression
(45%)

Figure 10.1: Relative frequency of extragroup versus intragroup problems in cases involving aggression towards human beings (n = 143 problems)

sense that it might react aggressively in a particular situation which it peacefully tolerated the day before.

- The attacks are often much more vicious than those associated with other aggression problems. The skin is usually broken, bites can be deep and leave scars, and owners often require medical attention or even hospitalization.
- During an attack, the dog doesn't act or look like its normal self. It has a strange look in its eyes which almost all owners notice. It may also show various offensive aggressive behaviors like erect ears and tail, hair standing up on the neck and back, and intense staring at the victim.
- Immediately after the attack, the dog may become very friendly, which people tend to interpret as apologetic behavior.
- The dog may show other behavior resembling dominant behavior directed towards another dog such as staring directly at family members until they look away or "standing over" them by putting its paws or chin on their lap or shoulders.
- Such dogs are often friendly and non-aggressive towards strangers, which is why veterinarians often get the impression that it's the people and not the dog which must have the problem. But this problem is only between the dog and members of its family. After a visitor has been in the home for a day or two, dominance problems usually begin to surface towards this newcomer as well.
- People who are very experienced in handling dogs like dog trainers and veterinarians

may never have any problems which these dogs. But this is not always the case: severely dominant-aggressive dogs which ultimately wind up in animal shelters may not be as impressed with an experienced handler's dominant behavior as most other dogs, and they may viciously attack shelter personnel for something as seemingly minor as trying to lead them in a direction in which they don't want to go.

- These dogs are not necessarily aggressive to all family members. It is almost always the case that the dog is much more frequently and/or seriously aggressive to some family members than others.
- Apart from the competitive or confrontational situations described earlier which are the hallmark of the dominance aggression problem, the dog is usually friendly to family members. While the dog is usually an obedient follower and begs for food and attention like any normal dog, it is almost invariably described by owners as being stubborn, strong-willed, and slow to obey. In some situations where the dog is highly motivated to do something else like play or fight with another dog, it tends to ignore the family members' commands entirely. All owners are conscious of the fact that a certain "respect" for them is lacking.
- Many owners learn to notice subtle signs that the dog is on the verge of becoming aggressive; for example, it may stiffen and give the owner a strange sideways look. Owners know then that it's time to stop whatever they are doing to avoid eliciting aggression.

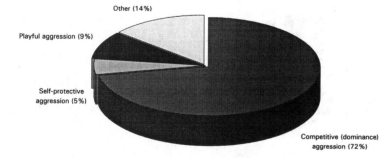

Figure 10.2: Relative frequency of different types of problems involving aggression towards human family members (n = 78 problems)

In general, family members learn to be extremely careful about what they do to or around the dog in certain key situations. And often the problem has existed for a long time before the counselor is contacted because owners have previously avoided being attacked by doing what the dog essentially demands in these situations.

- Physical punishment or severe scolding of such dogs for the threatening behavior is impossible, for it invariably elicits more intense aggression. In general, people usually try fighting force with force at a fairly late stage in the development of problem, and the dog's vicious reaction surprises them. Basically, owners are not prepared to really fight it out with the dog the way a police dog trainer might do. And they don't know how to physically fight with a dog without getting bitten. One or two bites convinces them to abandon this "get tough" approach entirely, perhaps leaving the dog's relatively high rank confirmed even more strongly than before.

- Family members usually admit to being afraid of the dog. They also say that this wasn't always the case, but things are different now that it sometimes becomes so viciously aggressive.

- Some of these dogs enforce arbitrary and sometimes rather bizarre rules concerning how family members must behave. For example, father is not allowed to open a certain drawer in the kitchen or mother is not allowed to get into bed unless father is already in it. These examples are from two cases where the people involved had to respect the dogs' rules to avoid being attacked. The woman who couldn't get into the bed before her husband was in it had to sleep on the sofa every time her husband worked the night shift in his job. In another case, a German shepherd would utter a low, throaty growl to "order" the family's teenage daughter to get up and open the back door of the house to let it out into the yard. Two serious bites for not obeying were enough to convince her that the dog meant business, and she always did as she was "told" thereafter.

- Not understanding the problem, and being shaken to the core by how vicious their otherwise affectionate and playful dog can suddenly become, owners often suspect that the dog is showing a form of insanity indicating that something serious must be physically wrong with its brain.

- In many of the most severe cases, treatment can only produce a limited improvement in the dog's behavior. Even with diligent owner application of the counselor's treatment recommendations, many dominant-aggressive dogs continue threatening and attacking family members and are ultimately far too dangerous to be kept in the family.

Pack theory

The predominant theoretical viewpoint among pet behavior problem counselors in the United States (Hart and Hart, 1985; Borchelt and Voith, 1986) and Great Britain (O'Farrell, 1992; Neville, 1991) is that dominant-aggressive dogs are behaving as if they regarded themselves as occupying one of the higher positions in the human family's version of a dog pack's dominance hierarchy by threatening or biting family members who (1) confront them over possession of some resource they value (e.g. bone, toy, sleeping place) or (2) behave towards them in a way which resembles a dominant dog's behavior towards a subdominant dog (e.g. touching them in certain ways, bending over them, threatening them). Presumably therefore the dog perceives its human family as it would a dog pack, is interpreting and reacting to human behavior in dog behavior terms, and is behaving in what would be a normal manner for one of a dog pack's more dominant adults when challenged by a subordinate dog. The leadership aspect of dominant dog (or wolf) behavior is also present in this model. For example, when enforcing arbitrary rules pertaining to family members behavior or pushing its way through doorways first, the dominant dog is presumably exercising its function as pack leader.

Why do some dogs behave this way? For one thing, most workers in the field suspect that dominant-aggressive dogs are predisposed for genetic reasons to display dominant behavior and strive to achieve one of the higher-ranking positions in their social group. In effect, as dogs go, they tend to be dominant or leader types which would probably end up becoming one of the "top dogs" in any dog pack. The facts that it is impossible to completely reform most of these dogs, the problem is much more prevalent in males than females, and a few of the most severely dominant-aggressive dogs cannot be safely managed even by the most highly-experienced dog handlers are consistent with this hypothesis.

Secondly, most counselors point out that certain types of owner behavior towards the dog play a major contributory role in the development of the problem. In particular, it is suspected that some kind of basic "misunderstanding" between the dog and family members is involved: the owner's positive, affection-motivated behavior towards the dog is misinterpreted by the dog as a confirmation of its high status. This in turn fuels the dog's dominant-aggressive tendencies and perhaps even creates the problem in some dogs. For example, family members feed the dog first before eating themselves. They allow the dog access to the furniture and family beds, the most coveted resting places which the most dominant members of any pack would reserve for their exclusive use. In their desire to be nice and fair to the dog, owners pet it and play with it on demand, essentially letting it control social interactions with them. They allow it to go through narrow passageways first and successfully defend its toys, bed, and food with aggressive growling. They let it win all tests of strength in tug-of-war games. They allow it to get more or less everything it wants by begging. They accept its pushiness and frequent disobedience without serious repercussions. They make a circle around it or step over it so as not to disturb it when it is lying in the way. And they may even routinely follow its lead during walks, letting it go where it wants, stopping when it stops, and just generally humbly tagging along behind. According to this perspective, it's no wonder that the dog gets the wrong idea and feels like

its one of the "top dogs" in the family rather than its lowest-ranking member.

Pack theory is probably an oversimplification of the view a genuinely scientific analysis of the problem might yield. Nevertheless, it has proven its practical utility by yielding the approaches to treatment discussed later in the chapter which are often very effective in reducing the severity of this very dangerous behavior problem.

Are owners responsible for the development of the problem?

To what extent are owners themselves responsible for the development of the dominance aggression problem? One popular view held by many veterinarians, breeders, dog trainers, animal shelter personnel, etc. is that by spoiling their dogs and treating them anthropomorphically in the ways described above, owners have essentially trained their dogs to be dominant aggressive. In effect, this view puts the burden of responsibility for the problem squarely on owners' shoulders.

But are the owners of dominant-aggressive dogs really responsible? Is their spoiling and anthropomorphizing really the root cause of the problem? Most pet behavior problem counselors don't think so. In the first place, pet behavior counselors know from their experience interviewing and observing the owners of hundreds of problem dogs of all types that most dogs which are spoiled and viewed anthropomorphically by their owners do not in fact turn out to be dominant aggressive. And secondly, pet behavior counselors also know from experience that the dominance aggression problem occurs in all kinds of family settings including those with sensible, experienced owners who seem to have done everything right as far as training their dog, being strict with it, making an effort to not spoil it, and trying to treat it like a dog and not a child is concerned.

Figure 10.3 presents some data from the survey of the owners of problem and non-problem dogs described in Chapter 3. It compares the answers to questions concerning spoiling and anthropomorphizing practices and attitudes of 55 owners of normal, non-problem dogs with those of the owners of the 31 dominant-aggressive dogs. Some differences between the two samples are indeed consistent with the popular view like: for example, the owners of dominant-aggressive dogs more frequently allow their dogs on furniture (20% higher) and share food with them from the table (12% higher). However, other differences like celebrating their birthday and confiding in them are less pronounced (8% and 9% higher respectively), and owners did not noticeably differ in terms of the answers to the six remaining questions. On balance therefore, the profiles of the answers given by the owners of these two drastically different types of dogs are surprisingly similar in light of the fact that it is here, for the dominance-aggression problem in particular, where the detrimental effects of owner spoiling practices and anthropomorphizing attitudes should be most clearly revealed.

This data therefore provides support for pet behavior problem counselors' impressions that while owner spoiling, permissiveness, anthro-

pomorphizing, etc. may well play a contributory role in the development or worsening of this problem in some families, it cannot be considered to be *the* cause of dominance aggression. As is the case of many other pet behavior problems, it is probably a matter here of certain kinds of inherently difficult animals turning into problem pets as a result of what are, statistically speaking, normal forms of owner treatment that need not and generally do not lead to the development of serious behavior problems.

Possible causal factors

The accompanying diagram presents a summary overview of the *causal factors* which are thought to play a role in some or all dominance-aggression cases as well as the various *treatment elements* which may be recommended by the counselor. Not all of the possible causal factors are relevant to each particular case. Rather, they should essentially be regarded as areas which the counselor must thoroughly explore during the consultation in

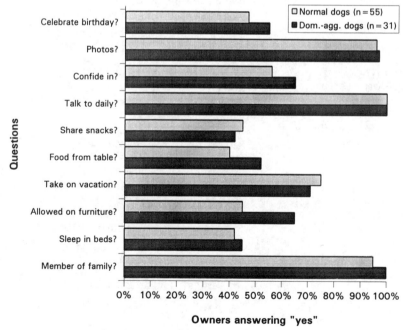

Figure 10.3: Comparison of anthropomorphizing and "spoiling" behavioral practices between the owners of dominant-aggressive and non-problem (normal) dogs

POSSIBLE CAUSAL FACTORS

Inherited predisposition
(suspected in serious cases)

Insufficient owner dominance
(i.e. owner-dog relationship problem)

Unintentional owner reinforcement
(rewarding pushy/aggressive behavior)

Erroneous owner beliefs
(e.g. normal for dogs to defend food/bed/toys;
treating dogs well means always giving them
what they want)

Hormonal influence
(much more frequent in males; castration
and progestin therapy sometimes effective;
problem sometimes worsens after
ovariohysterectomy)

Unintentional owner fostering
(dog inadvertently given privileges of
high-ranking pack member)

Lack of appropriate owner punishment
(e.g. of juvenile's aggressive defending of
food/objects)

DOMINANCE AGGRESSION

- Aggression directed towards family members in competitive situations or in
  response to what dog perceives as dominant behavior on the part of the owner

POSSIBLE TREATMENT ELEMENTS

**Increasing owner understanding
of problem**
(problem not pathophysiological; "pack
theory" explanation)

Increased owner authority
(getting tougher/being stricter advisable
if dog not potentially dangerous)

Change in care/maintenance conditions
(e.g. reduce dog's access to furniture/
bedrooms; no more bones/toys in home;
change bed/feeding location)

Specific training measures
(e.g. to improve obedience during walks)

Castration
(sometimes helpful in males; contraindicated
for females)

Physical aids
(e.g. muzzle, in-home leash)

Avoid confrontations
(e.g. avoid eliciting aggression; immediately
stop behaviors which elicit aggression)

**Changes in owner-dog interactive
ground rules**
(major changes in normal owner
behavior towards dog)

Correct owner misconceptions
(e.g. being nicer to dog will help; certain
treatment recommendations will make dog
more aggressive/are ethically questionable)

Systematic behavior therapy procedures
(e.g. to train dog to tolerate brushing
without growling/biting)

Medicaments
(progestins helpful in some cases)

order to develop a comprehensive understanding of why the dog is behaving in this way.

Inherited predisposition

As discussed above, it is often suspected that genetic factors are involved and the dog therefore would have probably turned out to be a problem in any normal family environment.

Hormonal influence

The three facts that (1) the problem develops much more commonly in males, (2) a dramatic worsening of dominance aggression problems is sometimes seen in bitches following ovariohysterectomy (O'Farrell and Peachy, 1990; Voith and Borchelt, 1982), and (3) castration and progestin treatment of males sometimes reduces the severity of the problem suggest that hormonal factors are in some way associated with the problem. However, the nature of this association is not clear, for castration alone is rarely an effective treatment. In many or most cases, it has no noticeable effect on the problem.

Insufficient owner dominance

Pet behavior problem counselors regard dominance aggression first and foremost as a symptom of an *owner-dog relationship problem* in which the owner's dominance is not sufficient to induce the dog to behave submissively in situations comparable to those in which dominance-related aggression occurs between dogs (i.e. where two dogs are directly competing over some resource or where one dog directs dominant behavior towards another).

Most dogs never aggressively challenge their owners in either type of situation. Owners can take the choicest bone away and physically manipulate the dog and threaten and punish it without eliciting the slightest hint of aggression. Essentially, in the normal family situation, owners' dominance position over the dog is supreme. To some extent, dominant-aggressive dogs are no different than other dogs: they are basically obedient, albeit often rather reluctant followers which would never dream of turning owners out of their beds or chasing them away from the dinner table so that they could eat the turkey themselves. But in the so-called confrontation situations in which aggression towards owners is common, such dogs behave as if they regarded owners as perhaps higher ranking but not so much so as to give them (the owners) the "right" to do what they are doing. Basically, as O'Farrell (1992) points out, such aggression usually has a defensive character in the sense that the dog is reacting aggressively towards what it perceives as a threat to its social position when owners go beyond what is appropriate to their higher, but not all that much higher position in the family "dominance hierarchy".

Unintentional owner fostering

Allowing dogs on the furniture, permitting them to sleep in family beds, petting them on demand, and letting them win in competitive and aggressive games do not necessarily lead to the development of serious behavior problems. Nevertheless, pet behavior problem counselors are convinced that such well-intentioned treatment fosters the development of the problem in animals which are predisposed towards becoming dominant-aggressive.

Unintentional owner reinforcement

Dominant-aggressive dogs are invariably described by their owners as strong-willed, stubborn, or even pushy. In most cases, the way owners have reacted to their dog's behavior in the past is partially responsible for the development of such undesirable traits. The dogs are often disobedient or slow to obey because owners have accepted refusals to obey or being slow to obey in the past without applying potent punitive consequence like scolding or hitting. Similarly, these dogs don't easily accept no for an answer and give up when they are begging for or demanding something by barking or tugging on the owner's sleeve because they have learned through experience that doing so will eventually pay off. Aggression itself has also often been rewarded in the past. The owner approaches the dog in possession of a bone, the dog growls menacingly, and the owner decides to leave the dog alone after all – thereby reinforcing the dog's aggressive reaction. The same can also be said for situations in which the dog bites and the owner simply accepts this without "fighting back" and abruptly stops whatever he/she did to provoke the aggression. Although such owner reactions are understandable and indeed necessary to avoid further injury, they nevertheless act to reinforce and strengthen the dog's tendency to behave aggressively in similar circumstances in the future.

Lack of appropriate owner punishment

In human relationships too, there are times when a youngster who has gone too far needs to be "put in his place" by being scolded, given additional work, or deprived of some rewarding privilege. Such appropriate types of punishment make for healthy parent-child relationships, and the parents who are lax in this regard may end up having unnecessary problems with their children. Similarly, pet behavior problem counselors are convinced that failing to punish young dogs for aggressively guarding objects or ignoring owner commands to stop undesirable behavior are potentially serious mistakes with dogs that are predisposed towards reacting in a dominant-aggressive way towards human beings. Although the most severely dominant-aggressive animals might have turned out to be dangerously aggressive even if punished when such problems first began to appear, not all dominant-aggressive dogs may be as highly motivated as this. Behavior specialists suspect therefore that at least some dominance-aggression problems are potentially preventable if owners were to make it clear to the young dog with effective punitive measures that such behavior simply will not be tolerated.

Erroneous owner beliefs

Owners who believe it is normal for their dog to growl and snap at them when they try to take food away from it or disturb it while it is sleeping are naturally inclined to accept this behavior without trying to counteract it. Similarly, many owners believe that ethical dog ownership means being polite or nice to their dog by giving it what it wants as much as possible, never ignoring it when it comes for attention, and petting it whenever it seems to need or want this. Basically, owners do many of the things they do to their animal – or refrain from doing certain things – for what they regard as good reasons which are, in reality, causing them to behave in ways which are exacerbating the problem or preventing them from taking much-needed corrective action.

Possible treatment elements

Here again, it is important to emphasize that in this and all other "possible treatment elements" sections in the book, the treatment elements may or may not be indicated in particular cases. Basically, the counselor must choose which of these possible treatment methods and approaches are most appropriate for each individual case.

Increasing owner understanding of problem

To allay owners suspicions that something may be physically wrong with the dog as well as lay the foundation for treatment recommendations, it is important to (1) point out that the problem is fairly common in dogs and generally not a sign of some medical disorder, (2) thoroughly explain the general nature of the problem, and (3) help owners understand that they must drastically alter the nature of the relationship they have with their dog to reduce the severity of the problem or eliminate it. It is also important in cases of dominance aggression to caution owners that in most cases, an improvement rather than complete elimination of the problem is the best that can be achieved, and that even after treatment, some dogs remain too dangerous to be kept as family pets. While Line and Voith (1986) reported an overall improvement rate due to a combination of behavioral treatment, castration, and progestin therapy of 88%, the problem was completely eliminated in only 1 of the 24 dominant-aggressive dogs in their sample.

Avoid confrontations

The first and most important recommendation given to the owners of dangerous or potentially dangerous dominant-aggressive dogs is to *temporarily avoid directly confronting the dog* as much as possible; that is, (1) refrain as much as possible from doing those things that often elicit aggression and (2) stop doing whatever one is doing when the dog starts behaving in a threatening manner. The importance of making it clear to owners that it is too dangerous for them to confront the dog directly cannot be overemphasized. During the consultation, owners may state that they are considering getting really tough with the dog and "beating it until it learns who's boss" as has been recommended to them by other owners or dog trainers. Even owners who have been seriously bitten while trying to punish their dog are often advised by others that their only hope for coping with the problem is to get even tougher with the dog when it threatens them again. In this connection, the counselor must convince the client that trying to show the dog who's boss or teach it a lesson in response to its threatening behavior will probably increase its aggression and could well precipitate an even more vicious attack.

Increased owner authority

The one exception to the above rule of avoiding confrontations is when the dog growls at the owner but never bites and always stops growling when scolded. In some of these cases, it can be assumed that it is safe for the owner to confront the dog directly by scolding or otherwise punishing the dog's threats as one should do with a puppy in this situation. Therefore, with some mildly dominant-aggressive dogs, advising the owner to stand up to the dog and "show it who's boss" is appropriate and may improve the problem or eliminate it. However, if it is suspected for any reason that the dog might escalate its aggression when confronted in this way, this get-tough approach is potentially very dangerous and essentially the worst advice that any behavior counselor can give to a client.

Changes in owner-dog interactive ground rules

Several recommendations are usually given to owners for altering their normal, everyday behavior towards their dog in order to modify the nature of the social relationship they have with it in ways which will ultimately lower the dog's tendency to react aggressively in problem situations. For example, the owner should make the dog follow a command to get everything it wants, never reward its begging or demanding behavior, completely ignore it whenever it comes to them for petting or attention, make it get up and move whenever it is lying in the way, and stop playing competitive or aggressive games with it. Seeing as how many or most owners find it difficult and unpleasant to treat their dog in this way, they may only comply with treatment recommendations if the logic of doing so has been thoroughly explained to them and they understand why each individual recommendation is helpful. They must understand, for example, that one is promoting submissive behavioral tendencies by making the dog follow commands to get everything it wants, dramatically demonstrating one's own position of dominance by controlling the time and duration of petting and other forms of social contact, and making the dog's more submission position clear to it by always insisting it move out of the way and not giving in to its requests or demands.

It is also important to prepare owners for how their dog might react to such new interactive ground rules: many dogs react strongly to them and act somewhat shocked, confused, or even withdrawn or depressed for a couple of days. In this connection, owners must be assured that these are only temporary reactions and that dogs do not find being treated this way nearly as aversive or traumatic as one might assume.

Change in care/maintenance conditions

A related strategy for essentially reducing the dog's dominance-related status in the family is to make certain key changes in the conditions under which it is kept or cared for. No longer allowing it on the furniture or in the family bedrooms is one example. Another is not to let it have any bones or toys in the house which it might be inclined to try and defend against family members. Sometimes such changes are advisable for more practical, safety-related reasons. Simply moving a dog's bed or feeding place to a more out-of-the-way place in the home may be a sensible way for family members to avoid confrontations with a dog that often becomes aggressive when lying in its bed or eating.

Correct owner misconceptions

One common owner misconception is that the dog's aggression is a sign that it is dissatisfied with something in its present life situation or not getting something it needs. This leads owners to try and cope with the problem by making a deliberate effort to be nicer and more attentive to the dog, which makes the problem worse and not better. A related misconception is that if they follow the treatment recommendations and start, for example, ignoring the dog when it comes for attention, turning it off the sofa, or locking it out of the bedroom, that the dog will become frustrated and dissatisfied and therefore perhaps even more aggressive. Some owners also believe that it is ethically questionable to treat dogs the way the counselor is suggesting. In answer to this, the counselor can argue that while treating a child this way would be ethically questionable, dogs do not in fact suffer under it and if anything usually seem noticeably more contented under the new regime than under the old one. It is as if underneath it all they expect this kind of treatment from their owners perhaps because it resembles the kind of treatment they would receive from higher-ranking members of a dog pack.

Specific training measures

Many dominant-aggressive dogs make problems during walks by being slow to come when called, ignoring other commands, or stubbornly straining on the leash. It is therefore sometimes appropriate to recommend measures to correct these minor problems as well. One might, for example, teach owners how to use food rewards and walking away to strengthen the dog's tendency to come when called (Chapter 18), or recommend that they carry out certain exercises like walking quickly and often changing directions suddenly to train the dog to be more of a follower and less of a leader when walking on the leash.

Systematic behavior therapy procedures

In some cases, it may be necessary for the counselor to work out systematic behavior therapy procedures for *desensitizing* animals to stimuli which normally elicit aggression while *counterconditioning* them to exhibit other, more acceptable behavior in such situations. Most common is when a long-haired dog which must be brushed daily reacts aggressively to brushing. An example of such a procedure is given in the sample recommendations box at the end of this section. The first step is to determine exactly how and where on the body the animal will tolerate being touched with a brush without growling. It is then frequently rewarded with tidbits every time this is done and it doesn't growl. Practicing in the context of several brief daily training sessions, the dog continues to be rewarded every time it is first touched lightly with the brush, then more firmly, then brushed with one stroke, two strokes, four, eight, etc. – in effect, gradually approaching the normal brushing situation over a period of several days or weeks.

Castration

Although there is no research evidence to support this, Borchelt and Voith (1986) and many other workers in the field are of the opinion that castration of dominant-aggressive males can sometimes help to reduce the aggressiveness. Given the gravity of the problem, the potential danger to family members, and the fact that castration has few serious side effects, it is probably wise to recommend this along with the behavior-oriented treatment measures which all behavior specialists agree are the key to treating this problem. Spaying is, however, contraindicated for dominant-aggressive females because clinical experience and survey results indicate that it can greatly increase this form of aggression in some bitches (Borchelt and Voith, 1986; O'Farrell and Peachy, 1990).

Medicaments

Many authors report that progestin therapy can sometimes reduce dominance aggression (Borchelt and Voith, 1986; O'Farrell, 1992). However, any effects are short-lived and accordingly this kind of drug therapy is usually recommended only as means of temporarily reducing aggression while corrective behavioral treatment measures are first applied. (See the "drug therapy" subsection in Chapter 8 for side effects and other important drug-related information.)

Physical aids

Finally, there are cases in which it is appropriate to recommend muzzling the dog in certain situations when family members are endangered and there is no way for them to avoid doing things which elicit aggression. Similarly, when a dog becomes dangerous when ordered or pushed off furniture, out of rooms, etc., it can sometimes be helpful to have it wear a short leash in the home which can be picked up by owners and used to physically move or control the dog at any time. O'Farrell (1992) suggests that this might help reduce the dog's aggressiveness for psychological reasons as well by making the dog "feel less dominant".

Sample recommendations box

The accompanying box presents a collection of sample recommendations. While some of them such as avoiding confrontation situations and ignoring the dog when it comes for attention are given in every serious case, others like not allowing dogs to have toys in the home or having some family members completely ignore the dog are only appropriate in some cases. Accordingly, these sample recommendation boxes which are presented throughout the book should *not* be regarded as a list of treatment re-

commendations which should be given in every case. Rather they are a list of *possible* treatment recommendations which may or may not be helpful or indicated. In effect, the specific treatment measures counselors recommend to clients are usually a selected subset of between 6 and 10 of the sample recommendations in the box plus one, two, or even more newly-designed, non-standard recommendations which are tailored to the specific problems, owners, animal, and living circumstances of the particular case. In writing a letter to clients several days after the consultation to summarize the various recommendations, I also often rewrite, qualify, or add to the standard recommendations in the box so as to make them apply more directly, personally, and effectively to the particular client's case. Basically then, the sample recommendation boxes provided throughout the book should be regarded as starting points which are intended to help the counselor work out the optimum treatment approach which is appropriate in each individual case.

Owners should continue following these recommendations as long as the dog is still growling. If and when the day comes when the dog stops growling and is as submissive, cooperative, and obedient as most other dogs, these recommendations can be gradually relaxed. But if the problem persists in spite of the new treatment regime – as happens in almost all serious cases – the owner must understand that the new relationship with the dog must always remain much like it is during treatment or the problem will worsen again. As O'Farrell (1991) points out, the dominance-aggression problem can be likened to alcoholism in humans in the sense that it can often be controlled but never really cured.

Maximizing compliance

The treatment approach outlined in the sample recommendations box is highly effective with many dogs. But there are often problems as far owner compliance with some of the recommendations is concerned. Essentially, it's one thing to advise owners to ignore their dog whenever it comes to them for petting or atten-

SAMPLE RECOMMENDATIONS

Dominance aggression towards family members

Scenario A: *very mild cases where dog growls but is not potentially dangerous*

- "Show the dog who's boss" whenever it growls at you by scolding or otherwise punishing it severely enough to immediately suppress the growling.

- Regular obedience training sessions, being more strict with the dog in general, and making sure never to reward the dog for pushy or demanding behavior by giving it what it wants are to be recommended.

Scenario B: *dog has bitten family members or seems potentially dangerous*

- Temporarily avoid all aggressive confrontations by avoiding doing things which often elicit aggression and/or by stopping whatever you are doing if the dog starts to become aggressive.

- Totally ignore the dog whenever it comes to you for attention, contact, to be petted, to beg for food, etc. without having been called.

- Never give the dog what it wants when it begs for or demands something.

- "Nothing in life is free": dog must follow a command like "sit, "down", "come", or "stay" before you give it something it wants (e.g. its dinner, petting, going in or out of the house, having its leash put on).

- Pet the dog only briefly as a reward for following commands. No more fondling.

- Dog should not be allowed on the furniture or in the family bedrooms.

- Whenever the dog is sitting or lying in the way, make it move to let you pass by.

- Don't let it have toys, chews, or bones in the home.

- Don't enthusiastically greet the dog when you come home. Act cool and disinterested while you "tolerate" its greeting.

- Avoid playing all competitive, aggressive, or test-of-strength games with the dog. Or better yet, don't play with it at all. Instead, take it to a park twice a day where it can play as long as it likes with other dogs.

- Be more strict with the dog in all situations where it accepts this without growling.

- Walk the dog on a leash for at least 30 min. a day. Change speeds and directions frequently without warning, pulling it firmly this way and that during the process if it accepts this without becoming even mildly aggressive.

- Train the dog to come more quickly when called when it is off the leash outside by rewarding it with food tidbits every time it comes when called and/or by turning and walking away without looking back or waiting for it if it doesn't come at this time.

- Don't let the dog push in front and go through doorways ahead of you. Train it to wait until you start through the doorway first.

- Family members who have no problems with the dog should temporarily ignore it entirely and not feed, pet, talk to, or play with it at all.

Example behavior therapy method for training a dog to tolerate brushing without becoming aggressive:

1. Use the dog's favorite tidbits to train it to come, sit, lie down, and stay on command in the situation in which it is to be brushed. Give the dog no food rewards whatsoever outside of these training sessions.

2. Determine how far you can go when brushing it or touching it with the brush without eliciting aggression: in effect, determine what specifically the dog will tolerate without growling and what it won't (e.g. very lightly brushing with 3-4 strokes is safe, but longer or harder than that isn't).

3. In several brief practice sessions spaced throughout the day, reward the dog for quietly sitting or standing in this brushing situation *without growling* when you brush or touch it in the way that it normally tolerates without growling.

4. As soon as the dog is used to playing this "game", start very gradually going a little beyond the limit of what it normally tolerates without growling (e.g. try brushing it slightly longer or harder than normal).

5. As soon as it has learned to tolerate this too without growling, change the rules again so that it must tolerate slightly longer and harder brushing to earn a reward.

6. If the dog growls at any stage during this procedure, don't give it a tidbit; wait a few minutes, and then resume the training at an earlier stage (e.g. with much lighter brushing). Remain at this level for quite awhile until it is time to start gradually increasing the number/pressure of brush strokes again – but this time increase the duration/intensity of the brushing much more slowly and gradually than you did before.

---

tion, but whether the owner will really do that consistently is quite another. Owners may not be entirely convinced that this is the best approach, they may not have enough self-discipline, they may resent having to go to so much trouble for the dog, or they may not want to give up the pleasures of allowing the dog in their bed, letting it up on the furniture, or petting in on demand. With owners who don't really want to be bothered or don't have the necessary self-discipline to carry out any kind of treatment which requires them to change their behavior in major ways, there is not much the counselor can do. But with owners who are well-motivated and theoretically able to carry out the treatment, the counselor's failure to convince them to carry it out diligently is disturbing.

The pack theory approach is appealing to owners. They accept it immediately and although it may be obvious by their mixed facial expressions that they have reservations about whether they can (or should) follow a few of the more extreme treatment recommendations, they nevertheless seem convinced that in general the nature of the problem is pretty much as the counselor explained and that the recommended treatment makes good, logical sense. But the problem is that owners often have difficulties in long maintaining the kind of competitive orientation towards the animal required by this treatment approach for any length of time. Basically, they feel like *parents* to their dog, not rivals. And so they are not very comfortable ignoring its friendly overtures, ordering or shoving it to the side whenever it's lying in the way, and just generally treating it in what feels to them to be a rather heartless, bullying, selfish way.

How can compliance be improved with these owners? There are cases in which it may be possible to improve compliance by modifying the explanation owners are given concerning the logic behind the treatment recommendations. The following paragraphs will discuss this modified conceptual "package" for what are basically the same set of recommendations. It is offered here not as necessarily closer to the truth or otherwise superior to explanations given by most other pet behavior problem counselors, but rather as an alternative approach which might help to improve compliance with some types of owners.

The classical approach is to explain to owners that they must start behaving more like the alpha dog or pack leader in the direct competition-over-dominance sense. In comparison, the alternative approach argues that treatment recommendations function to alter the owner's relationship to the dog in a way which makes it more resemble the kinds of adult-to-juvenile relationships a young dog would have with adult pack members in which dominance is never really an issue. Thus, it's not a question of promoting alpha dog behavior towards an aspiring beta dog on the part of the owner, but rather of promoting owner behavior resembling that which an adult dog might display towards a pack juvenile. In effect, it is explained to owners that the treatment is effective because it essentially reduces the dog's tendency to perceive family members as "equals" while strengthening its tendency to perceive and behave towards them as young juveniles in a dog pack might perceive and behave towards adult pack members.

This alternative view opens up new perspectives for convincing owners to treat their dogs in the unnatural, somewhat unpleasant way recommended. The following are some suggestions of how this view of the function of treatment recommendations could be presented to owners.

- *Most dogs always behave in some respects like perpetual puppies or juveniles towards the members of their family in the sense that they never think of threatening them in situations where they might threaten other dogs to show their dominance over them or to establish their rights to have certain things like toys or bones.*
- *Dogs which show the dominance-aggression problem, however, seem a little confused as to how to behave towards family members in the sense that in some situations they react towards them not as vastly superior adults whom they would never dream of challenging or biting but rather more like equals or the other dogs that they play with in the park. As result, they threaten or perhaps even bite them in the types of situations in which this kind of aggression often occurs between dogs.*
- *To successfully treat this problem it will therefore be necessary for you to change the nature of the relationship you have with your dog by having you behave more like an adult dog behaves towards young immature dogs in its pack and by having you avoid doing certain kinds of things that might encourage the dog to treat you more or less like its equal.*
- *The problem is not your fault. Most owners treat their dogs exactly like you do. But with some dogs, this normal kind of treatment creates problems. And these kinds of dogs need to have a more adult-to-youngster rather than friend-to-friend relationship with their people. Essentially, for the time being you will not be able to relax and do what comes naturally with your dog the way most other people do. For you happen to have a dog which is inclined to react to this normal kind of treatment by regarding and treating you more like a playmate or equal whom it competes with or tries to dominate in certain situations and less like a vastly superior pack member whom it would never think of threatening.*
- *Although you may find some of the recommendations harsh and unpleasant to follow, it helps at such times to remember that by doing things like not responding to your dogs social initiatives, or insisting that it move out of the way when you walk by, you are essentially imitating normal adult dog behavior towards young pack members and, hopefully, gradually changing the way the dog views you in the process.*

Comparing the two approaches to justifying treatment recommendations

In explaining both the general nature of the problem and the logic of the various treatment recommendations, the classical approach takes *interactions between adult dogs* as a model. Fundamentally, it is based on the same underlying assumptions as the brutal approach of some dog trainers who "hang" the dog by its leash to "break its spirit" and believe that "weak owners" are the cause of dominance aggression problems. Indeed, the classical approach is described as by most writers as *indirect* precisely because it is conceptualized as being a roundabout way of pursuing the same domination goal. The primary reason commonly given for using this indirect approach is not that it is more enlightened or effective, but rather that it is safer. In short, it is conceptualized as a substitute for the kind of "get tough" treatment which would be recommended by the counselor if it were safe to confront the dog more directly.

Instead of presenting recommendations to owners as a safe way of showing their dog who's boss, the alternative approach considered above is basically advising owners to act more like the dog's parent and less like its playmate. Psychologically speaking, the difference in the effect the two approaches produce on some owners could therefore be potentially quite significant. In conceptualizing the problem in adult-to-adult, dominance-submission terms, the classical approach tries to make owners aware of a competitive dimension that exists in their relationship with the dog. Thinking of the many test-of-wills situations they have experienced like, for example, when trying to get the dog to stop doing something, come when it's called, or surrender an object it has found while on a walk, owners are prepared to accept this competitive dimension viewpoint on principle. They are also prepared to accept the fact that some kind of dominance or leadership dimension is involved, for they know that their dog is more stubborn, strong-willed, and harder for them to control than other dogs in the neighborhood.

The problem lies, however, in applying the recommendations with the kind of consistency required. While owners have little difficulty in insisting the dog follow commands before they give it what it wants, they find it exceedingly difficult to maintain for days and weeks the kind of competitive orientation towards the dog which the treatment recommendations require. Not only does ignoring the dog every time it comes seeking attention seem cruel to them, but seeing this kind of situation competitively and feeling competitive enough themselves at this time to follow the recommendation consistently does not come easily. Perhaps part of the reason for this difficulty is the dog's motivation in this situation, which the owner senses is not at all competitive. Rather, it is quite clearly the type of affectionate, contact-seeking behavior that makes the owner feel liked or even loved by the dog. The same is also true with some of the other of the recommendations. Although the owner is asked to compete with the dog for who goes through doors first, the dog shows no signs that it perceives the situation as competitive. It just seems to be eager to get outside – behavior which owners view positively and not negatively.

The alternative approach has the potential of overcoming at least some of these psychological or emotional obstacles to compliance for several reasons. Firstly, it emphasizes competitiveness only over the issue of leadership. Feeling that they lack the respect of their dog and easy leadership capability that other owners have, owners see the need for this and are quite willing to diligently work on improving it.

Secondly, the alternative view is consistent with many attitudes and beliefs the owners already hold about their dog. It is indeed like a puppy or juvenile in many respects, and the relationship they have with it is indeed like that between adult and offspring, be it between adult dog and puppy or human parent and child. Owners are prepared to accept the classical model based on a "struggle for dominance between adults" to a certain extent, and in certain limited kinds of situations. But it is often not genuinely convincing, for the dog just doesn't act the part. Neither in its aggression nor in its more friendly behavior can one detect the kind of coherent strategy to achieve and maintain a maximally high position of dominance in the family that the model implies. It is indeed seldom that the dog acts overtly competitive or like it is in some sense trying to control the household. In becoming aggressive, it appears to be simply reacting defensively in response to something owners are doing to it.

Thirdly, this alternative approach may enhance compliance with some owners because it provides a more ethically acceptable rationale for the "necessary evils" aspects of treatment such as ignoring the dog whenever it comes to be petted. Essentially, this alternative approach tries to persuade owners to in some sense be better and more readily understandable (from the dog's viewpoint) parents rather than act in a way which might seem or feel more selfish by trying to teach the dog the lesson that they are the "top dogs" in the family. Thus, the model has the potential of engaging the parents in owners and exploiting their ability to act unselfishly in the interests of bettering their relationship with their child-like pet.

In practice, even the owners of these dominant-aggressive dogs can continue do what most owners do and treat their dogs like human children in many respects. But the treatment must be more that which is fitting for an older rather than younger human child – for example, by not lavishing so much attention and close physical contact on it, by being somewhat more distant and not showing so much interest in it, by not allowing it in their lap or bed, and by placing various behavioral requirements on it like rewards and privileges must be "earned" with obedience. By explaining the treatment in a way which emphasizes parallels between adult dogs' behavior towards young pack members on the one hand, and human parental behavior towards a somewhat older child on the other, treatment recommendations may therefore turn out to be less difficult to accept and follow than with the classical approach, which encourages owners to view their dogs as competitors which must either be forcefully put in their place or taught a similar less in a more subtle, psychologically sophisticated way. In effect, this new treatment perspective puts treatment recommendations in a new light which might help to convince some owners that the treatment is not so inhuman after all.

References

Borchelt, P.L., and Voith, V.L. (1982): Diagnosis and treatment of dominance aggression in dogs. *Veterinary Clinics of North America: Small Animal Practice* **12**, 655–664.

Borchelt, P.L., and Voith, V.L. (1986): Dominance aggression in dogs. *Compendium on Continuing Education for the Practicing Veterinarian* **8**, 36–44.

Hart, B.L., and Hart, L.A. (1985): *Canine and Feline Behavioral Therapy*. Philadelphia: Lea & Febiger.

Neville, P. (1991): *Do Dogs Need Shrinks?* London, Sidgwick & Jackson Ltd.

O'Farrell, V. and Peachy, E. (1990): Behavioural effects of ovariohysterectomy on bitches. *Journal of Small Animal Practice* **31**, 595–598.

O'Farrell V. (1992): *Manual of Canine Behaviour*. Shurdington, Cheltenham, Gloucestershire, UK, British Small Animal Veterinary Association.

11 Defensive Aggression Towards Family Members

This chapter deals with several forms of defensive aggression in which the dog is assumed to be responding to what it perceives as immediate and direct threats to its health and well-being – or that of its young offspring – posed by human family members. This includes two forms of *self-protective aggression* – aggression elicited by aversive stimuli and so-called fear aggression – *parental aggression*, and the often somewhat puzzling problem of aggression towards family babies and toddlers.

Pain or punishment-elicited aggression

As laboratory experiments with rats and pigeons have demonstrated, the administration of intense aversive stimuli can be a powerful elicitor of aggression even in relatively non-aggressive species. In one well-known "pain-elicited aggression" experiment, pigeons given painful electric shocks showed a tendency to attack others pigeon or even crude pigeon models that were in the cage with them.

It is not surprising therefore that a dog which has never previously been aggressive might bite a family member who is medicating a wound or giving it a painful beating. However, the fact that family dogs may tolerate such medication procedures or painful mistreatment without fighting back is a reminder that even such seemingly simple and straightforward problems emerge from the complex social behavioral dynamics of the interspecific family unit: the aggressive behavioral reactions of companion animals always depends at least in part on the nature of their social relationship with human family members.

Possible causal factors

Aversive stimuli

The nature and intensity of the eliciting stimuli themselves are relevant in the most direct way to understanding the problem. They are usually highly aversive to the animals and there is no mystery in animals' defensive aggressive reactions to them. By in large, owners are very understanding in such situations. They don't blame the dog for trying to defend itself against something painful or extremely unpleasant. As a result, they may simply refrain from punishing the dog this severely again or apply painful medical procedures more gently in future.

Past experience with similar aversive stimuli

Of course, pain- or punishment-elicited aggression which is out of proportion to the intensity of the aversive stimulus being applied can also be seen animals which have been experienced great pain or intense fear in similar situations in the past. In effect, such cases of pain- or punishment-elicited aggression can therefore be a form of conditioned, fear-mediated aggression, which will be discussed in the next major section.

Insufficient owner dominance

The nature of the dog's relationship with owners can have a great deal to do with determining its tendencies to bite or not bite in the kinds of defensive situations being considered. Many dominant-aggressive dogs react aggressively to having their bodies touched or manipulated in certain ways, being scolded, or being physically punished. And dogs which have shown tendencies towards dominant behavior without serious aggression in the past (e.g.

POSSIBLE CAUSAL FACTORS

Aversive stimuli
(e.g. punishment; painful medical treatment)

Insufficient owner dominance
(mild owner/dog dominance problem as contributing factor)

Lack of appropriate training
(e.g. growling/biting not punished in past)

Past experience with similar aversive stimuli
(i.e. conditioned hypersensitivity/fear due to past exposure to aversive stimuli)

Unintentional owner reinforcement
(owner's termination of aversive stimulus reinforces dog's aggressive behavior; calming/reassuring aggressive dog reinforces aggression)

PAIN-/PUNISHMENT-ELICITED AGGRESSION

- Growling at and/or biting family members as a defensive response to physical punishment or painful stimuli.

POSSIBLE TREATMENT ELEMENTS

Avoid problem situations
(abandon punishment method or punish with aversive sound rather than hitting)

Systematic behavior therapy methods
(e.g. food rewards to countercondition non-aggressive behavior in medication situation)

Standard obedience training
(increases owner control; teaches owner how to train animal)

Drugs
(analgesic, tranquilizer)

Cessation of ineffective treatment measures
(stop punishing aggression; stop soothing/reassuring/petting dog in response to aggression)

Increase owner authority/dominance
(e.g. be more strict with dog; dominance-increasing recommendations from Chapter 10)

Physical aids
(e.g. muzzle during medical treatment)

growling to defend food bowl or while grudgingly allowing itself to be pushed off the sofa) may be more prone to showing pain- or punishment-elicited aggression than other dogs. Indeed, in dogs where the aggressive reaction is out of proportion to the pain and where no conditioned fear seems to be involved, the problem is probably best regarded as yet another symptom of a dominance-related problem in the relationship between dog and owner.

Unintentional owner reinforcement

When the owner describes exactly what happens in situations in which a dog is being medicated on a daily basis, for example, it often becomes clear that the owner has been reacting in ways which are inadvertently training the dog to become increasingly aggressive with each passing session. One common scenario is that the owner is doing something like applying an ointment inside of the dog's ear, which the dog tolerates for a few seconds and then turns and growls or snaps at the owner's hand. Often the owner's response – essentially humanely motivated out of a concern that the snapping is an indication of just how painful the procedure feels to the dog – may be to immediately stop applying the medication and instead pet and reassure the dog until it seems relaxed again so that the medication process can be resumed. Essentially, from the dog's perspective, the growling and snapping pay off: its aggression is being consistently rewarded both by the owner's stopping of the unpleasant treatment and by his/her petting and sympathetic attention.

The same effect can operate with owner punishment as well. When the intensity of the owner's punishment increases above a certain threshold, the dog may stop reacting submissively and start defending itself with aggressive growling and snapping. This in turn may cause the owner to immediately stop, which essentially rewards the dog's aggression and would therefore be expected to make it more likely to react similarly in future when punished in this way. Additionally, the fact that learning effects tend always to generalize to other similar situations would lead to the related prediction that the threshold intensity which makes the difference between non-aggressive submission and aggressive self-defense might well decrease over time as well. In effect, if the dog learns that snapping stops owner punishment at a time when the owner punished the dog too severely, it may be inclined to use this behavioral strategy later in situations involving milder forms of punishment which it formerly tolerated without problems.

Lack of appropriate training

Most owners scold or physically punish dogs from puppy age onwards for aggressive growling or snapping at human beings. However, some are surprisingly tolerant of such reactions because either they view them as normal dog behavior or they may simply not take these incidents very seriously. Essentially, when questioning owners, it is worth exploring the owners' attitude towards minor aggression and what their approach has been in the past to control it. For some dogs threaten and bite human beings as easily as they do because owners have been too lax about counteracting aggressive behavior in ways which produce strong and lasting inhibition.

Possible treatment elements

Avoid problem situations

For punishment-elicited aggression, either the punishment method should be abandoned or another type of punishing stimulus should be administered which does not elicit aggression towards the owner. A blast from a compressed air horn or loudly shaking a metal can containing a few coins, for example, might frighten the dog without making it aggressive.

Most writers in the pet problem field agree with Hart and Hart (1985) in assuming that the related advantage of using something like a loud sound as a punisher is that it more anonymous than scolding or hitting the dog – that is, the dog doesn't perceive it as stemming directly from the owner. Accordingly, it is often recommended that the owner try to discretely administer the sound so that the dog isn't sure where it is coming from. However, other factors besides whether or not the dog sees the aversive stimulus being delivered by the owner may be involved here. In the first place, a loud sound may be highly aversive but not painful, and animals' responses to fear-arousing stimuli may be less likely to evoke aggression in certain situations than those producing pain or physical discomfort. A second major factor why fear-eliciting auditory stimuli may fail to elicit an aggressive response is the simple lack of owner aggression. Hitting a dog with the hand, its leash, or a rolled-up newspaper is in fact a highly aggressive act which is invariably accompanied by correspondingly aggressive owner facial expressions, body postures, and vocalizations. Although sounding a compressed air device or shaking a can of coins can also be done in an aggressive way, the combination of the strange sound and the owner's comparatively less aggressive behavior may not be perceived by the dog as the type of "attack" which requires an aggressive response.

One practical implication of this discussion: when applying such alternative types of punishers to dogs that tend to react aggressively to punishment, the owner should be advised to behave non-aggressively by, for example, smiling and attending to something else than glaring sternly at the dog.

Cessation of ineffective treatment methods

Punishing an animal more harshly for reacting aggressively to punishment may sometimes effectively suppress the aggression. But it is a risky tactic. More severe punishment may elicit more intense aggression or it may make the animal fearful of the owner – a potentially serious behavior problem in its own right (Chapter 15). Therefore, when a dog is reacting aggressively to punishment, it is usually more sensible to place more emphasis on behavioral training methods based on rewards rather than simply increasing the intensity of the punishing stimulus. Similarly, while punishing an animal for reacting aggressively to a painful, unpleasant, or fear-eliciting medical treatment may be effective in some cases, if such punishment must be more intense than mild scolding to suppress the aggression, it is better to use an alternative reward-based method like the one described below to accomplish the same objective of teaching the dog to peacefully tolerate the medical procedure.

Cessation of unintentional reinforcement for aggressive behavior is a potentially important treatment element as well. Although one cannot and should not avoid reinforcing the dog by stopping the aversive stimulation when it growls or snaps, one can easily avoid reinforcing it with well-intentioned soothing/reassuring measures like petting. Almost all owners make this mistake, probably because this strategy seems to work well in the situation itself – which of course reinforces the owners for employing it. But in the long run, soothing and calming an aggressive dog is likely to increase rather than decrease its tendency to become aggressive in similar situations in the future.

Systematic behavior therapy methods

Food rewards can often be effectively used to countercondition non-aggressive behavior during the time when an animal must endure some extended unpleasant treatment like being medicated or having its ears cleaned. The simple behavior therapy procedure for gradually training a dominant-aggressive dog to tolerate brushing discussed in Chapter 10 can be easily adapted to this situation. Here, the dog is both (1) gradually *desensitized* to versions of the aversive stimulus applied that are too mild to evoke aggression and (2) consistently rewarded for responding with non-aggressive behavior each time the aversive stimulus is presented. The intensity of the aversive stimulus is then very gradually increased over a number of days or weeks until the dog can be medicated or handled normally.

Increasing owner authority/dominance

Some dogs tolerate medical treatment and physical manipulation from certain people (e.g. veterinarians who behave in a confident, dominant manner) but not from others – like their owners, for whom a certain amount of respect may be lacking. When questioning of the owners reveals that, for example, dogs growl at them in other situations or are often disobedient or slow to obey, giving owners some of the dominance-increasing instructions discussed in the previous chapter may help. If this kind of dominance-related problem is minor and basically the fault of the owner being too lax in a variety of situations, simply advising owners to be more strict with dogs in insisting that they follow commands including those to stopping barking or growling when told to do so can often quickly increase the dog's dominance-related respect for its owner and, hence, lower its tendency to resist owner touching, handling, etc. with aggression.

Standard obedience training

This is another respect-increasing measure which is often recommended to the owners of dogs which, in addition to reacting aggressi-

SAMPLE RECOMMENDATIONS

Pain- or punishment-elicited aggression

Scenario A: *overly severe punishment is eliciting self-protective aggression in a basically non-aggressive dog*
1. Stop punishing the dog or at least stop punishing it so severely. Scolding which is severe enough to produce a submissive or very mild startle/fear response in the dog is sufficient to effectively punish undesirable behavior.
2. Punishing the dog for threatening or biting is not to be recommended, for it is likely to make the dog even more aggressive.
3. Instead of punishing the dog, use food rewards to train the dog to behave acceptably in problem situations using the following method:
(Recommend an appropriate reward-based training method)

Scenario B: *painful medical treatment is eliciting self-protective aggression in a basically non-aggressive dog*
(If some very painful medical treatment is involved which the dog can probably never be taught to tolerate without becoming aggressive, it should simply be muzzled during the treatment procedure. If, however, an unpleasant but not really so painful medical treatment is involved, the dog can be trained to react non-aggressively in this situation using some version of the method described in the sample recommendation box in Chapter 10 for teaching a dominant-aggressive dog to peacefully tolerate brushing).

Scenario C: *aggression is symptomatic of lack of appropriate training (i.e. to inhibit aggression) or a very mild dominance problem*
1. Stop hitting the dog or severely punishing it other ways which cause it to bite. However, in situations in which you are sure you can do so safely without running the risk of being bitten, counteract the dog's growling with scolding or some other mild form of punishment (e.g. leash correction, aversive sound) that is strong enough to suppress the threatening behavior.
2. Be much more strict with the dog in all situations in which it accepts this without becoming aggressive.
3. Use the dog's favorite food rewards to train it to come, sit, lie down, and stay on command.
4. "Nothing in life is free": Dog must follow a command like "sit", "down", "come", or "stay" before you give it something it wants (e.g. its dinner, petting, going in or out of the house, having its leash put on, etc.).
5. The dog should *never* be allowed to get what it wants (e.g. food, petting, playing, attention) when it shows begging or pushy, demanding behavior of any kind like, for example, barking, staring at you, whining, jumping up on you, or nudging, licking, or scratching you.

Scenario D: *punishment-elicited aggression is a symptom of moderate to severe dominance aggression*
(Recommend treating the dominance aggression problem as discussed in Chapter 10 and perhaps also recommend a reward-based method to improve the dog's behavior in situations in which it is now being punished).

vely to medication or punishment, are disobedient or difficult to control in other situations.

Physical aids

Some owners find that they can only medically treat their dog when it is wearing a muzzle. Where this type of highly situation-specific self-protective aggression is the only real problem owners have with their dog, this simple and direct approach may be all that is really needed. It is often recommended to owners who have not considered it before or have always refrained from taking this step because they feared it might in some way psychologically harm the dog. When such erroneous beliefs are involved, one should take plenty of time to address owners' fears and discuss the advantages of muzzling, its minor drawbacks, and how one should go about accustoming the animal to wearing one.

Drugs

Where painful medical treatment or some other kind of unpleasant physical procedure which causes an animal to become highly fearful is involved, some analgesic or tranquilizing medicament may be appropriate either as a temporary adjunct to a behavior therapy method or as a prelude to the physical procedure in cases where it must be carried out only occasionally. (See the "drug therapy" subsection in Chapter 8 for side effects and other important drug-related information.)

"Fear aggression" towards particular family members

So-called fear aggression is self-protective aggression directed towards a person or animal which the dog fears and is trying to drive away, keep away, or escape from. The fear component is very conspicuous in some dogs. For example, they attempt to escape and lower their ears, tail, and head when the feared person comes anywhere near them. In other dogs,

however, the aggressive behavior seems to lack a major or noticeable fear component. These dogs look friendly when approached, they might even approach the person with wagging tail and pleading eyes, but they snap without the slightest warning at the hand that reaches for them.

In this latter case, it is probably fair to assume that the dog is experiencing what psychologists would describe as an *approach/ avoidance conflict* in that it is motivated by friendly, contact-seeking and fearful, contact-avoiding motivations simultaneously. Animal experiments clearly illustrate this phenomenon. For example, if one separately measures the physical force specially-harnessed rats exert at various points in a long runway either to *get to* a food source or *get away* from a place where they are shocked respectively, one obtains the two approach and avoidance curves on the graph in Figure 11.1. Essentially, rats pull fairly hard to get at the food even when far away but are not very highly motivated at this distance to get even farther away from a shock location – which essentially results in the slope of the avoidance curve being steeper than that of the approach curve. When both motivations are brought into play by shocking hungry rats in a goal box containing food at the end of a runway, both of these approach and avoidance tendencies are presumably activated simultaneously. In this situation, the theoretical model predicts that the animal should approach the goal box fairly quickly when far away, slow down as it nears a point where the two approach and avoidance tendencies are about equally strong – and perhaps hesitate or vacillate there as if the "conflicting" motivations are pushing or pulling it in two directions simultaneously – but then primarily try to escape when placed nearer to the food/shock location, which is indeed what happens in these experiments (Walker, 1987).

The following discussion concerns the fear aggression problem as it commonly occurs within families. Similar problems directed towards human strangers or other dogs will be considered in Chapters 12 and 14 respectively.

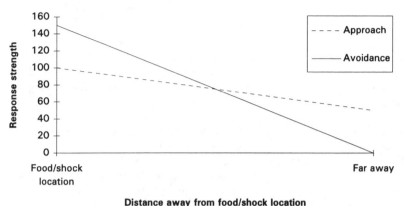

Figure 11.1: Relative strength of approach and avoidance tendencies as a function of the distance away from a food/shock location

Possible causal factors

Unintentional owner fostering

The most common cause of fear-related aggression towards family members is overly severe punishment. A common scenario is that the owner begins punishing the dog to try and stop some undesirable behavior like barking at visitors. If this method doesn't seem to be working well enough and the owner hasn't any idea of what else to do, increasing the severity of punishments may seem like the most logical approach. After all, the punishment may indeed have previously helped to reduce the problem barking somewhat.

Increasing the intensity of what appears to be a partially successful method of correction is therefore a natural owner response. But if the punishment becomes severe enough, some dogs react aggressively, growling and snapping to defend themselves when they are attacked in this way. And later, the aggressive response may generalize from a reaction to the punishment itself, to a reaction to the threat of punishment or even the close approach of the person who did the punishing.

Animals behave fearfully at such times, and it is therefore assumed that some kind of *classically conditioned fear* is involved. In classical conditioning (also called *Pavlovian conditioning*), a neutral stimulus is regularly and closely associated with a stimulus that instinctively elicits some behavior. This eventually results in the previously neutral stimulus acqui-

ring the capability to elicit this type of behavior as well. For example, if a bell (*conditioned stimulus*) is rung a number of times just as food (*unconditioned stimulus*) is put into a dog's mouth – a stimulus which instinctively elicits salivation – soon the dog will start salivating whenever it hears the bell alone. In the family situation we are considering, the approach of the person is analogous to the bell and the severe punishment to the food: as a result of the close temporal association between approach of the person and punishment, the person's approach comes to elicit some of the aggression and underlying fear which were formerly only elicited by the punishment itself.

From the behavioral science standpoint, this classically conditioned fear is only part of the story however. For each time the aggression is successful in keeping or driving a feared person away, the aggressive behavior is rewarded and thereby strengthened. Basically, many dogs which snap anyone who comes too close or reaches towards them are employing a learned defensive behavioral strategy. It is the end result of a long developmental history in which the behavior has proven itself again and again to be a genuinely effective means for the dog to drive or keep particular persons (or types of persons) which it fears away. Thus, for the dog which is afraid of someone and wants therefore to avoid contact, fear aggression pays off.

Finally, another dimension is often involved in cases of fear aggression towards family members. For someone who is basically very fond of

POSSIBLE CAUSAL FACTORS

Unintentional owner fostering
(e.g. conditioned fear resulting from overly severe punishment; feared person's reaction reinforces/strengthens aggression)

Traumatic experience
(single frightening/painful experiences can sometimes lead to intense and lasting fear)

Erroneous owner beliefs
(e.g. aggression should always be punished; punishment long after the problem behavior is still effective)

Unintentional reinforcement by other family members
(e.g. petting/distracting/reassuring aggressive dog reinforces aggression towards feared person)

"FEAR AGGRESSION" TOWARDS PARTICULAR FAMILY MEMBER

- Fear-motivated aggression towards particular family member when approached, touched, reached for, cornered, threatened, etc. by the person

POSSIBLE TREATMENT ELEMENTS

Increase owner understanding
(problem as normal behavior of highly fearful animal; treatment must focus on the underlying fear not the aggression)

Avoid problem situations
(e.g. feared person shouldn't force physical contact or do things which make dog fearful)

Change interactive ground rules
(e.g. feared person takes over feeding duties; others should temporarily ignore dog)

Avoid unintentional reinforcement
(e.g. fearful behavior should be ignored by other family members)

Systematic behavior therapy methods
(systematic desensitization/counterconditioning during "practice approaches" by family member)

Cessation of ineffective/counter-productive treatment methods
(severe punishment contraindicated, particularly for feared person)

Correct erroneous owner beliefs
(e.g. that fear aggression should be punished)

Conventional obedience training by feared person
(new, more positive way for dog to interact with person)

Training in problem situations
(reward non-fearful behavior in presence of feared person)

Physical aids
(e.g. muzzle)

Drugs
(tranquilizers as adjuncts in some cases; benzodiazepines contraindicated)

the dog, it can be extremely unpleasant to be treated like a monster who must be avoided at all costs. Realizing that they have obviously gone too far, family members may decide to stop punishing the dog entirely and attempt then to restore some of the damage their punishment has done. This may not be easy however. The dog may refuse to come when called and try desperately to keep a certain safe distance between itself and the person. In this situation, many people are impatient or don't realize that it is best not to hurry the process of fear reduction along. Instead they try constantly to approach the dog, pet it, and in other ways convince it that their intentions are now only the best. Children too may not accept the dog's rejection and avoidance. Wanting to pet and play with the dog, they may chase, corner, and attempt to pet it – here again, with the best of intentions: simply to show the dog that they mean no harm. To the dog, however, these active attempts to reduce the distance at which it feels safe are perceived as a form of threatening harassment which keeps the animal nervous and on its guard rather than encouraging it to relax in the feared person's presence.

Erroneous owner beliefs

When overly severe punishment has produced the problem, erroneous beliefs are usually partly responsible for the owner's behavior. A few common ones are as follows:

- Aggression towards human beings should *always* be punished.
- The more serious the aggression, the more severe should be the punishment.
- When mild punishment has proven helpful, more severe punishment should function even better.
- If applied correctly, punishing a dog long after it has done something wrong like eliminated in the home will teach it a useful lesson which will eventually solve the problem.
- A dog's "guilty" look long after it has done something wrong is a sign that the lesson the owner is trying to teach it with punishment is starting to show results.

Obviously, identifying such erroneous beliefs and explaining to owners why they are erroneous is often crucial to convincing them to abandon the counterproductive punishment method in favor of some reward-based alternative.

Traumatic experience

There are other possible sources of fear aggression towards family members besides overly severe punishment. Most common, a child may have teased the dog or in some way unintentionally mistreated it by, for example, pulling its tail or poking it in the eye. The child need not be young. Sometimes older children quite maliciously tease or mistreat (e.g. with fireworks) a dog to show off in front of friends. Use of the term *traumatic* emphasizes the possibility that single experiences can sometimes exert powerful effects on the animal's behavior. In the extreme case, only one very frightening experience is enough to produce a relatively great and lasting fear.

Unintentional reinforcement by other family members

The feared person comes too close, the dog growls, and someone else in the family immediately pets and talks reassuringly to it to try and convince it that the feared person means no harm. While one may succeed in encouraging a fearful animal to relax in the situation itself by petting it, talking to it, giving it something to eat, or getting it to play, doing these things as an immediate response to the dog's fearful or aggressive behavior is an additional source of reinforcement for the problem behavior.

Possible treatment approaches

Increase owner understanding

It is important to explain two general aspects of this type of problem to owners. First: the dog is showing what is basically normal behavior for an animal which is fearful and feels genuinely and seriously threatened. And second: it is the underlying fear and not the aggression itself on which the treatment measures must be focused. Once owners understand these two aspects, they become receptive to the required treatment approach and easily understand the logic of each of its recommendations.

Cessation of ineffective/counterproductive treatment methods

Obviously, severe punishment is contraindicated even in cases where punishment itself is not the cause of the fear problem. This applies particularly to the persons the dog fears. For them, even milder sorts of punishments like scolding should be refrained from except where absolutely necessary to, for example, stop the dog from attacking a stranger. It may still be appropriate or necessary in some circumstances for other family members to punish certain behaviors with scolding and leash correction. But with animals which are inclined to become fearful and therefore aggressive towards persons who treat them somewhat harshly, it is better that family members learn to correct other behavior problems and control the dog's overall behavior primarily with reward-based training methods while employing mild punishments like scolding only as an adjunct to temporarily suppress problem behavior so that positively-rewarded alternatives can be elicited and rewarded.

Avoid problem situations

The feared person is advised to refrain as much as possible from doing the types of the things that make the dog fearful and aggressive. Aside from not punishing the dog, this mainly means leaving the dog alone and not approaching it and trying to pet it when this makes it react fearfully. Basically, the best approach is for the feared persons to simply sit back and patiently wait until the dog discovers on its own that they are no longer a threat and begins to relax in their presence. Calling the dog and giving it a food reward when it comes is permissible and sometimes even helpful as far as reducing the

seriousness of the problem is concerned, but approaching the dog when it is showing any signs of nervousness or fear should be avoided at all costs.

Correct erroneous owner beliefs

Naturally, when erroneous beliefs/attitudes/opinions are standing in the way of abandoning overly harsh punishment or accepting and implementing alternative approaches to correcting a behavior problem, these must be dealt with directly during the consultation. The counselor should politely but firmly point out that certain beliefs are erroneous and, most importantly, explain what is the better, more accurate, more productive way of viewing things. Telling people that they are wrong about something can be a touchy and difficult matter. But it often must be done. One can, however, do so tactfully: for example, "although most people would agree with you there, the problem is that ....." or "one would think that's the way things work – I mean at first glance it seems logical – but the problem with that is ...".

Change family-dog interactive ground rules

Some changes in how, when, and where various family members interact with the dog can be quite helpful in some cases. In the case example of Bernard described in the sample recommendations box at the end of this section, the advice given was that Bernard should refrain from punishing the dog, take over the daily duties of feeding and walking the dog, be the only one who is allowed to give the dog food rewards, and that other family members should ignore the dog entirely until it showed signs of losing its fear of Bernard. Potentially, this strategy of increasing the dog's dependence on the feared person and perception of the feared person as the sole source of life's most valued rewards (food, going outside, attention, petting) can have a dramatic beneficial effect in some cases.

Not surprisingly, however, compliance with such recommendations is often poor. Although other family members are usually more than willing to turn some duties of dog ownership over to the feared person, they may not be as willing to refuse to interact with the dog even on the temporary basis for several reasons. In the first place, ignoring the dog feels like one is punishing it, for it shows obvious signs of becoming disturbed when first treated in this way. Secondly, the fact that the problem is directed at someone else and not themselves means that family members may not be willing to go as far as they might if they themselves were suffering. In effect, they can live with the problem more easily than the feared person, and it is natural therefore that they might not be as inclined as he/she is to take drastic steps to solve it. Finally, if they have felt all along that the dog was being mistreated by the feared person and sympathized with it, they may feel that the feared person is getting exactly what he/she deserves, and – in spite of their expressed willingness to help solve the problem – they might secretly have no intention of doing much to change things.

Essentially, like the treatment of dominance aggression, the personalities, attitudes, emotional needs, etc. of the various family members, and the interpersonal dynamics between family members, play a major role in determining the level of compliance with what is, for most families, this very demanding and unpleasant treatment approach.

Conventional obedience training by feared person

If close contact is possible in some situations (e.g. outside during walks where the dog might not feel so cornered) without arousing aggression and/or fear, the feared person can also carry out conventional obedience training with the dog by rewarding it for following the basic sit, down, stay, and come commands with at first only food tidbits, and then later, after the problem has improved substantially, with brief petting combined with food rewards. If carried out correctly, such training sessions are a source of great pleasure for the dog and can therefore represent a new, more positive way for it to interact with the feared person.

The potential efficacy of this approach is based on two behavioral science principles. Firstly, being the sole dispenser of highly-prized food rewards encourages the development of more positive "emotional responses" in the dog towards the feared person due to simple classical conditioning association learning. And secondly, the coming, sitting, and lying down without acting aggressively or fearfully that are being strengthened during practice sessions are alternative behaviors whose increase in frequency and intensity necessarily reflect a decrease in frequency and intensity of the aggressive, avoidance, and escape behaviors. In effect, the feared person him/herself is counterconditioning behaviors which "compete" with the problem behaviors – one of the most powerful methods for solving many kinds of behavioral problems.

Avoid unintentional reinforcement

Other family members must learn to be careful about how they react whenever the dog growls, barks, or snaps or shows any kind of fearful behavior (e.g. avoidance, coming to other family members for protection). Basically, they should stop trying to end the dog's growling, calm it down, or soothe its fear by petting it, talking to it, or distracting it with playing. For these can all function as positive reinforcements and strengthen the dog's tendency to behave aggressively and/or fearfully in these situations in future. People rarely perceive this danger on their own, for these calming, reassuring, distracting measures do seem to work at the time: the animal may indeed stop growling or act less fearful when being petted by someone. Obviously, it must be thoroughly explained to owners here that in the long run, an animal which is petted and fussed over every time it growls or comes for protection is being trained to do such things more readily not less so.

The proper reaction for other family members is, of course, to consistently ignore such problem behavior by not reacting to it in any way. However, with regard to growling or barking, there are cases where other family members should react more actively to scold and thereby suppress such behavior rather than ignore it. This is particularly true when, for example, a young child is being growled at and parents are using their dominance-related authority over the dog to suppress the problem behavior. While it is true that in general one must be careful with the use of punishment methods with animals whose problem behavior is motivated by fear, this does not mean that all forms of punishment are contraindicated in every case. Mild punishment like scolding of a dog which is accustomed to be scolded need not arouse much fear and yet may carry with it the powerful and useful message that the owner does not approve of the behavior and there will be further trouble if the behavior is not stopped. As is the case with fear problems generally (see Chapter 15), being too reluctant to scold fearful dogs can sometimes also be a serious mistake that allows other problems to develop or stands in the way of eliminating them.

Training in problem situations

Rather than being part of the problem, other family members should try to be a part of the solution by fostering desirable behavior with petting, attention, praise, playing, and so on. In this case, desirable behavior on the part of the dog means not behaving aggressively or fearfully towards the feared person in situations in which such behaviors are often exhibited. Particularly when the treatment measures start showing results and the dog is tolerating progressively closer contact with the feared person without showing signs of aggression or fear, others in the family can help the process along by deliberately rewarding the dog in these specific situations where, not too long ago, it was behaving fearfully.

Systematic behavior therapy methods

The classical behavior therapy method of *systematic desensitization* has received much attention in the literature as a way to treat dogs which are fearful of specific persons. However, it is generally less useful and appropriate for treating fear aggression reactions towards family members than the above-described measures because it is so time-consuming, difficult to correctly carry out, and represents an overly elaborate and somewhat unnatural way of addressing problems which are embedded in the interpersonal dynamics of the family situation. In general, classical systematic desensitization behavior therapy – which is always combined with counterconditioning of non-fearful behavior using food rewards – is probably most appropriate and useful against fear aggression towards young children or severely handicapped people in the family. For in these cases, the feared persons themselves cannot play the kind of active role recommended for Bernard in the sample recommendations box below.

Young (1982) gives an excellent detailed description of a systematic desensitization/counterconditioning behavior therapy procedure which could be used to reduce the dog's fear and, therefore, fear-aggression towards a young child.

Physical aids

As with other forms of canine aggression, when the family situation and family-dog interactive ground rules cannot be changed sufficiently to protect a family member who is at risk of being bitten, the dog should be muzzled in all potentially dangerous situations. Particularly when children are at risk, muzzling the dog when it is in their presence is a wise precaution. And in cases where very young children simply won't keep away from the dog, it is absolutely essential.

Drugs

Anxiolytic medicaments can be a useful adjunct in a few cases where, for example, the degree of fear is particularly great and/or very close physical contact with the feared person cannot be avoided. Detailed information about medicaments used to treat fear problems in dogs is provided in Chapter 15. In the experience of some American veterinarians, benzodiazepines can sometimes make fear-aggressive dogs more aggressive. It is theorized that they may act to reduce an animal's fear and fear-re-

SAMPLE RECOMMENDATIONS

Fear-related aggression towards a particular family member

Case example: Bernard, the family's 16-year-old son, has been bitten twice while punishing a 2-year-old West Highland white terrier, once by hitting it with his hand and the other time by hitting it with its leash. The dog is noticeably fearful of Bernard and growls when he comes too close, particularly in the home, but it is not fearful of other family members and reacts much less fearfully towards Bernard outdoors.

- Bernard should take entirely over the duty of regularly feeding the dog.
- To the extent his school schedule allows, Bernard should also take over the duty of regularly taking the dog for walks.
- During walks, Bernard can be calmly firm with the dog, but never threatening. Bernard should not punish the dog physically (hitting, leash correction) under any circumstances.
- The use of overly severe punishment (i.e. which elicit more than a very mild startled or submissive reaction) should be avoided by all other family members.
- Bernard should never approach the dog to pet it or elicit playing. Instead, he should wait until the dog comes to him of its own accord even though it might take days or weeks before this happens.
- It may also help if Bernard gives the dog two or three short, 5-min. obedience training lessons everyday during walks. He should call the dog and then reward the dog with its favorite food tidbits for following commands like "come", "sit", "down", and "stay". Commands should be given in a quiet, calm voice, and he should not reprimand the dog for making mistakes.
- To accelerate the process of reducing the dog's fear of Bernard, all other family members should *completely ignore* the dog until the problem with Bernard shows signs of improving. Essentially, during the next two or three weeks, Bernard should be the only one in the family who pets the dog, talks to it, takes it for walks, gives it food tidbits, and plays with it.

lated inhibition against behaving aggressively. If this is the case, they should be contraindicated for fearful dogs which show aggressive behavioral tendencies of any sort. (See also the "drug therapy" subsection in Chapter 8 for side effects and other important drug-related information.)

Defensive aggression towards young family children

It is understandably alarming for parents when the family dog growls and snaps at babies or toddlers. In comparison to owners with other sorts of problems, they are especially anxious to have a expert's opinion on how dangerous the situation really is for their child and how to deal with this new, extremely worrisome and stressful development.

This problem seems to fall into two general categories. Firstly, it can be purely self-protective in the conventional sense in that the dog growls and snaps at a young child who approaches it too closely, pets it, pulls its hair or tail, bangs on its back, or steps on its foot. In most of these cases, the dog acts suspicious of the child when it comes too close and tries to avoid it whenever possible. Often, the dog appears fearful when approached, tries always to stay away from the child, and growls and snaps only when prevented from moving away – the typical fear aggression pattern. But in other cases, the element of overt fear is much less pronounced. Here the dog tolerates and perhaps sometimes even approaches and interacts normally with the child except when the child does something it finds painful or aversive, which elicits threatening growling or snapping – the typical aversive stimulus-elicited aggression pattern.

In the other type of case, the problem appears to be a form of competitive or dominance-related aggression in the sense that the dog reacts with menacing growling to being touched or approached by the child when, for example, it is lying in one of its normal resting places. It may also growl at the child in other competitive situations as when both child and

dog are playing with one of the parents on the floor. In this form of aggression, the dog shows no signs of fear of the child and does not appear to be reacting to behaviors which are aversive in the physical sense of the term. Rather, it seems to be reacting towards the child like a higher-ranking adult pack member might towards a lower-ranking juvenile which is violating one of the unwritten rules of the dog pack social order.

Essentially, the various problems which Hart and Hart (1985) treat together under the general heading of "competitive aggression towards children" or "sibling rivalry" seem to be appropriately distinguished from one another using the following sort of scheme:

Self-protective aggression:

- Elicited by genuinely *aversive stimuli* from the child which can range from very painful or fear-arousing like hitting the dog hard, yanking on its fur, jabbing it in the ear, etc. to relatively mild (e.g. repeatedly thumping on its back or grabbing hold of its tail).
- *Fear-related aggression* elicited by the feared person's approach/reaching/touching due to:
  - fear of the *particular child* acquired as a result of mistreatment from the child or having been frightened by child's noisy playing, hectic behavior, screaming, etc., or
  - fear of *all young children* reflecting either past mistreatment by young children or the lack of experience early in life interacting with young children.

Competitive (dominance-related) aggression:

- In response to *dominant behavior* on the part of the child (e.g. touching dog, bending over it) or in *competitive situations* (e.g. during play with family adult; child touches dog's toy or approaches dog when it is eating).

Several things should be noted about this classification system. Firstly, it is an empirical system based primarily on the present author's impressions from a number of cases of this sort. Accordingly, it is therefore best regarded as a preliminary working hypothesis intended to guide the counselor's questioning of owners and observation of the dog's behavior towards the child in the rather diverse set of cases that fall into this general category. Secondly, it emphasizes that the dog's motivation for growling or snapping can differ considerably from one case to another. The child may be a source of

aversive stimuli, a fear-eliciting stimulus, or viewed as a rival or ill-mannered subordinate. And finally, the different categories are not mutually exclusive. It is possible, for example, that some dogs growl for reasons related to both self-protective and dominance-related motivations. It is also possible that the dog's reaction may be differently motivated at different times as if the dog is somehow uncertain as to how it should treat the child and therefore vacillates from time to time. This latter impression is one the author has gotten in several cases. And perhaps it is revealing. Perhaps some dogs are rather "confused" as to how to behave towards this small, pushy, noisy, friendly, but dangerous and unpredictable family member who is given such preferential treatment by others in the family. The child may pull the dog's fur while laughing, start crying when the dog tries to play with it, and not at all be deterred by a threatening growl the way any other normal human being would. Perhaps it is understandable therefore that the dog's relationship to the child is far more complex and unstable that those it has with the family's older children and adults. Basically, the child may be perceived and treated by the dog as a playmate, ill-mannered subordinate, competitive rival, object of fear, torturer, or source of stress depending on the situation.

Table 11.1 presents some statistical information taken from 11 cases of this type. Interestingly, the 3 males and 1 female which also showed mild dominance aggression towards other family members were *not* the same animals as those which showed a history of being aggressive to children outside of the family – which seems consistent with the classification scheme's distinguishing between self-protective and dominance aggression.

Possible causal factors

Response to aversive stimuli

In some cases, the aggression is a direct response to aversive stimuli stemming from the child. For example, the child may be growled or snapped at while in the act of pulling on the dog's fur or slapping it repeatedly on the back. Then too, very young children are often extremely insistent and make it impossible for the dog to avoid or escape from them. They may follow the dog whenever it tries to go away and grab it by the leg or fur to prevent its further avoidance. Of course, this is also a kind of aversive treatment that makes the dog feel cornered and in need of putting up a stronger defense.

Traumatic experiences

Often the key to why particular animals react this way lies in the past. A dog that has had some particularly painful experience with a young child (e.g. poked in the eye, having a sore part of the body roughly pulled or prodded) may react hypersensitively when the child grabs it, pulls on its fur, or corners it. This sort of problem would be appropriately con-

Table 11.1: Statistical information from eleven cases of aggression towards very young family children

Male dogs (n = 7):	
Age of child:	*7 mo. – 2 years (median: 1 1/2 years)*
Other major behavior problems?	*4 dogs*
Mild dominance aggression towards family adults?	*3 dogs**
Mild/serious aggression towards children outside of family?	*3 dogs**
(6 different dogs)*	
Female dogs (n = 4):	
Age of child:	*7 mo. – 3 years (median: 11 months)*
Other major behavior problems?	*2 dogs*
Mild dominance aggression towards family adults?	*1 dog***
Mild/serious aggression towards children outside of family?	*1 dog***
*(** 2 different dogs)*	

POSSIBLE CAUSAL FACTORS:

Aversive stimuli
(e.g. child hits dog, pulls on its fur or tail,
etc.)

Restricted early experiences
(possible source of basic mistrust/fear
of all children)

Genetic predisposition
(e.g. tendencies towards dominance aggression, fearfulness, noise hypersensitivity,
low growling/biting thresholds)

**Unintentional reinforcement by other
family members**
(e.g. pet/distract animal to stop growling)

Traumatic experience
(e.g. fear of child after particularly painful/
frightening experience with it)

Dominance-related aggression
(aggression parallels dominance
aggression towards human adults or other
dogs)

Unintentional fostering by owner
(e.g. reduced attention/petting/playing
when child present may turn it into aversive
discriminative stimulus)

Lack of appropriate training
(growling and snapping at human beings
tolerated by owners in other contexts)

DEFENSIVE AGGRESSION TOWARDS YOUNG FAMILY CHILDREN

- Barking, growling, or biting directed at family children between 6 months and
3 years of age in self-protective or competitive, dominance-related contexts

POSSIBLE TREATMENT ELEMENTS

Avoidance of problem situations
(e.g. keep dog and child separated when
unsupervised)

**Cessation of counterproductive
treatment methods**
(e.g. paying more attention to dog
when child absent)

Training in potential problem situations
(combination of rewards for non-aggressive
behavior and mild punishment for aggression
towards child in some cases)

Conventional obedience training
(e.g. to increase owner control over dog in
potential problem situations)

Physical aids
(muzzle in potentially dangerous situations)

Increase owner understanding
(e.g. possible severe consequences for
child; growling is aggressive threat behavior
which must be taken seriously)

Change family interactive ground rules
(e.g. feeding, attention, playing, tidbits,
privileges given to dog only in presence of
child; recommendations from Chapter 10 to
lower dominant-aggressive dog's status in
family)

**Avoid unintentional reinforcement of
problem behavior**
(stop petting/soothing/distracting as direct
response to aggression towards child)

Systematic behavior therapy methods
(e.g. desensitization/counterconditioning to
reduce fear of child possible in some cases)

sidered to be fear aggression. In these cases, the fear aspect may be quite clearly seen in the animal's avoidance and other fearful behavior.

Restricted early experiences

In some cases, the dog's reaction to young children in the family mirrors its reaction to young children in general: the dog is suspicious and fearful and possibly aggressive to all young children under any and all circumstances. One possibility for accounting for why some dogs just don't seem to like young children and always react suspiciously, fearfully, and perhaps aggressively towards them is that the animals may have had little or no experience with children during the first few months in life. Indeed, questioning owners often reveals that the dogs spent the first 3 or 4 months of life in some secluded rural situation where they were only exposed to one or two human adults. Children and their noisy, hectic, and extremely active way of behaving may therefore always seem alien, threatening, and therefore basically aversive to such dogs.

Dogs whose negative reactions to children seem to stem from lack of early experiences with them may show two kinds of reactions towards young family children. The dog may fearfully avoid them and be aggressive towards them as if responding to some kind of threat. Or it may simply avoid them and be aggressive towards them as if, for example, to shoo away a playful young kitten that keeps pouncing on its foot. This would essentially represent a form of interspecific aggression which might parallel, for example, the occasional aggressive interactions between the members of different species which share the same outdoor enclosure in a zoo. Basically, this view postulates that the dog is treating the owner as a conspecific while behaving towards the child as if it were a member of an alien species. Although such a theoretical speculation may seem overly extreme, so too is the difference between an animal which treats older family members like gods while barely acknowledging the existence of the family's youngest member.

However, the fact that babies and toddlers are pretty much ignored by a family dog does not in itself necessarily indicate that it has had inadequate experience with young children early in life and therefore excludes them from being suitable partners for species-typical social behavior. Many dogs may act disinterested essentially because the young child is incapable of the kinds of interactions which the dog has with the other family members. Its attempts at eliciting normal social behavior may always be ignored by the child or elicit a variety of much different, sometimes aversive sorts of behaviors than those elicited in older family members. But most of these dogs are not aggressive, presumably because the young child is indeed viewed as an immature conspecific and fellow group member whose occasional unpleasant behavior must be tolerated or avoided without aggression.

Dominance-related aggression

Thus there may be several different ways in which dogs can perceive and react to a family's basically innocent, ignorant, and friendly one-year-old. Some young children are bitten in self-defense by dogs which fear them, some are roughly driven away like unpleasant but basically insignificant pests, and others are threatened and bitten by an animal which seems to view them as juveniles who are old enough to be put and kept in their place in the family's dominance hierarchy. As with dominance aggression generally, these latter problem situations are of two sorts: either the dog is reacting to dominant gestures from an individual which it considers to be a subordinate (e.g. being touched in certain ways, bent over, or intensely stared at) or it is reacting aggressively in competitive situations over some limited resource (e.g. a bone, a toy, a place on the couch next to the owner, or the owner's petting or attention itself).

Genetic predisposition

Genetic differences of various sorts may interact with the complex human family environment and help account for why particular dogs react aggressively to young children. Most behavior specialists strongly suspect that fear problems and dominance aggression may have a genetic basis in some dogs. It is also reasonable to suspect that phenomena which may often be associated with aggression to young children such as a dog's noise hypersensitivity or low barking, growling, or biting thresholds might also be partly genetically determined. And finally, gene-based "personality" differences in how playful, calm, excitable, etc. dogs are might greatly influence how, for example, the playfully rough and therefore often unpleasant approaches by an uninhibited and uncoordinated young child are dealt with by the family dog. There is no way to assess the role such possible genetic factors are playing in the real-world situations being considered. However, it is not unreasonable to suspect that such factors may indeed be involved and helping to give particular problems their distinctive forms and set limits on what can or cannot be achieved by the various treatment methods.

Unintentional fostering by owner

A contributing factor in some cases may be the difference in attention given to the dog by family adults in the presence and absence of the child. Anxious to prevent the development of "jealousy" problems between a dog which has been the center of attention of the family for years and a baby, many parents make an extra effort to give the dog its fair share of attention. The problem is, however, that whether by design ("It's fair that he has his special time with us too") or by accident ("I only have time for him when my daughter is asleep'"), the amount of attention, petting, and playing given to the dog turns out to be substantially greater in the absence of the child. This in turn can add up to a situation in which the dog may learn to perceive the appearance of the baby as a signal indicating that less in the way of rewarding interactions with adults is now possible. Animal research indicates that stimuli which are associated with the termination or reduction of positive reinforcement conditions is aversive and may elicit active avoidance behavior. For example, a pigeon will learn to peck a disc on the wall for no other reward than turning off a light which signals to it that no or fewer rewards for pecking another disc are now available (Rilling, Askew, Ahlskog, and Kramer, 1969). Interestingly, Azrin, Hutchinson, and Hake (1966) showed that at the beginning of periods in which reward availability was temporarily suspended, pigeons showed a heightened tendency to be aggressive to a nearby pigeon – so-called *displaced* or *redirected aggression*. This is a further indication of the inherent aversiveness for the animal of the ending of circumstances in which it has had the opportunity of obtaining highly-valued rewards.

Whether such an effect really results in a child becoming a conditioned aversive stimulus that is thereafter "disliked", avoided, and perhaps attacked is unknown. But the fact that this kind of effect is theoretically possible – and the related possibility of intentionally using such a discrimination learning effect to advantage and turning the child into a *positive discriminative stimulus* by giving dogs substantially more attention than normal when the child is present – is enough to justify inclusion of deliberate manipulation of attention from family adults as a standard treatment measure in these cases.

Unintentional reinforcement by other family members

Another causal, learning-related factor is invariably found to be operating in almost all dog aggression and fear cases: namely, the unintentional rewarding of problem behavior by other family members who are trying to stop it either by calming or reassuring the animal (e.g. by talking to it or petting it) or distracting it (e.g. with food rewards, toys, or playing). That such owner attempts at coping with the problem behavior are so ubiquitous is a measure of their short-term effectiveness: they often do stop the problem behavior in the situation itself. However, the long-term effect of such measures is quite different. By coping with problem situations in this way, owners are essentially rewarding problem behavior and hence inadvertently training animals to act even more aggressively or fearfully in similar situations in the future.

Lack of appropriate training

Some owners have been surprisingly lax about controlling their animals' aggressive barking, growling, and snapping in a variety of contexts. This may have started when the dog was being playfully aggressive when young and continued throughout its life when, for example, it reacts aggressively to passersby on the street. This lack of training is not a major factor in most cases of aggression towards young family children. But there are cases in which the failure of owners to take steps throughout the dog's life to produce a strong inhibition against displaying aggression towards human beings can result in an animal which shows a low threshold for barking, growling, and snapping at anything and everything it doesn't like – young family members included.

Should treatment be attempted?

In 5 of the 11 cases summarized in Table 11.1, it was strongly recommended that the owners find a new home for the dog in a family without young children. In 3 of these cases, this was the only recommendation, and in the other two where it was clear that owners were not prepared to part with the dog under any circumstances, it was strongly recommended that the dog be kept muzzled when in the presence of the child until the child was older and less at risk. In the remaining 6 cases in which the degree to which the problem was treatable was uncertain and a set of treatment measures were recommended, it was strongly pointed out that at present the child is in great danger of being bitten, muzzling the dog when in interacts with the child was essential, and that another home should be found for the dog if the treatment measures did not completely eliminate all signs of the problem. In general, however, when one is quite sure that the problem is not entirely soluble in the sense there is no way that this particular dog (e.g. dominant-aggressive, aggressive to all children) can be made really safe for the child, the behavior counselor should strongly emphasize how seriously the child might be injured by the dog, strongly recommend giving the dog to a family without small children, stress the present necessity for muzzling the dog in the child's presence, and discourage the idea that the problem can and should be treated. In short, considerations of the child's safety should be placed clearly above parents' desires to keep their dog at whatever cost even at the risk of sometimes overreacting and convincing owners to find a new home for a dog which may in fact never have injured the child.

Another relevant aspect of these problems is what might be termed the stress factor. By the time the behavior counselor is contacted, families have usually lived through several extremely stressful days or weeks which began the first time the dog growled at the child. Even parents who appear to take such aggression lightly are affected. While they may try to tell themselves that such behavior does not indicate the dog is really dangerous, they are nevertheless on their guard from that time onwards, watching the dog more carefully when the child is present and remaining ready to quickly intervene if the dog becomes aggressive again. But most parents react more strongly than this. For them, the dog's behavior is extremely alarming and the complete trust they have always had previously that it would never be aggressive towards the child is gone. In short, a dimension of constant worry, uneasiness, and stress enters into family life which does not entirely subside even after several days or weeks have passed since the incident. In a way, it represents a kind of irrevocable loss of innocence – a realization that their much-loved pet is capable of behavior which they would have never dreamed possible before the incident occurred.

It is against this background of constant stress, of no longer being able to completely trust the dog around the child, of always fearing the worst, and last but not least, of being constantly in turmoil as to whether to keep the dog, try to find it another home, or have it euthanized that the consultation takes place. Basically, not only the physical safety of the child is a stake, but so too is the whole fabric of family life. And somehow the counselor must respond to this family stress aspect too by, for example, showing empathy, discussing how such a problem inevitably brings worry, stress, and uncertainly along with it, and if necessary by pointing out to owners that keeping a dog which is potentially dangerous not only means that their child will be constantly at risk, but also that the kind of worries they have now will continue and until the child is much older. In short, this dimension of severe family stress is a feature of these cases which also must be dealt with openly during the consultation and taken into account by the counselor when making recommendations.

Interestingly, many of those parents to whom the counselor has strongly recommended finding a new home for the dog in a family without small children are afterwards extremely grateful for his/her firm and unambiguous advice, and write or call later to express this: their dog is now living with a nice family with only older children, it seems to have adjusted to the new situation perfectly, and they realize now that this was the best and indeed only real solution.

Possible treatment approaches

Avoidance of problem situations

Owners are always advised to keep the dog separated from the child in situations in which the two cannot be closely supervised, and under no circumstances to leave the two alone in the same room, not even for a minute or two. Although parents usually have been doing this ever since their dog began showing signs of aggression towards the child, sometimes they are uncertain as to whether they are being overprotective and exaggerating the real danger to the child or, on the other hand, whether they are underestimating it and should not in fact have kept the dog as long as they have. Exactly how dangerous is the dog for the child? In many cases, the sole purpose of contacting a pet behavior problem counselor is to get an answer to this question from an expert they can rely on.

As discussed above, avoiding situations in which the child may be bitten and perhaps seriously injured by the dog is the primary goal in such cases. And this in turn requires that owners take the risk extremely seriously and take steps to rule out such an attack even in those borderline cases in which it appears to both owner and counselor to be unlikely. Basically, "unlikely" is simply not good enough under these circumstances. Having 5 or 3 or even 1 out of 100 of these young children seriously injured is unacceptable, for both owners and counselor were forewarned by the dog's growling and the attack was therefore preventable.

Increase owner understanding

The counselor must usually explain or emphasize several things to owners in such cases. The first is that even mild growling is aggressive threat behavior which should be taken very seriously. In some cases, people are so convinced that the dog would never harm the child that they regard the dog's growling, barking, and even snapping as minor signs of the dog's discontent rather than as alarming signs that the child may be in danger. Accordingly, the counselor should point out in no uncertain terms that otherwise friendly, non-aggressive family dogs have indeed been known to attack and seriously injure children under similar circumstances. It should also be pointed out that young children are especially at risk because for one thing, they don't understand the danger they are in and tend to simply ignore the dog's threat rather than stop whatever they are doing to it as an adult or older child would. And for another, they are often injured more seriously than adults. As hospital bite statistics indicate, facial injuries are especially common in young children presumably because they are often down on the floor with the dog or have the tendency to come close to it with their faces.

Practically speaking, very young children are best viewed as being untrainable as far as learning to keep away from or be careful around the dog is concerned. Of course, from the behavioral science viewpoint they are not really untrainable. They could, for example, be conditioned to stay away from the dog by, for example, punishing them every time they approach the dog. Indeed, Hart and Hart (1985) propose doing just this by spraying the child with a plant water sprayer. However, this suggestion seems somewhat naive. Animals draw small children like magnets: they are extremely attractive playmates that only the most frightened youngster will stay away from. And if even being bitten doesn't teach the child to stay away from the dog – many children are indeed bitten more than once for doing the same thing to the dog – being squirted with water is obviously not going accomplish this objective. Basically, unless one is prepared to punish the child severely enough to teach it to really fear the dog, an entirely unacceptable alternative to most parents, this method has little to recommend it. Furthermore, it may be strongly contraindicated in cases where an emphasis on training the child diverts client attention from taking effective bite prevention measures.

Cessation of counterproductive treatment methods

When the dog's reaction is not easily explicable as an understandable reaction to some kind of mistreatment from the child (e.g. fur-pulling, ear-poking), parents usually assume that the dog is aggressive because it is jealous of the child or the affection and attention which the child is getting. This assumption leads many parents to try and cope with the problem by making a special effort to give the dog more attention especially when the child is absent so that the dog can enjoy the treatment to the full without having to share it with the child. For the reasons discussed above, this association of attention with the absence of the child – and less or no attention with the presence of the child – may make these problems worse and not better.

Change family interactive ground rules

Two sorts of changes in how family members routinely interact with the dog may be useful here. In the first place, where the dog seems to

have a general aversion to or "dislike" of the child, things should be arranged so that many of the good things in the dog's life like attention, petting, playing, tidbits, etc. are provided only when the child is present. At other times, the attention and other rewards given to the dog are either drastically reduced or eliminated altogether. Related recommendations such as first allowing the dog some privilege (e.g. being allowed into the living room) when the child appears on the scene are also appropriate in some cases.

The second major type of potentially helpful change in family interactive ground rules involves dogs which show minor dominance-aggression symptoms towards other family members and whose aggression towards the young child seems to be a manifestation of this problem (i.e. the dog is warning or teaching a lesson to what it perceives as a subordinate). Here, it may be desirable to reduce the dog's status in the family as a whole by applying some of the recommendations which are given in cases of dominance aggression (see Chapter 10).

Training in problem situations

The application of conventional training strategies in potential problem situations in which the dog sometimes growls or barks at the child can be as helpful here as they are with many other kinds of behavior problems. Basically, petting, praise, and perhaps even food rewards for non-aggressive behavior (i.e. any kind of friendly or quiet behavior) in the presence of the child is combined with mild punishment (e.g. scolding) for aggression. While one does not want to be frequently punishing the dog in the presence of the child – which might increase the dog's tendency to react negatively towards it – parents should not be too hesitant to use their authority as "pack leaders" to make it clear to the dog on these occasions that such behavior is unacceptable.

Avoid unintentional reinforcement of problem behavior

During the process of discussing how owners should react to growling/barking, owners must obviously also be explicitly warned against un-intentionally rewarding problem behavior. As with the previous aggression problems, it is explained to owners that although petting, reassuring, or distracting (e.g. with a toy) the dog in response to growling at the child may indeed be effective in stopping the problem behavior in the situation itself, these reactions essentially function as rewards which might well increase the animal's tendency to behave in a similar way in the future. From the dog's perspective, the message conveyed by such owner behavior may be one of tolerance and even approval rather than disapproval and warning of the possibility of punishment.

Conventional obedience training

To increase overall obedience and owner dominance, give owners a greater capability of controlling the dog's behavior in potential problem situations, and carry out the preliminary training required for some dominance-reducing (e.g. dog must follow a command to "earn" everything it wants) or systematic behavior therapy procedure, it is sometimes recommended in these cases that owners teach their dogs to respond appropriately and quickly to the basic sit, down, stay, and come commands.

Systematic behavior therapy methods

Hart and Hart (1985, p. 41) gave clients the following set of recommendations for carrying out a systematic behavior therapy procedure to teach their 2-year-old Samoyed, Plucky, to tolerate having its hair pulled by the family's toddler, Janey, without growling and snapping (the key recommendations have been rephrased rather than quoted directly):

1. *Begin by patting Plucky and giving her a favored food reward. During the course of a few brief daily sessions, gradually increase the patting pressure until hair pulling is introduced. Continue rewarding non-aggressive behavior in response to gradually stronger and stronger hair-pulling, and eventually let another adult also carry out the*

training. Continue with this procedure until the dog's response to even relatively strong hair-pulling is positive and non-aggressive.
2. *Introduce Janey by having her in the dog's view when its hair is being pulled.*
3. *Finally, have Janey be the one who pulls the hair.*

Whether or not a systematic behavior therapy procedure such as this is appropriate or practicable depends on the specific nature of the problem situation. In this case, the dog was reacting to one specific stimulus, hair-pulling, which it was possible for the parents to systematically vary (i.e. from patting, to mild hair-pulling, to stronger hair-pulling, to hard hair-pulling) during the training procedure. These characteristics make it feasible to design a systematic *desensitization/ counterconditioning* procedure to gradually train the dog to react non-aggressively to the problem-eliciting stimulus. Another element which makes this behavior therapy approach feasible is that the animal had learned to fear only one specific child – as opposed to all children of that age.

However, in the real-world family situations in which serious behavior problems like these occur, such behavior therapy procedures are rarely appropriate and rarely successful. They are complex and time-consuming, difficult for the average person to carry out correctly, usually require the constant supervision of the counselor during the early phases, and the basic requirements for the successful implementation are often not met. For example, if it was Janey's approach rather than her hair-pulling that was eliciting the aggression, successful fear reduction using systematic desensitization would require that the dog never comes in closer contact to Janey than it had learned to tolerate while remaining entirely relaxed and non-fearful – a precondition which would be impossible to meet in most family situations in which aggression towards toddlers occurs.

Physical aids

As with other forms of canine aggression, when the family situation and interactive ground rules cannot be changed sufficiently to protect

SAMPLE RECOMMENDATIONS

Defensive aggression towards babies and toddlers

In all cases:

• *Never* leave the child alone with the dog – not even for a minute or two.

In all cases where dog potentially dangerous and close contact with child unavoidable:

• The dog should *always* wear a muzzle in the presence of the child. However, it should also often wear the muzzle when the child is absent, and never put the muzzle on or take it off just before or after the child enters or leaves the room so that the muzzling process will not appear to the dog to be directly connected with the child.

Scenario A: *dog is displaying potentially dangerous self-protective or dominance-related aggression which does <u>not</u> appear to be sufficiently treatable to completely eliminate the danger to the child. The following recommendations are from two separate cases.*

• The dog represents a danger to your young child which cannot be entirely eliminated by carrying out some kind of treatment. Therefore to guarantee your child's safety, another home for the dog should be found in a family without small children. *(Case involving probable dominance aggression towards child)*

• The dog should *always* wear a muzzle in the presence of young children. This should be regarded as a permanent and not a temporary measure. There is simply no way through behavioral training or some other kind of treatment to sufficiently reduce the danger that the dog may again bite a child. *(These clients stated categorically that they were determined to keep the dog in spite of the danger to their son and other young children)*

Scenario B: *dog is displaying potentially dangerous but still relatively mild aggression which appears to be treatable.*

• The growling is a sign of potentially dangerous aggression. Therefore never leave the child – not even for a moment – alone with the dog.
• Growling at the child or other human beings should always be scolded severely enough to immediately end this behavior.
• Praise and pet the dog frequently, play with it, and reward it with tidbits for following commands when the child is in the same room.
• Over the course of the next few months, ignore the dog completely during times which the child is out of the room.
• For the time being, do not allow the dog to come into the living room when the child is absent. Then let it in just as the child is brought into the room.
(In the case from which this last recommendation was taken, a few additional recommendations from Chapter 10 were also given to reduce the dog's dominance-related status in the family as a whole and increase overall obedience and controllability such as having it follow commands to earn everything it wants, never rewarding begging/ demanding behavior, controlling social contact by ignoring its approaches, and being more strict with it in a variety of situations)

someone who is at great risk of being bitten, the dog should be muzzled in all potentially dangerous situations. Particularly when young children are involved, muzzling the dog when it is in their presence is a wise precaution. In cases where the children simply won't or can't keep away from the dog, it is indispensable.

When recommending this, the counselor should point out that the dog will never like being muzzled but that it will quickly get used to it. Of course, the counselor must also explain how to do it without running the risk of increasing the dog's aggressiveness towards the child: essentially, by avoiding a direct and obvious (to the dog) connection between the presence or appearance of the child and the putting on or wearing of the muzzle by, for example, having the dog sometimes wear the muzzle when the child is absent, never putting the muzzle on at the same time the child appears, and never taking it off when the child is leaving or has just left the room. One can also manipulate attention, petting, or special privileges to make wearing of the muzzle more tolerable to the dog by making an effort to give the dog substantially more attention, petting, play, etc. when it is wearing the muzzle than otherwise.

Parental aggression

Sometimes a bitch with young puppies becomes aggressive towards family members when they attempt to approach the nest area. Some females which have gone through pseudopregnancy show a similar form of defensive aggression – guarding the nest area and surrogate puppy objects (e.g. stuffed toys or other small objects) she has collected there.

Possible causal factors

Genetic predisposition

Given the two facts that (1) there seems to be no obvious experiential factor which leads to the behavior and (2) some bitches always behave this way during pseudopregnancies while others never do, it is generally assumed that the presence or absence of a genetic predisposition towards aggressively defending puppies, surrogate puppies, and/or nest area is one of the most important causal factors determining this form of intragroup defensive aggression.

Elicitation by victim

Such aggressive reactions usually only become dangerous when children or other family members don't heed the dog's warning and come close to the nest to try and pet the female, handle the puppies, or remove the surrogate puppy objects. Another possible source of danger is when the nest area is somewhat inconveniently located and difficult for family members to avoid.

Hormonal influence

To the extent that the pseudopregnancy phenomenon is under hormonal control, so too is this form of aggression, which can essentially be regarded as a normal feature of the pseudopregnancy phenomenon in some bitches.

Possible treatment approaches

Increase general owner understanding

Basically, it should be explained to owners that the aggression is an inherited maternal behavior which is much more pronounced in some females than in others for unknown reasons.

Avoid problem situations

Generally, one does not attempt to treat this problem in the sense of training or otherwise inducing the dog to react otherwise. Rather, family members simply make it a rule to avoid going close to the nest area until the dog's reaction to their approach has normalized.

Correct owner mistakes

Attempts by family members to ignore the threats and approach the nest in order to convince the female that there is nothing to fear may succeed in some cases. But in others, this may worsen matters or be more dangerous than owners suspect. Certainly when this has been tried without success, owners should be cautioned against trying it again.

Change maintenance conditions

Simply moving the nest to a more secluded, out-of-the-way location in the home can often help make it possible to live safely with this temporary problem.

Drug therapy

According to Allen (1986), pseudopregnancy is sometimes successfully treated with estrogens, androgens, progestagens, the synthetic ergot alkaloid, *bromocriptine*, and *prostaglandin F₂ alpha*. Although Voith (1989) states that *mibolerone* is the current drug of choice, she recommends treating the pseudopregnancy syndrome with *megestrol acetate* at 2 mg/kg orally for five to eight days given early during the course of pseudopregnancy, but also cites results with indicates that 10 to 15 percent of dogs again experience pseudopregnancy when the drug is withdrawn. Johnston (1991), however, reports that such treatment is of little value because there is usually a relapse of the pseudopregnancy signs after cessation of therapy. (See the "drug therapy" subsection in Chapter 8 for side effects and other important drug-related information.)

Systematic behavior therapy methods

If approaching the nest is necessary for purposes of examining or medicating the puppies – or if the owner and dog live essentially in one room with no out-of-the-way place in which to relocate the nest – it may be appropriate for the owner to carry out some form of *desensitization/counterconditioning* behavior therapy: food rewards are given for non-aggressive behavior in response to "practice approaches" by family members using a procedure that parallels in major ways the fear-aggression procedure discussed earlier in the chapter.

When sheer lack of space in the home is the problem, simply *habituating* the bitch to repeated approaches is another possibility. Here one makes it a rule to come just close enough to the nest to elicit a slight negative reaction (i.e. suspicion, nervousness) in the female. And during the course of the day, one deliberately comes this close many times until the female becomes accustomed to it and no longer reacts negatively. The distance can then be progressively and gradually decreased over a number of days until the bitch has learned not to react negatively to even close approaches to the nest area. As a rule, this procedure will only be successful if, during the training, the owner makes sure never to go any closer to the female than she will tolerate without becoming more than *slightly* uneasy.

The difference between these *desensitization* and *habituation* procedures may at first glance seem slight. However, there is a major conceptual and procedural difference between the two. Whereas the desensitization procedure is designed and carried out in such a way that even the mildest types of negative reactions never occur, the habituation procedure focuses on the gradual reduction of mild negative reactions which are, in effect, intentionally elicited many times in a context where the animal can eventually learn that the eliciting stimuli are harmless or without real significance (Leibrecht and Askew, 1980).

Castration

Such problem behavior in females with puppies or during pseudopregnancy is often one of the major grounds for spaying them, which prevents repetition of the problem for obvious reasons.

References

Allen, W. E. (1986): Pseudopregnancy in the bitch: the current view on aetiology and treatment. *Journal of Small Animal Practice* **27**, 419–424.

Azrin, N. H., Hutchinson, R. R., and Hake, D.F. (1966): Extinction-induced aggression. *Journal of the Experimental Analysis of Behavior* **9**, 191–204.

Borchelt, P.L., and Voith, V.L. (1982): Classification of animal behavior problems. *Veterinary Clinics of North America: Small Animal Practice* **12**, 571–585.

Hart, B. L., and Hart, L.A. (1985): *Canine and Feline Behavior Therapy*. Philadelphia, Lea & Febiger.

Johnston, S.D. (1991): Questions and answers on the effects of surgically neutering dogs and cats. *Journal of the American Veterinary Medical Association* **198**, 1206–1214.

Leibrecht, B.C., Askew, H.R. (1980): Chapter 12: Habituation from a Comparative Perspective. In Denny, M.R. (ed.): *Comparative Psychology: An Evolutionary Analysis of Animal Behavior*. John Wiley & Sons, New York.

O'Farrell V. (1992): *Manual of Canine Beha-viour*. British Small Animal Veterinary Association. Shurdington, Cheltenham, Gloucestershire, UK.

Rilling, M., Askew, H. R., Ahlskog, J. E., and Kramer, T. J. (1969): Aversive properties of the negative stimulus in a successive discrimination. *Journal of the Experimental Analysis of Behavior* **12**, 917–932.

Voith, V.L. (1989): Behavioral disorders. In Ettinger, S. (ed): *Textbook of Veterinary Internal Medicine*. Philadelphia, WB Saunders.

Walker, S. (1987): *Animal Learning: An Introduction*. London, Routledge & Kegan Paul Inc.

Young, M.S. (1982): Treatment of fear-induced aggression in dogs. *Veterinary Clinics of North America: Small Animal Practice* **12**, 645–653.

12   Defensive Aggression Towards Human Strangers

The conventional ways of classifying aggressive behavior towards human strangers or humans which the dog recognizes but does not treat as fellow group (i.e. family) members into, for example, protective (or territorial/protective) and fear aggression (Borchelt and Voith, 1982; O'Farrell 1992, Voith, 1989), or territorial and fear-related aggression (Hart and Hart, 1985) are in need of revision. Consider the following facts:

- So-called territorially aggressive dogs – that is, dogs which are aggressive to strangers only when they enter the yard or home – vary in the degree to which they also show signs of fear. Some are boldly aggressive without showing the slightest trace of fear whereas others are noticeably fearful, reacting to the encroachment of a stranger into their home site area with vacillation between aggressive advance and fearful retreat and, perhaps, also showing more exclusively fearful behavior towards strangers away from home.

- Aggression to strangers away from home often seems to have a self-protective element rather than being, as is commonly implied by the term "protective", a case of the dog's simply defending owners. When the dog is by the owner's side, it is often not possible to decide what the dog is defending – itself, the owner, or "the group" (i.e. itself *and* the owner simultaneously). However, these dogs sometimes react aggressively to the approach of a stranger when the owner is some distance away, and often they do not react aggressively when the owner is approached by a stranger in this situation. Finally, the situation may be further complicated if the dog only seems to have the "courage" to aggressively threaten strangers when it is close to its owner (or being held in the owner's arms or lap). When some distance away, however, it might silently avoid the stranger and scurry back to its owner – its big, protective, all-powerful ally. While owners like to assume in this situation that the dog is primarily motivated to protect them, this therefore may not be the case at all.

- Like so-called territorially aggressive dogs, dogs which are aggressive to strangers away from home also vary greatly in the degree to which a fear element is apparent. Some are boldly aggressive and show little or no overt fear while others clearly show a combination of aggressive threatening with fearful retreat (e.g. in response to any sudden or forward movement of the stranger).

- Both dogs which are aggressive to strangers only at home and those which are aggressive to strangers everywhere may be especially or exclusively aggressive to only certain types of strangers such as men or children. One possible interpretation for this is that dogs perceive certain types of strangers as more potentially dangerous – perhaps because of certain negative experiences with them in the past. Thus, such problems too may involve conditioned fear in some way.

- Revealingly, many owners of even the seemingly least fearful dogs which are aggressive to strangers in public places or only in or around their home are convinced that the problem developed because of the dog's underlying fear of strangers. In many cases, they remember the dog's fearful or suspicious reactions towards strangers when it was young and have therefore always assumed that the present problem was a manifestation of this basic mistrustful/fearful orientation towards strangers which the dog exhibited from the start.

Taken together, this combination of observations suggests that rather than defining a special "fear aggression" category, fear is better regarded as a variable aspect (from dog to dog) or underlying dimension which is present to a greater or lesser extent – or in more overt or covert forms – in most stranger-elicited aggression cases.

Table 12.1 presents some data from two surveys which provide suggestive support for this view. The answers are to the question "Does the dog show excessive fear reactions?" put to a number of owners of both dogs with severe behavior problems and dogs without major problems. It can be seen here that as a group, the protectively/territorially aggressive animals (i.e. "group-defensive aggression" in the table) tend to be described as sometimes or often reacting excessively fearfully to almost as great an extent as dogs showing the classical fear-aggression pattern (i.e. "self-protective aggression"), to a lesser extent than dogs showing non-aggressive fear problems, but to a considerably greater extent than (1) dogs with pro-

blems unrelated to either fear or aggression towards strangers and (2) normal, non-problem dogs. Of course, this is not to say that the aggression problem need necessarily be directly related to the fearful behavior the owner was referring to when answering the question. But the difference between both groups of dogs which are aggressive to strangers and, for example, the sample from the normal dog population is considerable. It may well indicate that many or most animals which are aggressive to strangers tend to be, as dogs go, somewhat fearful types and not, as the popular stereotype of the territorially aggressive dog implies, courageous fighters that are basically not afraid of anything.

As indicated in the table, extragroup defensive aggression cases involving aggression towards human beings outside of the family are primarily classified into *self-protective* and *group-defensive* aggression in the present discussion. In self-protective aggression cases, the animal appears to be acting to defend itself by, for example, trying first to avoid or escape

Table 12.1: Answers of the owners of various types of problem dogs and normal, non-problem dogs to the question "Does your dog show excessive fear reactions?"

"Does dog show excessive fear reactions?"	Survey 1 "Yes"	Survey 2 "Often"	"Sometimes"	"Never"
Self-protective aggression (classical "fear aggression" pattern)	70% (n=10)	40%	60% (n=5)	0%
Group-defensive aggression (classical "protective" or "territorial" aggression patterns)	69% (n=23)	54%	25% (n=24)	21%
Non-aggressive fear problems (e.g. phobias, separation anxiety)	91% (n=11)	63%	37% (n=8)	0%
Other serious problems (e.g. not involving fearful behavior or aggression towards human strangers)	52% (n=33)	19%	33% (n=21)	48%
Normal animals (without major behavioral problems)	No data collected	4%	42% (n=55)	55%

from the stranger, and then reacting aggressively only when cornered, suddenly reached for, or threatened. Although traditionally referred to as "fear aggression", the degree to which there is an overt fear component to this form of aggression actually varies widely. Some dogs act extremely fearfully to the approach of strangers while others only snap when touched by a stranger without showing any prior overt signs of fear such as lowered head and tail, laid-back ears, or attempted avoidance. In contrast, group-defensive aggression is a more overtly offensive form of aggression seen, for example, when a dog barks at and attacks the mailman. Here, presumably the biological function is not simply to protect oneself against some immediate physical threat, but rather to both keep or drive an undesirable stranger away while simultaneously warning (loud barking) and perhaps recruiting fellow group members (via the social facilitation effect) to join into a group aggressive display. As mentioned above, there are considerable differences between animals here too with regard to the degree to which a noticeable fear component accompanies the group-defensive display. Some will boldly and seemingly fearlessly attack an intruder without a moment's hesitation while others threaten strangers in a more ambivalent and "cowardly" manner by hastily retreating when the stranger makes a move in their direction, trying to keep a certain safe distance between themselves and the stranger, or only trying to bite the stranger when his/her back is turned.

One could further subdivide the group-defensive aggression cases into territorial and non-territorial forms analogous to the distinction drawn by many workers in the field between "territorial" and "protective" aggression. However, this may be going too far. As considered in Chapter 9, the territoriality of domestic dogs seems to be a remnant of the wolf's tendency to defend the core or den area of a pack's territory more fiercely than other areas rather than directly paralleling the full scope of the phenomenon of territory-related aggression in wolves. Then too, the many complications encountered when trying to apply this territori-

al versus non-territorial distinction make it less useful than most workers acknowledge. While it is true that some dogs which attack strangers in their yards are friendly to strangers away from home, this may not be the rule. Many owners of dogs that are primarily aggressive to strangers in the yard and home also report that the dog sometimes threatens strangers on the street, never permits a stranger to touch it or approach it closely then, and in general just do not seem to care much for human beings outside of those in its family.

Basically, the approach taken in this chapter is not to use differences either in the degree of overt fear displayed or variation between the intensity of aggression shown at home versus on the street to define separate forms of aggression problems. Rather, these will be treated as important dimensions along with the various self-protective and group-defensive aggression cases vary. This is not, however, diminishing the importance of these dimensions in any way. To the contrary, considering how fearful the animal is and in what specific settings the aggression occurs is just as critical to understanding specific problems and deciding how they should be treated as before.

Group-defensive aggression towards human strangers

In contrast to the self-protective aggression pattern where a dog tends to remain quiet, tries simply to avoid the threatening stranger, and only reacts aggressively when cornered or reached for, dogs displaying the group-defensive aggression pattern tend to boldly threaten strangers who approach them on the street or enter their yard or home. Rather than trying to avoid the types of human beings which elicit the aggression, such dogs may go out of their way to threaten and attack them – running towards them when they are spotted from a distance and attacking them in a boldly offensive, seemingly fearless way. Included in this general category are not only what are conventionally referred to as "territorial" and "protective" aggression, but also many cases of what is often

POSSIBLE CAUSAL FACTORS

Early experience deficit
(lack of contact with strangers/types of
strangers early in life)

Traumatic/negative experience(s)
(fear-/pain-eliciting experiences with
strangers in past)

Intentional owner fostering
(young dog's aggression towards strangers
approved of/intentionally rewarded by owner)

Unintentional owner reinforcement
(attempted control of aggression by petting/
reassuring dog or distracting it with playing,
tidbits, etc.)

Erroneous owner beliefs
(if problem corrected, dog won't defend
home/owners when necessary)

Lack of basic obedience training
(results in dog which is difficult to control
and owner who hasn't learned how to train
dog)

Insufficient owner dominance
(results in dog which is disobedient/slow to
obey and hard to control/reform)

Reinforcement/elicitation by victims
(e.g. victim aggression can increase dog's
fear/aggression; victim stopping/retreating
when threatened reinforces aggression)

Social facilitation
(one dog's aggression often leads to group
display when more than one dog in family)

Inadequate maintenance conditions
(e.g. too much time chained up outside
alone)

GROUP-DEFENSIVE AGGRESSION TOWARDS HUMAN STRANGERS

• Barking at or attacking human strangers in public or when they enter the yard or home.

POSSIBLE TREATMENT ELEMENTS

Avoid problem situations
(e.g. keep dog on leash during walks/
separated from visitors at home)

Correct erroneous owner beliefs
(e.g. correcting problem will reduce dog's
value as family/home protector; normal for
dogs to be aggressive to people who fear
them)

Conventional obedience training
(increases owner control/dominance;
preliminary training required for counterconditioning measures; teaches owner
how to train animal)

Increase owner dominance
(to increase owner control in potential
problem situations)

Correct owner mistakes
(stop unintentionally rewarding aggression)

Training in problem situations
(e.g. combining punishment of aggression
with rewards for non-aggressive behavior;
early intervention method)

Systematic behavior therapy methods
(e.g. special outdoor training locations; staged
"practice visits" by series of strangers;
systematic manipulation of attention)

Physical aids to control aggression/dog
(e.g. leash, muzzle, head collar)

inappropriately labeled as "predatory" aggression like, for example, when dogs chase, bark at, and bite joggers or bicyclists.

Possible causal factors

Early experience deficit

Many dogs which show group-defensive aggression tend to avoid contact with human strangers under any and all circumstances. In some animals, this basic negative orientation takes the form of an apparent deep-seated fear or mistrust of strange humans which is the long-term result of a lack of experience with a variety of types of human strangers early in life. Questioning owners often reveals that such dogs were bred in a rural kennel environment where one or two family members were the only human beings it had contact with during the first 3 or 4 months of life.

Traumatic/negative experience(s)

An underlying fear or all strangers or certain type of strangers like men, children, or blond girls between about 5 and 10 years old can also be acquired later in life as a result of negative experiences with human beings of this type. The experiences which result in dogs later treating all strangers or certain types of strangers as threatening can be a series of negative ones or one single, traumatic one in which the animal was very badly frightened or mistreated.

Intentional owner fostering

When the puppy or juvenile reaches an age when it begins growling and barking at strangers who enter the yard or home, most owners realize that this could become a problem and therefore start suppressing the behavior by scolding the dog every time it occurs. However, some owners do the opposite: they reward the behavior with petting and praise because the dog has done what they want it to do – defend their home against strangers. Indeed to most pet owners, mild aggressiveness towards strangers when they first enter the yard or home is understandable, acceptable, and even desir-

able. It is only when the aggression becomes more severe than this and can no longer be easily controlled that the behavior counselor is contacted.

Although intentional owner fostering of aggression towards strangers away from home is less common, some people who themselves tend to be mistrustful or suspicious of strangers encountered on the street find the dog's occasional aggressive barking at strange persons during walks reassuring – particularly if they assume that the dog is primarily trying to defend them rather than itself. Especially in situations where the dog has just succeeded in intimidating some formidable-looking stranger, rewarding owner attention and petting is likely to convey the message of approval. In many cases, dogs tend to be aggressive only during walks after dark. Although the owners (usually women) tend to assume that perhaps the dog can't see as well in the dark and is therefore more nervous and insecure at this time, one suspects that the dog's behavior is basically more a reflection of owner nervousness and insecurity, which would translate itself into less in the way of scolding and more in the way of intentionally or unintentionally rewarding aggression at this time.

Another revealing developmental scenario is sometimes seen in cases where puppies show fearful behavior towards strangers from the start. Concerned that the dog is going to develop into a fearful adult, owners welcome and heartily reward the initial transformation of this fearful behavior into aggression, for this seems to them to be a definite step in the right direction. In such cases, the connection between a basic underlying fear of strangers and later development of the group-defensive aggression problem can be seen especially clearly.

Unintentional owner reinforcement

If one asks owners how they cope with aggression towards strangers at home or during walks, most will reply that it usually helps to pet and talk to the dog – to calm and reassure it – or distract it by throwing something that elicits play or by giving it a food reward. Such unintentional owner rewards are a feature of virtually all of these cases, even those in which the owners sometimes react correctly by scolding the dog for its aggression. Unfortunately, the price paid for such short-term, partly-successful calming or distraction measures is a progressive increase in the severity of the problem over time.

While not a reinforcement effect, owners may unintentionally make things worse when the dog is threatening a stranger by scolding or screaming at it in a way which is not only ineffective in suppressing the behavior, but may be misinterpreted by the dog as indicating that the owner behind it is in fact joining in the aggressive display. Another possibility here is that the dog is not as stupid as this and understands full well that the owner is "barking" at it and not the other person, but this unpleasant owner treatment adds an additional negative element to the situation which acts to intensify its aggression due to something akin to a displaced aggression effect.

Erroneous owner beliefs

"But if I train him to be friendly to strangers, will he still defend our home when we're not there or protect me when I really need protecting?" Most owners tend to have mixed feelings about aggression towards strangers. On the one hand, their dog is becoming increasingly dangerous and hard to control in the presence of strangers. But on the other hand, if they succeed in making their dog less aggressive to strangers, will it still protect home and family as effectively as it is obviously doing now? In effect, owners know they have a serious problem, but they are reluctant to do anything effective against it because they fear the dog might become too tame and lose its value as a watchdog and family protector.

Convincing owners that this fear is ungrounded can therefore be critical to maximizing compliance with the treatment recommendations. In these cases, whole-hearted compliance can only be achieved if the anxious owner can be convinced that solving this kind of inappropriate aggression problem will not affect the dog's tendency to recognize situations in which the threat to the home or family members is real and react appropriately.

Lack of basic obedience training

Not only do many owners fail to train animals not to overdo their aggressive reception of strangers, they don't train their animals at all and, accordingly, may also have other major and minor behavioral problems with them. Essentially, lack of basic obedience training which results in a dog which is difficult to control under any circumstances and owners who know next to nothing about how to train their animal to do or not to do anything is a feature of many of these cases.

Insufficient owner dominance

Sometimes owners are not in a position to control or train their dog because their relationship with it is such that all of their commands and control attempts are ignored by a dog which shows little or no respect for them under any circumstances. In effect, insufficient owner dominance results in a dog which is difficult to control, slow to obey, and difficult or impossible to reform when it is showing behavioral problems which must be reduced or eliminated. According to statistics from 47 cases involving group-defensive aggression towards strangers on the street or in the home, owners' replies to the behavior problem section of the client information form described in Chapter 6 indicated that 22 of these dogs (i.e. 46.8%) showed either moderately severe or severe dominance aggression (13 dogs) or two or more symptoms of at least a mild dominance problem (9 dogs which sometimes growled at family members to defend bed/food/toys, when brushed/dried off, when punished/scolded, etc.). Given that the mild dominance problem figure was 20% in a sample of 55 animals which displayed no major behavior problems, this is suggestive evidence for insufficient owner dominance being a contributory factor in a great many cases of aggression towards strangers.

Reinforcement/elicitation by victim

The behavior of the victim of the dog's aggression is another contributory factor which plays a role in the development of this problem. If the persons who are being threatened are separated from the dog by a fence, or if the dog is tied up, they may react to the dog's aggressive display with an aggressive display of their own – scolding the dog or perhaps threatening it with an object or throwing something at it. Persons threatened by the dog on the street may react similarly and try to end the dog's barking by frightening it. Such victim reactions may essentially confirm the dog's presumed perception of them as potentially threatening enemies who must be driven away, thereby strengthening the dog's tendency to react similarly to these types of persons in the future. And finally, if victims must stop in their tracks or turn around and walk away to avoid being bitten, this too can reinforce the dog's aggressive behavior for obvious reasons.

Apparently, some people are often barked at by dog's on the street or when visiting people's homes while others rarely have this problem. Owners generally assume that these are people who are highly fearful of dogs, and that the dog somehow senses this and reacts aggressively to it for some reason. If this is indeed the case, one would suspect that these people must be behaving differently than other people and perhaps doing something like staring worriedly or intently at the dog which it might interpret as threatening.

Social facilitation

When one dog in a family with two or more dogs begins barking at a stranger, it is likely that the others will join in too. And many owners report that in end effect, this aggression problem turns out to be infectious, with even the friendliest and least aggressive dog in the family eventually tending to also become increasingly aggressive towards strangers. Social facilitation can also lead to a kind of snowballing effect: barking stimulates barking in other dogs, and their barking stimulates the initiator and causes it to escalate its aggression.

This social facilitation effect underscores the fact that in dogs, defense is often a group activity in which members of a group join forces in a cooperative group threat display or group attack to drive intruders away. In effect, it reveals the fundamental *group-defensive* character of the kinds of behavior problems being considered.

Inadequate maintenance conditions

Many dogs which spend a great deal of time chained up outside alone become highly aggressive to strangers. One reason may be teasing or threats from passersby who take advantage of the dog's lack of mobility. Another may be so-called frustration-induced aggression due to the drastic restriction of mobility: animal experiments indicate that a common proximate cause of aggression are conditions involving the blocking or thwarting of an animal's attempt to engage in some kind of behavior or achieve some kind of desired goal. "Boredom" is also commonly cited as a contributing factor in the sense that the restricted environment and movement possibilities result in a lowering of thresholds for reacting to any and all new stimuli and cause animals to react much more strongly to them than would otherwise be the case.

Possible treatment elements

Avoid problem situations

Keeping dogs on a leash during walks when other people or the type of people which elicit aggression from the dog such as children or joggers are nearby is indispensable in most cases. Not only does this protect the safety of others, but it keeps the dog next to the owner who is then in a position to effectively intervene and suppress the aggression.

Simply keeping dogs separated from visitors is one common solution with dogs which react aggressively towards visitors in the home. Owners often express concern here that perhaps being locked away in another room when guests are in the house may make the dog even more aggressive or be psychologically harmful to it for some reason. Although the locking-in procedure usually immediately follows or occurs simultaneously with the appearance of a visitor and, therefore, might indeed tend to increase the aversiveness of visitors (and hence the dog's aggressiveness to them), this is the lesser of two evils. In general, owners should be reassured that this is a sensible response to the problem which won't psychologically harm the dog.

Correct erroneous owner beliefs

Before treatment measures are discussed, owners who have mixed feelings about correcting the problem may need to be reassured that no matter how well the dog is trained to remain non-aggressive in the presence of strangers, this does not necessarily mean that it won't defend family members if they are threatened by a hostile stranger. Dogs are good observers of human body language and behavior generally, and it is therefore reasonable to assume that they would in fact be able to easily discriminate between a friendly and hostile stranger – and react accordingly to protect family members. Basically, when owners voice this fear, it is best to take it seriously and discuss the matter at some length. For compliance is likely to suffer if the counselor cannot succeed in convincing the owner that correction of the aggression problem will not reduce the protective value of the dog in genuinely threatening situations.

Another erroneous view which some owners have is that it is normal for dogs to be aggressive to people who fear them. In this case, it is important for the counselor to firmly point out that such behavior is definitely not normal for dogs and requires correcting.

Conventional obedience training

Owners should be advised to carry out basic obedience training (either using the methods described in Chapter 8 or by attending an obedience training class) as a first step in the treatment process for several reasons. It increases owner control over the dog in all potential problem situations. It trains the dog to respond correctly to the commands which are most commonly used to countercondition the dog to behave non-aggressively in situations where they are now threatening and attacking strangers. It tends to increase owner dominance. And it teaches the owner some exceedingly valuable lessons in how specifically to train and control dogs which can be applied in most any kind of future problem situation.

Increase owner dominance

As mentioned previously, almost half the dogs presented for this problem also show dominance aggression towards owners or two or more mild dominance problem symptoms. In these cases, applying some of the recommendations from Chapter 10 can increase the owner's capability for effectively intervening and preventing or suppressing aggression.

Correct owner mistakes

As is the case with most other dog aggression problems, many owners of dogs which show group-defensive aggression towards strangers during walks or in the home have learned to rely on various kinds of calming, reassuring, or distracting measures to control the dog's aggression. Here it must be clearly explained to owners that although these measures may at times help to end aggression, they reinforce the problem behavior, will increase its future probably and intensity, and are therefore to be avoided at all costs. If owners are skeptical in this regard, simply reminding them how the problem has continued to worsen in spite of their application of these measures can help convince them.

Training in problem situations

Owners must essentially learn to react entirely differently in problem situations than they have in the past. On the one hand, they must cease doing anything which is rewarding for the dog such as petting it or distracting it with playing.

Instead, they must begin consistently punishing the aggression by, for example, severely scolding the dog or making a loud startling sound which the dog finds aversive and will eventually learn to inhibit or stop its aggressive behavior to avoid. How specifically owners should punish the dog depends on the dog, the situation, and the owners themselves. The guideline is that the owner must find some way to punish the dog severely enough to stop the aggression *immediately* and *every time it occurs* without, however, making the dog unnecessarily fearful. For most dogs, this can be achieved by having owners loudly and firmly scold the dog with much more authority than they have in the past. Hart and Hart (1985) recommend hitting the dog when no milder sort of punishment suffices. However, most other pet problem counselors prefer alternative methods (e.g. a loud startling noise) to physical punishment with dogs which ignore owner scolding because the motivation to perform the problem behavior is too high or the owner is not the type of person to be able to put much in the way of real authority behind it. In defense of Hart and Hart (1985), however, it is fair to point out that many owners have used physical punishment effectively at certain times in the past without experiencing the kind of side effects (e.g. dog will learn to fear its owner) many counselors warn against. Dogs do bite each other from time to time, and an occasional "bite" from the owner may sometimes be a highly effective way to quickly teach a dog to behave somewhat more respectfully towards him/her and in effect, set up conditions in which future scolding (without hitting) may be more effective than previously.

Animal learning research with laboratory animals clearly indicates that punishment is most effective when the animal is provided with a rewarded alternative behavior which it can perform instead of the punished behavior. In effect, simply punishing a behavior is a far less effective means of lowering its future probability than is combining the punishment with a counterconditioning procedure to reward and thereby strengthen a competing behavior (i.e. another behavior that the animal can only perform instead of and not in combination with the punished behavior).

Basically, owners must do more than just punish problem barking and growling, they must also learn to notice and reward – with petting and, initially, also with food rewards – quiet, non-aggressive behavior in the presence of strangers. There are several ways in which this can be done. One can simply begin periodically rewarding the dog for remaining quiet during the few minutes after punishment has temporarily suppressed the problem behavior. Alternatively, choosing a time where the animal is not so highly motivated to bark and growl, one can employ a more active training approach by giving and rewarding a few of the commands in the presence of strangers which one has been practicing with the dog when alone. In cases where the dog is not so highly motivated to continue being aggressive, and the family has made it hard and fast rule that food rewards are only given to the dog at such times, this can be a highly effective method to get and keep the dog out of an aggressive mood and essentially begin conditioning more acceptable behavior in the presence of strangers.

Many behavior counselors also recommend the use of a distraction or *early intervention method* to facilitate the counterconditioning process. With this method, a loud or unusual sound is used to distract the dog in potential problem situations just at the moment when the dog notices the stranger. This essentially redirects the dog's attention towards the owner who can then call it and reward it for some desirable alternative behavior like sitting down, lying down, or staying *before it begins being aggressive.* Timing is therefore of paramount importance here. If the owner interrupts and distracts the animal before it has even noticed the potential target, the problem may be prevented but the animal will obviously not have learned anything useful from the experience. But if one waits too long and the animal is already barking at the stranger, it will be the problem barking which is being reinforced.

After repeating this procedure many times, the loud or unusual sound used by the owner to distract the dog or attract its attention comes to function as what is referred to by experimental psychologists as a *discriminative stimulus* which essentially signals to the dog the availability of food rewards for other behavior. Ideally, after successfully employing this procedure for several weeks, the sound may no longer be necessary. By then, the appearance of the stranger itself may have also become a discriminative stimulus signaling the availability of food rewards for some specific desirable behavior like going to the owner and sitting down. When, for example, a dog which has formerly chased joggers is always distracted from orienting towards a jogger it has just noticed and then called and rewarded with tidbits for coming, it may eventually become accustomed to looking around for the owner and then running expectantly to him/her without having been called as soon as it sees a jogger. Therefore if successful, the method has the potential of changing the nature of the dog's reaction towards and presumed perception of the former target of its aggression. Instead of being a threatening intruder which must be driven away, the stranger may become something much more positive to the dog – a sign or signal indicating that one of the best things in life is soon to come.

Naturally, how specifically these kind of training principles are put into practice differ greatly depending, for example, on whether the problem involves aggression towards approaching strangers on the street or visitors in the home. Outdoors there is usually more space, and when the owner chooses areas for walks which facilitate this kind of training, approaching strangers can be detected at a distance which makes it relatively easy to elicit the desired alternative behavior from the dog before it has become aggressively aroused. In the home, however, there is little space and everything happens too quickly: the doorbell rings and the dog is racing barking towards the door before the owner has time to react in any way. In this situation, the treatment emphasis must usually be placed solely on punishment-produced suppression of aggressive behavior combined with frequent rewarding of the dog for remaining quiet in the presence of visitors.

Systematic behavior therapy methods

For severe cases or those in which the physical constraints of the surrounding neighborhood are not conducive to improving the dog's behavior during the normal walks, some kind of behavioral therapy method could be devised to carry out this training at special times, in a special setting, and in a special way. One might, for example, drive twice a day to a local park and practice quiet non-aggressive obedience behavior in the presence of passing strangers at a location which has been specially chosen for these sessions (i.e. very open, just the right distance away from the pathway used by passing strangers, not too many dogs or other distractions, etc.). Over time, the distance to the path can then be gradually decreased, the training can be carried out in a series of locations which involve increasing closer proximity to strangers, more strangers, more distractions, and so on. An extendible or unusually long leash can also be used to train a dog that is presently too dangerous to be let loose to come back to the owner from some distance away when called at the time a stranger is sighted.

Similarly, in some extremely severe cases of aggression towards visitors in the home, the dog's reaction may be so intense that the application of aggression-suppressing punishment measures when a visitor walks in through the door is not effective. Here too, it may sometimes be useful to work out and apply a special behavioral therapy method which allows the dog to be gradually trained to react differently under these circumstances.

One method commonly described in the pet behavior problem literature is to arrange for a series of practice visits by someone playing the part of a visiting stranger. This can first be a family friend or neighbor the dog knows well who rings the doorbell, comes in and takes his/her coat off, and sits down in the living room several times during daily practice sessions. Starting at the time the doorbell rings, the dog is commanded to sit or lie down, and then is periodically rewarded for staying (and remaining quiet) in a particular place or for following other commands which have been

SAMPLE RECOMMENDATIONS

Group-defensive aggression towards human strangers

Scenario A: *where owner can safely scold or physically punish the dog to effectively stop aggression towards strangers in the home:*

- Barking and growling at strangers in the home should always be scolded or otherwise punished severely enough so that the dog *immediately* stops *every single time* it is punished. It should be scolded/punished just at the moment it *begins* being aggressive.
- Generously reward the dog for good behavior (i.e. quiet, non-aggressive, friendly, obedient) with petting, praise, and most especially food tidbits in situations where the aggression often or sometimes occurs. Outside of these situations, don't give the dog any tidbits at all.
- Avoid unintentionally rewarding the aggressive behavior towards visitors by trying to bring it under control using calming or distracting tactics like, for example, petting the dog, talking to it, picking it up, or distracting it with a bone, toy, or playing.
- The dog should be muzzled in the presence of visitors until the problem has been completely solved. *(Particularly appropriate in cases where dog especially unpredictable, attacking guests quickly and without warning after showing no signs of aggression for some time)*

Scenario B: *where owner can safely scold or physically punish the dog to effectively stop aggression towards strangers during walks:*

- The dog should wear some kind of choke collar or head collar during walks so that you will be able to physically control it. If it tries again to attack someone, you must have enough physical control over it to hold or pull it back. *(Required in cases where pure physical control of an aggressive dog is a problem)*
- The dog should be muzzled in situations like riding on the subway where close contact with strangers is unavoidable.
- Initially, the dog should always be kept on a leash in potential problem situations during walks so that it is physically controllable and always near enough to you so you can take steps to end its barking.
- Barking and growling at strangers on the street should always be severely enough scolded or otherwise punished by a severe "No!", a sharp tug on the leash, or a startling noise so that it *immediately* stops *every single time* it is punished. The right moment to punish it is just when it *begins* being aggressive.
- Generously reward the dog for good behavior (i.e. quiet, non-aggressive, friendly, obedient) with petting, praise, and most especially food tidbits in the presence of the types of strangers towards whom it is often aggressive. Outside of these special training situations, don't give the dog any tidbits at all.
- Avoid unintentionally rewarding the aggressive behavior by trying to bring it under control using calming or distracting tactics like, for example, petting the dog, talking to it, picking it up, or distracting it with a bone, toy, or playing.
- However, it is acceptable and often advisable to distract the dog by, for example, calling it or giving it a command *before* it begins actually being aggressive towards an approaching stranger in order to elicit and then reward acceptable behavior when the stranger is passing by.

(In cases where it is desirable to sometimes let the dog run free or clients are unwilling to keep it on a leash, some additional recommendations for training the dog to come more quickly and reliably when called during walks may also be appropriate).

thoroughly practiced often during the few days prior to the visitor training. If the dog becomes aggressive at any time, it is scolded or otherwise punished intensely enough to immediately suppress the aggression. When the dog is performing well, the visitor can then be a neighbor the dog knows less well but still well enough so that the aggression which is elicited will be less intense and more readily controllable than in the case of a complete stranger. Finally, other people whom the dog doesn't know at all can be recruited to play the visitor role.

An entirely different sort of special training method to cope with aggression towards strange visitors in the home is suggested by Hart and Hart (1985): one attempts to condition the dog to "like" strangers by having family members totally ignore the dog by withholding all attention, petting, and playing from it except when visitors are present. As soon as a stranger has entered the house, however, the dog is petted, talked to, and given food rewards often – particularly from the stranger if the dog will accept such things from him/her. Naturally, when first applying this method, many friends are contacted and asked to help so that many visits take place during the first few days of the procedure.

Theoretically at least, this method could be extremely effective if it were to be consistently applied over a long enough period of time. But the problem is, of course, that many or most owners are unwilling to treat their dog in this way. Compliance with recommendations can be problematic under the best of circumstances, but where the recommendations require that owners basically stop interacting with the dog entirely for days or perhaps even weeks on end, the compliance problem is likely to be insurmountable. While the various other methods described above may not have the same potential for getting the dog to really "love visitors" – which is the stated goal of the Hart and Hart (1985) method – they too can be very effective without demanding that owners treat their dogs in ways which they (the owners) find distasteful, unethical, or psychologically impossible to consistently implement.

Physical aids to control aggression/dog

If problems occur during walks, owners are advised to keep the dog on a leash in all potential problem situations in which it is likely that the dog will come in contact with the types of strangers which elicit aggression. This protects other people and keeps the dog physically close to the owner so that the aggression can be effectively suppressed. Muzzling is another option for times in which it is desirable to let the dog run free to play with other dogs. In cases where physical control of an aggressive dog is a problem even when it is on the leash – as it often is with large dogs owned by not so large women or elderly persons – some additional aids to control such as collars which tighten uncomfortably when the dog strains on the leash or so-called head collars which also do something uncomfortable for the straining dog like pulling its head to the side may be essential.

In the home, keeping the dog on a leash or muzzling it in the presence of visitors is often advisable. Although the barking and growling is not prevented, the fact that the dog is prevented from biting allows both owner and guest to relax much more than would otherwise be the case, and this in turn may allow the owner to concentrate more effectively on remedial training measures which might eventually make the leash or muzzle unnecessary.

Group-defensive aggression towards familiar human beings

Group-defensive aggression can be more personal as a result of the dog's repeated encounters with particular neighbors who pass by yard regularly, neighborhood children who live on the same street, owners of other pets who are often encountered during walks, or people who regularly approach the home like mailmen. Essentially, enemy-like relationships can develop between the dog and particular people to the extent that the dog reacts more aggressive to them than it does to complete strangers.

The development of this problem can take several forms. Victims may be angered by the dog's barking and react with threatening gestures, shouting, or throwing something – which tends to increase the dog's aggression towards them. Another possibility which produces the same effect is teasing, usually by children. The dog's barking attracts the children's attention, and provoking it becomes a game which is repeated every day on the way home from school. If a person reacts usually fearfully to the dog, this too can provoke increased aggression which is elicited every time the two meet. Why particularly fearful people appear to be so often threatened by group-defensive aggressive dogs is not clear. As discussed previously, one suspects that such people stare more intensely at the dog than others or otherwise behave strangely from the dog's perspective. A final example involves the owners of neighborhood dogs with which the dog has had problems in the past. In trying to prevent or break up fights, other owners may directly confront the dog by scolding it, or their attempts to pull or keep the dogs apart may have involved some other type of behavior which is threatening to the dog.

Understanding and treating such problems is not much different than in cases involving complete strangers. However, there is the additional potentially very important element here of possible modifications in the victim's behavior. The parents of the teasing children can be talked to. And those regular passersby who react either fearfully or aggressively to the dog can be talked to and convinced that the best approach to the problem is to simply not react to the dog's threats, for ignoring such reactions can mean eliminating possible eliciting stimuli or sources of reinforcement which have been maintaining or strengthening the behavior.

Self-protective aggression towards human strangers

As discussed earlier, there are several reasons why the term *self-protective aggression* seems preferable to the conventional label of fear aggression for problems where animals reactive defensively by growling and/or snapping when approached closely, reached for, or touched by a person. In the first place, self-protection is a straightforward description of the biological function of the behavior and, therefore, superior on this count alone to the fear aggression label. Secondly, fearful body postures, facial expressions, and general escape/avoidance behavioral tendencies may also be seen in connection with other types of defensive aggression problems or, conversely, be highly abbreviated and difficult to detect in the cases of some "fear biters" which appear friendly to strangers but snap when touched. Thirdly, a self-protective aggression category also subsumes aggressive reactions towards aversive stimuli like, for example, punishment- or pain-elicited aggression towards strangers whom the dog did not fear prior to the incident. This makes good biological sense: here too the dog is reacting both aggressively and fearfully to what it obviously perceives as immediate threat to its personal safety. And finally, the self-protective label is advantageous in that it emphasizes the solitary nature of the aggressive behavior which, in contrast to group-defensive aggression, seems to lack a pronounced social facilitation element.

As in the case of self-protective aggression towards family members considered in the last chapter, the various types of self-protective aggression scenarios involving human strangers can be summarized with the following sort of scheme:

- Elicited by genuinely *aversive stimuli* from strangers which can range from painful or intensely fear-arousing events such as being attacked to being grabbed or restrained by the person.
- *Fear-related aggression* elicited by the approach of or touching by a feared person involving one of the following:
  - Fear of *particular individuals* acquired as a result of having been threatened or mistreated by them in the past,
  - Fear of *all strangers* reflecting lack of experience early in life interacting with unfamiliar human beings.
  - Fear of *particular types of strangers* (e.g. children, men, darkly-clothed men with canes, etc.) due either to past aversive experiences with these types of people or insufficient experience with them during the first 3 or 4 months of life.

POSSIBLE CAUSAL FACTORS

Restricted early experience
(possible source of fear of strangers/
types of strangers)

Elicitation/reinforcement by victims
(victim aggression can increase fear/fear-
aggression; victim stopping/retreating when
threatened reinforces aggression)

Genetic predisposition
(some dogs more fearful or have lower
growling/biting thresholds than others
for genetic reasons)

Fear-/pain-eliciting experiences
(fear acquired as result of fear-/pain-
eliciting experiences with strangers in past)

Unintentional owner reinforcement
(e.g. owner reacts to aggression with
petting, reassurance, distraction with
playing, tidbits, etc.)

SELF-PROTECTIVE AGGRESSION TOWARDS HUMAN STRANGERS

- Aggression towards human strangers when approached too closely, reached for, touched, cornered, etc.

POSSIBLE TREATMENT ELEMENTS

Avoid problem situations
(avoid taking the dog into situations where
close contact with strangers unavoidable;
advise people not to touch dog; do not
leave dog unattended in public)

Correct owner mistakes
(e.g. stop unintentionally rewarding
aggression; punishment of aggression
sometimes contraindicated)

Systematic behavior therapy methods
(e.g. desensitization/counterconditioning
using "practice approaches" by feared
persons; flooding)

Physical aids
(e.g. muzzle dog when contact with
strangers unavoidable)

Training in problem situations
(possible owner scolding of aggression
and/or rewarding non-aggressive behavior
towards strangers in some cases)

Conventional obedience training
(increases owner control in potential
problem situations)

Increase owner dominance
(increases owner control in potential
problem situations)

Possible causal factors

Restricted early experience

Fear of strangers resulting in self-protective aggression can sometimes be traced back to a lack of experience with a variety of unfamiliar human beings – or certain types of human beings – during the first 3 months of the dog's life. It is important to explore this possibility when questioning owners, for such fearful tendencies are particularly resistant to modification and the prognosis and approach to treatment can therefore be substantially different than in the case of fear which was acquired at some later time.

Fear-/pain-eliciting experiences

Although knowing when and how fear acquired later in life developed may not be critical to determining how the problem should be treated, it can certainly help to assess the severity and possible modifiability of the problem. In general, the prognosis is most favorable when the animal's fearfulness is not too intense and of recent origin.

Elicitation/reinforcement by victims

The behavior of the victim is always relevant in self-protective aggression cases. Pain-elicited aggression towards veterinarians who touch a painful area on an animal's body is an obvious example. Likewise, a common scenario is where a person who is unaware that the dog is fearful of strangers reaches for or touches it when it is tied on a leash outside a supermarket. Another is when a stranger walks by too close to where the animal is lying (e.g. under a restaurant table) without even seeing it. In both situations, the animal has little room to maneuver and easily feels cornered.

Victim behavior can also affect the problem in other ways. He/she may react aggressively to being threatened by trying to frighten or punish the dog, which is likely to produce an escalation of the aggression and perhaps greater fear of the person and other similar persons in future. And when victims immediately withdraw by pulling their hand back or stepping away in response to growling or snapping, this reinforces the dog's aggression and thereby helps to maintain or strengthen the dog's tendency to react aggressively under similar circumstances.

Unintentional owner reinforcement

As is the case with most aggression problems, owners often make the mistake of petting, reassuring, or trying to distract the dog when it reacts aggressively to a stranger. These owner reactions are another possible source of positive reinforcement which can greatly affect the problem.

Genetic predisposition

Some dogs are much more fearful than others under a variety of circumstances. In some cases, there is nothing out of the ordinary in the dog's history such as restricted early experience or negative experiences later in life to account for this. In addition, some dogs seem much less inhibited about growling and snapping at anything which disturbs them than other dogs even though owners have not been unusually permissive in this regard. In effect, genetic differences between dogs in fearfulness or aggression thresholds may sometimes account for why some dogs show self-protective aggression in situations which most other dogs tolerate without becoming aggressive.

Possible treatment elements

Avoidance of problem situations

Since these dogs do not go out of their way to bite human beings, avoiding problem situations usually amounts to the owner's (1) avoiding certain kinds of key situations like dense crowds, or restaurants where it is inevitable that the dog will be in close physical proximity to unfamiliar human beings, (2) refraining from leaving the dog unattended (e.g. tied up outside a supermarket) where someone might approach and try to pet it, or (3) explaining to guests, children, other pet owners, etc. that it is not safe to try and touch the dog.

Physical aids to control aggression

In situations where physical contact with unfamiliar persons cannot be avoided or controlled by the owner, muzzling the dog is a sensible approach. Most German clients do not like to do this because it causes their dogs to be stared at by persons in public and because they themselves are sometimes berated by strangers for "mistreating" the animal. Nevertheless, in some cases it is the ideal solution to how to avoid problems in specific situations. Dogs certainly don't like wearing muzzles, but they get used to wearing them. By putting the muzzle on just before much-loved walks, and perhaps by giving the dog clearly more than the normal amount of attention when wearing the muzzle, owners can help counteract the dog's negative reaction to it.

Correct owner mistakes

There are two common mistakes which must be avoided. The first is punishing fear-related aggression so severely that one essentially adds fear of punishment to the animal's fear of strangers – and makes the problem worse. The second mistake is doing something positive which might function to reward and strengthen the behavior when the dog is growling or has just snapped at someone.

Training in problem situations

While many behavior counselors rule out in principle the use of punitive measures in all self-protective aggression cases, this may be going too far. Although one certainly doesn't want to do anything which might substantially increase the animal's underlying fear, there are some cases in which animals are abnormally quick to react aggressively towards strangers whom they do not appear to find all that threatening. In these cases in particular, it may be a mistake to let the aggression occur unchecked without trying to give the animal some

sort of clear message of owner disapproval, which might strengthen the animal's tendency to inhibit aggression in future. Then too, given that the owner is not the feared person, the risk that unpleasant owner scolding is going to substantially increase the dog's already deep-seated suspicion or fear of unfamiliar persons may be minimal. In short, sometimes the benefits to be gained by having owners exercise their authority over the dog to teach it to inhibit aggression in all but those situations in which its fear is genuinely intense outweigh the potential risk of this kind of owner reaction causing an increment in the dog's fear.

There is another somewhat more psychological factor operating in many of these cases. Owners who know that their animal reacts unusually fearfully compared to other dogs in a variety of situations often have a tendency to feel sorry for it, not be as irritated and impatient with it as the normal owner might, and most importantly, be much more hesitant to be strict with the dog and use scolding and other punitive measures to control its behavior. It is often the case, therefore, that a dog which reacts fearfully in one type of situation becomes a problem in a wide variety of other situations as well because owners are just not as strict with it as they might be with a normal, non-fearful animal. In general, it is probably best to advise owners of all fearful dogs that it is better where possible (i.e. in all situations in which it is not specifically contraindicated) to treat the dog as one would treat any other dog and expect from it the same kind of obedience and inhibition of problem behavior. In many cases, this implies that it is appropriate to emphasize to owners that fear or no fear, dogs must be trained to behave acceptably in a human-oriented environment with human-oriented requirements and human-oriented prohibitions by employing a balanced combination of rewards for desirable behavior and punishment for undesirable behavior.

In summary, although owners who tend towards being overly heavy-handed with their dog, and those whose punishment of a highly fearful dog for reacting aggressively towards strangers is obviously making the problem worse, should be advised in no uncertain terms to stop punishing the dog at this time, there are many cases in which carefully dosed owner scolding may help increase the dog's inhibition of aggression without substantially increasing the severity of the underlying fear problem.

This lengthy discussion of the rather complex issue of whether or not punitive measures are appropriate in the treatment of self-protective aggression is only one side of the coin. The other concerns what sorts of positive measures owners might apply in potential problem situations to help reduce the severity of these problems. The fact that the aggression is directed towards strangers who approach the dog or try to pet it often makes it difficult to devise some kind of informal counterconditioning procedure which can be used during everyday life to gradually train the dog to react non-aggressively in potential problem situations. Nevertheless, it is possible to use this kind of approach in certain cases. For example, where dogs sometimes tolerate petting from guests and sometimes not, one can recommend that the owner ask guests who wish to pet the dog to offer it a few tidbits before trying to pet it, then only slowly react out their hand and touch the dog's head while offering it a tidbit, and only later give it tidbits while petting it lightly and briefly.

Systematic behavior therapy methods

There are two possible behavior therapy approaches to the self-protective aggression problem. The first is a straightforward application of the desensitization/counterconditioning procedure using a series of staged practice approaches by the person or type of person the dog fears. The person approaches repeatedly, and stops at a certain prespecified distance away from the dog while the owner rewards the dog with a food tidbit for relaxed, non-fearful behavior. The person is instructed to come no closer to the dog each time than the dog has learned to tolerate without showing any signs of fear or uneasiness. As the animal learns to remain relaxed when the person approaches to a certain distance, the distance can be gradually

reduced until finally the dog can be closely approached and perhaps even lightly touched and petted by the feared person. If carried out correctly, the dog never becomes fearful during the entire process.

This behavior therapy procedure is potentially most useful when the animal fears only one specific person or type of person (e.g. blond girls between 5 and 10 years old). Here practicing with a number of blond girls of this age might produce results which would transfer to other similar children. However, when the dog fears all strangers or all unfamiliar men, the procedure is less useful. While the fear of certain individuals might be reduced during the training sessions, transfer to other strangers or unfamiliar men is likely to be a problem.

The second behavior therapy method is *flooding*. It can be used if there is some way to more or less continuously expose the dog to the type of person it fears for several hours at a time. If, for example, the dog reacts fearfully to strangers in crowds, the owner could spend several hours with the dog in one of the main passageways of a bustling shopping center (with the dog muzzled) where the dog could be exposed to hundreds of closely approaching strangers per hour. The key to the proper application of this method is that the owner must remain long enough in the situation each and every time for the dog's fear to have substantially diminished, which can sometimes take several hours. (See Chapter 15 for details concerning the flooding procedure and its applications and limitations.)

In summary, although systematic behavior therapy procedures to counteract self-protective aggression towards strangers may be feasible in certain specific types of cases, these methods are extremely time-consuming, difficult for owners to implement correctly, difficult for owners to arrange and coordinate given that persons unfamiliar to the dog must be involved in the training, and often lack the necessary generalization to ensure that the dog no longer represents a danger to the types of strangers it will encounter in the future. In short, such behavior therapy procedures are useful from time to time, but they do not offer

SAMPLE RECOMMENDATIONS

Self-protective aggression towards human strangers

Scenario A: *animal's fear when approached or touched by strangers probably cannot be substantially reduced, and the recommendations therefore focus on preventing aggression by other means.*

• The dog should always be muzzled when taken into situations like a crowded restaurant, around young children, or when using public transportation where close physical contact with strangers is unavoidable.

• There is no way to completely eliminate the dog's deep-seated mistrust, fear, or dislike of strangers. It will therefore always be necessary for you to caution guests in your home or strangers who approach the dog on the street not to suddenly reach for, touch, pet, or too closely approach the dog.

• Either carry out daily obedience training at home or attend an obedience training class. This will give you more control over the dog in situations where it might become aggressive to strangers. (*Some additional recommendations to increase owner dominance may also be helpful in this regard.*)

• Refrain from unintentionally rewarding aggression towards human beings by responding to the dog's growling/snapping by, for example, petting it, talking to it, picking it up, or distracting it with a bone, toy, or playing. Although such measures may seem to work at the time, in the long run they make the problem worse.

• Growling and snapping at human beings should always be severely scolded. (*Appropriate in cases where this is likely to be beneficial in training the dog to inhibit aggression without substantially increasing its fear of strangers.*)

Scenario B: *the problem is fairly mild with the dog only sometimes reacting fearfully and aggressively towards strangers.*

• Generously reward the dog with petting, praise, and most especially food rewards for good behavior (i.e. not acting fearfully or aggressively) in the presence of the kind of strangers towards which it is sometimes aggressive. Outside of these situations, don't give the dog any tidbits at all.

• Fearful behavior without aggression should always be completely ignored; that is, all petting, talking to, looking at, distracting, picking up, etc. of the dog when it shows signs of fear should be stopped.

• As far as training, controlling, or scolding the dog is concerned, view it as being entirely normal and treat it accordingly. Among other things this means that growling and snapping at human beings should always be severely scolded.

practical and genuinely effective solutions to the vast majority of these cases.

Conventional obedience training

If a dog has been well-trained to reliably come, sit, lie down, and stay on command, the owner is in a position to be able to control the animal's movements in certain potential problem situations and thereby often prevent problems entirely.

Increase owner dominance

Measures for increasing owner dominance may also be important for similar reasons. A dog which shows, for example, a conflicting tendency to approach strangers in an apparently friendly way but then snaps when reached for must be kept away from them, which is difficult for owners to do with dominant dogs which are often slow to obey or downright disobedient.

Intraspecific versus interspecific aggression

As we have considered previously, most dogs in some sense "imprint" on humans early in life, they grow up as a member of a human social group, their daily contact with other dogs is comparatively limited, and they live with their owners in a world populated primarily with human beings. It is not surprising therefore that this combination of continuous social contact with human beings, early imprinting, and partial deprivation of contact with conspecifics facilitates the elicitation of intraspecific social behavior by human beings. In effect, most domestic dogs behave towards human beings to some extent as if they were other dogs, and all of the aggression problems which have been considered in this chapter and the last assume that the dog is in some significant sense perceiving and responding to human family members or strangers as conspecifics.

But imagine how a dog which grew up in a pack situation in the wild without any contact at all with human beings might react in the self-protective problem situations which are being considered. Here, it seems reasonable to take the extremely fearful and aggressive reactions elicited by humans who approach or try to handle dogs which have always lived wild or been experimentally isolated from all contact with humans during the first few months of life (Scott and Fuller, 1965; numerous studies cited in Fox and Bekoff, 1985, and Voith and Borchelt, 1985) as a model for *interspecific* self-protective behavior. In practice, the issue of whether forms of defensive aggression towards human beings are fundamentally intra- or inter-species behavior may therefore relate directly to the source of the animal's underlying fear of human beings. In particular, it seems fair to assume that dogs which have always been in close contact with humans from birth onwards basically perceive humans as conspecifics and, hence, all aggression towards them can be rightly considered to be one or another of the intraspecific forms of aggression. On the other hand, where the aggression is a manifestation of intense and apparently irreversible fear which is clearly related to the absence of the kinds of early experiences during the first 3–4 months of life – which are regarded by animal behaviorists as being critical to determining species identification and therefore the later focus of adult social behavior – then fundamentally interspecific aggression may at least in part be involved.

The well-known example of dogs displaying the "kennelosis" syndrome may represent something of an in-between case. On the one hand, fear of strangers is extremely intense and the dog may behave during walks as if it is being forced by its owner to move about in a world full of potentially dangerous predators. And yet, the behavior of the dog towards family members may not be different than that of any normal dog. The question is, of course, how such a dramatic difference in the behavior and inferred perception of human beings is indeed possible, for any simple conception of lack of species identification due to extremely restricted early experiences would predict an all-or-none result. One possible explanation may be that the "world full of dangerous predators" assumption is unjustified. That is, the dog has in fact experienced the minimum amount of contact with humans required for normal human-directed social behavior, but the lack of contact with unfamiliar human beings has resulted in the dog placing them in that totally alien and therefore threatening category to which traffic noises belong for a dog that has spent its early months in a relatively isolated rural environment. In effect, the tendency to react fearfully to anything and everything unfamiliar overrides whatever tendency the dog might have to approach and interact with a conspecific. Of course, this view would be consistent with the observation of how quickly and completely some of these animals can lose their fear of familiar human beings.

As far as the treatment of specific behavior problems is concerned, this speculative discussion is of academic interest only. Whether it is a case of restricted early experiences resulting in a dog which can live normally within a human family in spite of its deep-seated fear of unfamiliar human beings or, alternatively, virtually complete isolation from human beings early in life comparable to that in the Scott and Fuller studies resulting in a dog that will never be able to perceive and behave towards even familiar human beings as conspecifics, the prognosis for any kind of resolution of the underlying fear problem must be the same: only the most limited sorts of progress are possible. And as far as the ability to become a normal pet is concerned, the dog must be regarded as irreversibly damaged.

References

Borchelt, P.L., and Voith, V.L. (1982): Classification of animal behavior problems. *Veterinary Clinics of North America: Small Animal Practice* **12**, 571–585.

Fox, M.W., and Bekoff, M. (1975): The Behaviour of Dogs. In E.S.E Hafez (ed.), *The Behaviour of Domestic Animals*, 3rd Edition. London: Bailliere Tindall.

Hart, B. L., and Hart, L.A. (1985): *Canine and Feline Behavior Therapy*. Philadelphia, Lea & Febiger.

O'Farrell V. (1992): *Manual of Canine Behaviour*. British Small Animal Veterinary Association. Shurdington, Cheltenham, Gloucestershire, UK.

Scott, J.P, and Fuller, J.L. (1965): *Genetics and Social Behavior of the Dog*. Chicago: Chicago University Press.

Voith, V.L. (1989): Behavioral disorders. In Ettinger, S. (ed): *Textbook of Veterinary Internal Medicine*. Philadelphia, WB Saunders.

Voith, V.L., and Borchelt, P.L. (1985): Fears and phobias in companion animals. *Compendium on Continuing Education for the Practicing Veterinarian* **7**, 209–221.

13 Other Forms of Aggression Towards Human Beings

Play aggression towards human family members

The aggressive play of some dogs can be a problem for family members. The dogs charge at owners during walks, jump up at them, nip at their hands, and bite and tug on their pants legs. If the victim is a young child who becomes frightened, starts crying, and tries to run away, or a frail elderly person who becomes flustered and tries to push the dog away or swat it, the behavior of the victim may stimulate the dog to intensify the attack. Basically, being caught up in an aggressive game which it is highly motivated to play – and perhaps being a rather active, unruly type to begin with – anything the owner does in response to the aggressive behavior other than the most severe type of scolding may be misinterpreted by the dog as playful (Voith 1989).

While in many cases owners are fully aware that the dog is just being playful, sometimes they are not so sure. In one of my cases, a young cocker spaniel was on the verge of being euthanized for its playful aggression towards the family's 4-year-old boy because both the family veterinarian and owner suspected that this was one of those especially dangerous, unicolored cockers that they had heard about. Simply explaining to owners that such rough play is normal for many dogs – and that victim reactions may be misinterpreted by the dog as playful – helps them to understand both the behavior and the reasons for the kinds of recommendations which are necessary to control it.

Possible causal factors

Genetic predisposition

These dogs tend to be highly active, extremely playful, and show a strong preference for the more aggressive types of play – presumably for genetic reasons.

Inadequate care/maintenance conditions

Dogs which are highly motivated to play in some sense need to play. And if they are deprived of the opportunity to play with other dogs, they have no other choice but to direct their play and play invitation behavior towards human beings. For some dogs, the play aggression problem is therefore a symptom that the dog's basic play and related activity and social needs are not being satisfactorily met.

Unintentional owner fostering

Before the behavior becomes a problem, owners may have played with the dog often and perhaps even encouraged the dog to play aggressively by play-fighting or playing games like tug of war in which the dog's strength and tenacity are pitted directly against that of the owner.

Unintentional owner reinforcement

Each time the owner joins into a game which the dog has initiated, this reinforces the dog's behavior and makes it more likely that it will try to initiate playing in this way in future. Trying to cope with the dog's increasingly bothersome attempts to initiate play by giving in and doing what it wants can therefore be a serious mistake. Another mistake of this general type is to try to end playful aggression by throwing a toy or giving it a tidbit to distract the dog. This may indeed stop the assault at the time. However, it may essentially train the dog to be even more aggressive in future for obvious reasons.

POSSIBLE CAUSAL FACTORS

Genetic predisposition
(e.g. to be highly active/playful)

Inadequate care/maintenance conditions
(lack of exercise/opportunities to play with
other dogs)

Unintentional owner fostering
(playing aggressive or competitive games
with dog like chasing, tug of war, play-
fighting, etc.)

Unintentional owner reinforcement
(playing with dog in response to its
play soliciting behavior; distraction control
measures)

Victim elicitation/stimulation
(victim pulling away, chasing, or trying
to hit dog intensifies dog's assaults)

Lack of appropriate training
(e.g. to inhibit unacceptable behavior on
command)

Lack of owner dominance
(dog disobedient/hard to control in many
situations due to dominance-related
problem)

Erroneous owner beliefs
(e.g. assumption that aggression potentially
dangerous or symptomatic of disease
prevents effective remedial action)

PLAY AGGRESSION

• Playful aggression which is a problem for family members

POSSIBLE TREATMENT ELEMENTS

Correct erroneous owner beliefs
(e.g. explain that dog not showing
dangerous form of aggression)

Changing care/maintenance conditions
(provide more opportunities for
exercise/play with other dogs)

Avoid problem situations
(e.g. don't play with dog at all)

Correct owner mistakes
(stop unintentionally rewarding problem
behavior; stop fostering/eliciting aggressive
play)

**Cessation of ineffective treatment
methods**
(e.g. ineffective scolding; chasing dog
to try and hit it)

Conventional obedience training
(to increase dog's obedience and teach
owner how to control/train dog)

Increase owner authority
(e.g. be more strict with dog)

Training in problem situations
(combination of punishing problem behavior
with eliciting/promoting acceptable games)

**Change owner-dog interactive
ground rules**
(to increase owner dominance)

Victim elicitation/stimulation

By the time the dog's aggressive play has reached a stage where it is no longer tolerable, owners discover that there is seemingly little they can do to stop it. The dog ignores the owner's refusal to play and is even stimulated to more intense play by scolding and attempts to chase and swat it. And if the owner becomes fearful and tries to pull or go away, the game enters what may seem from the dog's point of view to be a new and even more enjoyable stage. In short, when things have developed this far, anything relatively mild the owner does to combat the problem just makes it worse.

Lack of appropriate training

Owners with these kinds of undisciplined, uncontrollable dogs are often those which have been permissive for the first few months of the dog's life by more or less accepting the dog's unruly behavior like jumping up on the furniture, barking demandingly, or tugging at clothing or hands to get what it wants as normal rather than actively combating it. In comparison, owners who from the start have both a strong conception of how the dog must be trained to behave – for example, to have enough respect for a sharply uttered "No!" to immediately stop whatever it is doing – and the determination to train the dog to be this way have little difficulty in coping with an animal whose playful aggression is becoming a problem.

Lack of owner dominance

The dog's disobedience and uncontrollability in the play-aggression situation can also reflect more general disobedience and control difficulties which are symptomatic of a dominance problem between the dog and family members.

Erroneous owner beliefs

Sometimes owners are fully capable of coping with the problem, but have not taken the obvious steps to do so simply because they didn't recognize the basically playful nature of the behavior. Essentially, assuming or fearing that the dog is becoming dangerously aggressive, or is exhibiting signs of some medical or psychological disorder, prevents the application of effective problem-solving measures.

Possible treatment elements

Correct erroneous owner beliefs

It must be explained to owners that it is normal for some dogs to play in an aggressive way, it is common for most dogs to play like this with other dogs, and therefore any fears they might have that the dog is showing a potentially dangerous form of aggression, exhibiting disturbed or neurotic behavior, or displaying symptoms of some pathophysiological disorder are unfounded. This reduces owner anxiety and establishes the right perspective to enable owners to understand the logic of the various treatment elements which are required to solve this highly treatable problem.

Changing maintenance conditions

Owners of playfully aggressive dogs should be closely questioned about what sort of opportunities the dog is being given daily to run or play with other dogs. If these are insufficient, owners should be strongly urged to find a way to give the dog what it needs. It should also be explained to them that when the animal is deprived of opportunities for much-needed exercise and play in normal settings (i.e. outside with other dogs), it has no choice but to make do with what it has and drive family members crazy with its unruly behavior and continuous pestering for play.

Avoid problem situations

One possible approach in some cases is for the owner to refuse to play with the dog at all. This is particularly so in cases where playing starts out on a kind of mild, innocent level and then gradually becomes more aggressive and difficult to stop when the owner has finally had enough. Providing that the dog has sufficient opportunity to play with other dogs once or twice a day, it is likely that it will accept the owner's lack of interest in playing quickly and easily.

Correct owner mistakes

An obvious mistake is for owners to engage in rough aggressive play with a dog which is becoming a problem in this regard. Owners should also understand that every time they give in and play the kind of aggressive or competitive game which the dog seems to want to play – thinking, perhaps, that this is the only way to end bothersome pestering – they are rewarding the dog's pushy, demanding behavior and aggressive style of play. Basically, it should be made a hard and fast family rule that no games of this sort should be played with the dog and all of the dog's efforts to initiate such games should either be ignored or punished.

A further mistake which needs correction is, of course, the owner's reliance on distraction tactics like throwing a ball or giving the dog a tidbit to end the aggression. These too reinforce and thereby strengthen problem behaviors.

Cessation of ineffective methods

Although owners may think that they are punishing the dog by shouting at it or running after it to try and swat it with something, this may be just the kind of game the dog really loves. Even if the owner eventually succeeds in getting close enough to the dog to actually swat it, the dog may simply accept this as being part of the game. As a general rule, effective punishment always immediately suppresses ongoing behavior. This must be clearly explained to many owners, and those who have been relying on ineffective or counterproductive punishment measures should be encouraged to either abandon them entirely or increase the effectiveness of the punishment procedure by, for example, scolding the dog with much more authority or activating some noise-making device which it finds extremely aversive.

Conventional obedience training

Playfully aggressive dogs often have permissive owners who see no particular value in training

their dog to do or not do anything. To solve the problem, this passive owner attitude must change. One approach is to have owners train their dog to sit, lie down, stay, and come when told to do so (either by using the methods described in Chapter 8 or by attending an obedience training class). As discussed previously, this kind of training not only teaches the dog something useful, but it teaches owners a very valuable lesson about how to go about controlling and modifying their dog's behavior in other contexts as well.

Increase owner authority

Another approach with some owners is to encourage them to be much stricter and firmer with the dog under all circumstances, including the play aggression situation. Sometimes this is all that is required. Armed with new insight into the playful and basically harmless nature of the problem, the owner who has been previously tolerating playful attacks out of a sense of helplessness or fear may now be able to effectively confront the dog and dramatically demonstrate to it that such behavior will no longer be tolerated. This can result in a complete, virtually instantaneous solution to the problem in some cases.

Training in problem situations

Some problems are not as easily solved as this. Owners may be unwilling or unable to take the dog to a place where it can play with other dogs every day. Or they may be the type of people who have difficulty asserting themselves with sufficient authority to make much of an impact on the dog's behavior, which results in a situation where trying to suppress the dog's playful aggression is a never-ending battle that owners can never quite seem to win. What is needed in such cases is (1) the consistent application of punishing stimuli which are strong enough to temporarily suppress the problem behavior every time it occurs combined with (2) a procedure which essentially trains the dog to engage in acceptable types of play behavior in the problem situation. One way to do this is

SAMPLE RECOMMENDATIONS

Play aggression

- The dog should always be immediately scolded or punished in some other way (e.g. with a loud startling sound) for aggressive biting of hands, legs, pants, shoes, etc.
- This scolding or other punishment should be administered just at the moment the aggressive behavior begins.
- Punishment must be severe enough to stop the problem behavior *immediately* and *every time* it is punished, but it should not be so severe that the dog becomes extremely fearful and takes some time to get over it.
- Games involving tests of strength (e.g. tug of war), direct competition between you and the dog (e.g. chasing), and play-fighting should not be played with the dog.
- As a general rule, the dog should never be allowed to take a person's hand, arm, or clothing in its mouth either playfully or to get something it wants.
- Encourage the dog to play in more acceptable ways by, for example, throwing a ball, stick, or Frisbee *before* it starts being aggressive.
- Avoid unintentionally rewarding aggression by playing with the dog or distracting it by throwing something or giving it a tidbit after it starts jumping up on you, nipping at your hands or pants legs, etc.
- Take the dog to a place at least twice a day where it can play with other dogs as long as is necessary for it to become disinterested in further play.

When the victim is a young child:

- Never leave the child alone with the dog. Even though the dog's motivation is purely playful, for the child such attacks can be extremely frightening, and potentially serious facial, eye, etc. injuries could result.

(If there is also a concurrent mild dominance problem between owner and dog, some of the recommendations from Chapter 10 should also be given. Recommending conventional obedience training may also be appropriate in the case of particularly unruly dogs.)

have the owner carry some noise-making device in potential problem situations to be able to punish the dog every time it launches an attack on clothes, arms, or legs. At the same time, the owner is instructed to try and consistently elicit other, more acceptable, but equally active forms of play like chasing a ball or Frisbee (Voith 1989). The owner must be cautioned, however, to make sure to elicit these new games *before* the animal starts being playfully aggressive – and not during or after the aggression – for otherwise something like throwing a ball may well reward and thereby strengthen the aggressive behavior.

While it may not be easy initially to decide what kind of punisher to use, what kind of alternative games to promote, and how exactly one should go about administering and timing both, owners usually have little difficulty in developing satisfactory solutions on their own. Essentially, although owners may not know immediately what kind of new game they can encourage the dog to play, if they know that they must encourage the development of a more acceptable game of some kind, they can then experiment with various possibilities and quickly find something appropriate. Obviously, the same applies to the problem of what noise-making device can be used to punish the dog. Some experimentation is often needed here too because of individual differences between dogs in their reactions to various sounds. But knowing that some such aversive sound must be found is enough: it usually doesn't take the owner long to find something effective.

Change owner-dog interactive ground rules

Sometimes questioning the owner reveals that the dog's unruliness and disobedience in the play situation is symptomatic of the existence of a mild dominance problem between owner and dog. In addition to stubbornly continuing to attack the owner in the play context in spite of scolding or commands to stop, the dog might, for example, aggressively defend toys, be slow to obey or disobedient under a variety of other circumstances, or react with growling when brushed, dried off, or lying in its bed. If such a concurrent dominance problem exists, some of the recommendations given in Chapter 10 for improving the dog-owner relationship by changing the general way the dog is treated by family members should be given to the client in addition to those for controlling the play aggression problem itself.

Redirected aggression

Borchelt and Voith (1982) define so-called redirected aggression as a "growl or bite redirected to a person or object other than that which evoked the initial aggression". In the typical scenario, a dog which is engaged in fighting with or threatening another dog bites either its owner or the owner of the other dog when the person tries to break up or prevent a fight by stepping in between, pulling the two apart, or pulling one or the other away from the fray. Dogs may also become aggressive towards their owner in situations where they are being aggressive towards human beings if, for example, the owner tries to stop the dog's growling or biting by grabbing it, restraining it, or pulling it away from the victim.

Although owners prefer to assume that

these bites happen "by accident" – that the dog is so excited that it is just biting anything than moves – close questioning of the owner concerning the dog's behavior in other situations often makes another explanation more plausible: the dog's bite is its way of telling its not-all-that-dominant owner to stop interfering in what is, from the dog's viewpoint, serious business. And potentially dangerous business, which suggests that basically a form of self-protective aggression might be involved here. For interference by the owner at this time might distract the dog or hinder its movement or defensive capabilities to the point where the other dog might temporarily gain the upper hand. Thus, the aggression would not actually be "redirected" in the psychological sense that, for example, an animal which has backed down from a fight with a superior foe might then turn and attack some less formidable group member.

Essentially, no separate aggression category appears to be required. The behavior seems primarily understandable as self-protective aggression which is usually symptomatic of a dominance problem between dog and owner: in effect, owners who have not established a position of clear dominance over the dog are much more at risk – which is also the case, for example, in the pain- and punishment-elicited aggression settings.

The fact that owners are so ready to believe that such bites (even the fifth or sixth one) are accidental is interesting. Essentially, owners have the tendency to give their basically loyal, trustworthy, and obedient dog the benefit of the doubt by assuming that it was so excited that it didn't know what it was doing. This is apparently more comforting to believe that the opposite (i.e. that the dog's bite was deliberate and intentionally directed towards them). Explaining to owners that it is not abnormal for a dog to treat other members of its pack this way in certain highly arousing and potentially dangerous circumstances can be important in most cases. And as far as compliance with the recommended treatment is concerned, it is critical to convince the owner to abandon the accident theory in favor of the more realistic view that the dog knew exactly what it was doing.

Although it is a case here of a special type of problem situation scenario in which self-protective and/or dominance-related aggression is evoked – rather than another type of aggression problem entirely – nevertheless a few treatment elements will be discussed below. Interference in aggression confrontations with other dogs is a leading cause of owners being bitten by their dogs, and it is therefore particularly important that the behavior counselor is able to provide sound advice in this regard.

Possible treatment elements

Correct owner/victim mistakes

Some anxious or overly protective owners routinely intervene in aggressive confrontations between dogs before it is really necessary – in some cases, to the point of having always prevented any sort of fighting with or even serious threatening of other dogs. In this latter case, owners may not only be running the risk of being injured, but they may also be depriving the dog of valuable social experiences which could help it to learn how to get along with and even enjoy interacting with other dogs in the neighborhood. Therefore, in some cases it is best to advise the owner to stop intervening. Even though overprotective owners are often skeptical that this is the best way for them to avoid getting bitten again – or that being allowed to fight with another dog could be in some way good for their dog – they can usually be persuaded to at least try it a few times in situations where, for example, the other dog is of equal size and not a particularly aggressive type.

Correct erroneous owner opinions

To lay the groundwork for such a change in owner behavior, it is necessary to give owners an account of the function and normal course of canine aggression. This discussion should emphasize the following: aggression towards conspecifics is normal canine behavior. It is not always negative and need not always be suppressed or prevented. Such aggression often looks more vicious and dangerous to human beings than it really is. Submissive behavior on the part of the loser usually completely inhibits further aggression by the winner – which prevents the serious injuries that the owner fears. And it can do some dogs good to end up on the losing side of such an encounter and thus to experience the full, rather uncomfortable force unleashed by their overly self-confident, basically inappropriate provocation of other dogs. In short, getting more or less what they deserve from other dogs can be good medicine for some basically inexperienced or incompletely socialized dogs which are constantly provoking problems with their most peaceable and playful neighbors.

Physical aids

In cases where the dog's fights are often vicious, result in serious injuries, and therefore must be prevented, simply putting a leash on the dog when passing through certain areas or when a known enemy, or type of dog with which it often fights, is first spotted down the street can be a sensible precaution which prevents fighting and, hence, the need to intervene. Some owners who are accustomed to letting their dog run free are reluctant to do this. Either they rule out the use of a leash on principle or they lack good judgment and need reminding that dog ownership also carries with it the responsibility to protect other dogs and dog owners in the community from their dog's potentially dangerous aggression.

Using a long, retractable leash (i.e. to be able to pull the dog away from a safer distance), or having the dog wear some kind of head collar which makes it easier to physically manage, may be helpful in some cases where aggression towards owners occurs when they try to pull the dog away as soon as its greeting and related checking of the anal region of another dog has turned aggressive. Muzzling the dog is another option which might be appropriate in some cases.

Conventional obedience training

If the dog is disobedient and difficult to control under a variety of circumstances, conventional obedience training should be recommended. If the training is to be carried out by owners themselves, training the dog to follow commands when no other dog is in the vicinity is the first step which precedes training it to follow the same commands when other dogs are nearby. In some cases, gaining much more control over the dog by carrying out this kind of basic training is the owners' only real hope for preventing the development of situations where they must intervene and risk being bitten.

Change family interactive ground rules

As previously mentioned, low owner dominance is often a feature of cases in which clients have been repeatedly bitten when trying to break up fights between dogs or suppressing aggression towards human beings. Therefore the nature of the relationship between owner and dog should be thoroughly explored during the early stages of the consultation. Even mild tendencies in this direction indicate that some of the recommendations from Chapter 10 for increasing owner dominance should be given to the client.

Predatory aggression towards human beings

Three types of aggression behavior problems are commonly either referred to as predatory aggression or suspected to be this type of interspecific aggression by writers in the dog behavior problem field. The first and most common is when a dog chases after and barks and snaps at bicyclists, joggers, or cars. The second type of problem is the extremely rare case where packs of dogs chase, attack, and injure or perhaps even kill and eat part of a human being. Also rare is the third type of problem where a family dog attacks and sometimes kills a newborn infant – usually within a few hours after it has been brought home from the hospital.

Chasing and biting of moving bicyclists, joggers, etc.

There are two possible ways to interpret this problem behavior. O'Farrell (1992) assumes that it is basically interspecific predatory behavior – that the dog begins chasing the moving object and, if the predatory sequence runs its full course, will attack the "quarry" without growling or threatening and continue biting it until it is motionless. O'Farrell suggests two possibilities to account for why it seldom comes to an attack: either the eliciting stimulus is too weak (i.e. dog starts chasing then simply loses interest and turns back) or the dog stops when close to the quarry and starts barking at it rather than attacking. O'Farrell hypothesizes that this barking is a displacement activity reflecting the underlying conflict between the motivation to attack and the motivation to stay away because the object presents an "anatomical puzzle" (bicycle) or looks too threatening (a hissing cat).

While this account may be plausible in some cases, there is another possibility which can be raised by asking the question of whether the dog essentially goes after the target in order to catch and eat it or to chase it away? As Campbell (1992) implies, most of these cases of so-called predatory aggression probably do not involve predatory behavior at all, but rather group-defensive aggression; in effect, an attempt to drive an undesirable/feared individual away with an aggressive display which would, biologically speaking, function both to warn other group members and recruit them to join in the group-defensive effort. Why is the walking human acceptable but the slowing running one not? As was discussed in Chapter 12, it may be a question here too of fear – at least initially, when the problem behavior was first elicited. The young dog may have been fully accustomed to walking people and then was startled and perhaps felt threatened to suddenly see the first running human being it had ever seen bearing down on it. Many dogs do indeed react like this to strange-looking or strange-acting human beings such as men with canes, women pushing squeaky baby carriages, people in wheelchairs, or retarded or handicapped people whose movements are jerky and unco-ordinated. Another possible source of fear is that as a puppy or young juvenile, the dog might have playfully chased a jogger who stopped and threatened and frightened it. In any case, once a dog begins to react this way towards joggers, the threatening reactions of some joggers and the fact that the dog's threatening always works in the sense that the jogger jogs away every single time – is enough to explain why the problem worsens over time.

But even if this second view of the group-defensive rather than predatory nature of the problem is sound, the analysis of these problem situations turns out to be more complicated than situations involving the group-defensive aggression towards other human strangers on the street. For true predatory behavior may eventually become involved in such cases. Not because the dog is basically stalking and chasing a surrogate prey object, but rather because part of the reason why chasing itself can develop into a self-rewarding pattern of behavior may be related to the dog's lack of opportunity of being able to use its genetically-pre-programmed hunting behavioral repertoire. Perpetually deprived of the opportunity to hunt, chasing things like balls, sticks, Frisbees, or birds (which always escape) is a popular game with most domestic dogs which never have a chance to chase things in a natural hunting context. And after years of tangling with joggers or bicyclists and learning how basically harmless and helpless they are, this same "sport" element may eventually become pronounced in some dogs.

Regardless of whether or not this predatory behavior element is or finally becomes involved in specific cases of jogger, bicycle, or car chasing, the primary factor which seems to account for the initial development of the problem and continuing resistance to modification in many cases involves what might be loosely described as the dog's basic negative perception or underlying fear/dislike/mistrust of the chased target. Thus, the resemblance to genuine predatory behavior appears to be largely superficial. It is typical group-defensive aggression which seems to be mainly involved, with the only difference with the group-defensive aggression cases discussed in the last chapter being that the target happens to be moving and may, therefore, elicit potentially self-rewarding chasing along with the usual kind of barking, growling, and biting behaviors.

True predatory behavior of dogs packs towards human beings

Borchelt et. al. (1983) report rare cases in which groups of dogs engaged in what is clearly predatory behavior towards humans – chasing, attacking, and sometimes killing and eating some of the flesh of the victim. In general, such packs are usually small temporary groupings of predominantly owned, free-ranging dogs which are usually non-aggressive to human beings. In some cases, it seemed to be the combination of the three elements that which elicited this predatory pack behavior: the dogs had just been chasing a small animal, the victim was a child, and the child's reaction to the dogs was to start screaming and/or running away.

Wright (1991) cites statistics from a number of studies which indicate that most severe and fatal dog bites are due to owned dogs and not strays. Children are especially at risk. Two studies cited in this article reported that children younger than 12 years old were the victims in 64 of the 74 (86.4%) deaths from dog bites in the United States from 1966 to 1980, and children younger than 9 years old in 110 of 157 (70%) of fatal attacks from 1979 through 1988 respectively. Probably few of these were, however, due to what could be regarded as genuine predatory behavior.

Fatal attacks on neonates by family dogs

Wright (1991) cites a study which reports the following USA statistics:
"...the annual death rate for infants younger than 1 year was 68.3 deaths/100 million population/year. The rate for neonates was particularly high: 295 deaths/100 million population/year, almost 370 times that of adults 30 to 49 years old." (p. 307).

According to Voith (1984), attacks on newborns seem to most commonly occur during the first day after the baby is first brought into the home "when the dog unexpectedly comes upon the new baby in an unsupervised situations". In the same article, Voith describes one such attack which proved fatal for baby:

"One unfortunate case involved a dog with no known history of aggression to people. However, the dog had an unusual background. The original owners had the animal from puppyhood until it was 1 1/2 years old, when they gave away or sold the dog because it frequently killed rabbits, squirrels and birds.

Five years later, a few months before their second child was born, the original owners came upon the dog and resumed ownership of it. The dog had been neglected and abused during its 5-year absence, but was friendly with the family and played with children in the household and neighborhood. However, while the dog was accustomed to small children, it had not been exposed to infants.

When the mother returned from the hospital with her new baby, she took the precaution of putting the dog outside when she left the baby. A few hours later, the dog was allowed inside and was very attentive to the baby. The infant was in a bassinet, and the mother stepped 6-8 feet way to speak to her husband in the next room. The dog suddenly leaped up, grabbed the baby by the head, and carried it across the room. It dropped the child as soon as the parents set up a cry, but the baby was fatally injured.

This was a particularly sad case because the mother had conscientiously followed the rule of never leaving a dog and a new baby alone. It did not occur to her (nor would it to most people) that the dog would attack the infant in her presence, since it was friendly with small children and had shown no aggression towards people. Unfortunately, this dog was particularly predatory; few people are aware that some dogs view infants as potential prey......Before this dog was euthanized, we observed its reactions to small mammals and birds. It consistently tried to chase every small animal it saw." (pp. 540–541)

It is Voith's (1984) view that this behavior is the result of the dog's reacting to the baby as if it were a new, strange animal species rather than a human being – essentially that true predatory behavior is involved.

Voith (1984) warns that there are three types of dogs which may be especially dangerous in this regard:

"...those which have already manifested aggressive tendencies to babies, those that are, in general, also aggressive to adults, and those that have a history of predatory behavior, i.e. they chase and kill squirrels, birds, cats, goats, sheep, or other mammals". (p. 539)

The sample recommandations box is based largely on Voith's various suggestions for safely introducing a family dog to a neonate. It also contains advice for maximizing the chances that the dog will not become aggressive to the infant during the course of the following months.

Idiopathic aggression or so-called "rage syndrome"

Hart and Hart (1985) define a special category of aggression which they refer to as idiopathic vicious attacks on people characterized as "unpredictable and unprovoked vicious attacks on people the dog knows well". These attacks are relatively infrequent (i.e. less than once a month) with the dog giving little or no warning before the attack. Owners sometimes notice, however, that the dog "no longer seems to recognize people in the family, and may even get a glazed or distant look in its eyes". Referring the problem as "rage syndrome", O'Farrell (1992) agrees that such attacks are sudden, savage, and without warning. But she also suggests that although the attacks seem "crazy and unprovoked" to the owner, "careful investigation usually reveals that he did something (often involving touching the dog or brushing against it) which it could have interpreted as a dominance challenge or threat of some kind. These dogs usually show other signs of dominance within the family" (p.88).

Voith (1989) agrees with O'Farrell in this regard and suggests that the "histories available

SAMPLE RECOMMENDATIONS

Suggestions for safely introducing the dog to a neonate

1. Starting before the baby is born, use the procedures described in Chapter 8 to train the dog to come, sit, lie down, and stay for a relatively long period of time when it is told to do so. *(This helps ensure that the parent will have relatively good control over the dog's behavior when the baby and dog are together in the same room in the hours, days, and weeks after the baby has been brought home from the hospital.)*

2. Be especially vigilant and careful during the first day or two after the infant is first brought home and the dog is still aroused by or curious about it. *(Voith (1984) suggests that it is only when the dog has become fully accustomed to the child's presence/ sounds/movements (i.e. pays little attention to them, baby's sounds and movements do not make dog restless or curious, dog remains relaxed and relatively disinterested in baby under all circumstances) that parents can start to relax supervision of the dog in the baby's presence.)*

3. Keep the dog separated from the baby when mother and baby first come home from the hospital. Let the dog greet the mother when she is alone first, and let it become accustomed to the odor and sound of the baby for a few hours before bringing the two together.

4. Keep the dog on a leash during the introduction process.

5. Ask it to sit, show it the baby at a great enough distance away so that it could not reach the infant if it snapped at it, and reward it with food tidbits for remaining sitting and quiet.

6. Repeat this introduction process several times and reward the dog for following commands and remaining quietly staying in one place in the presence of the baby for extended periods of time.

7. Eventually, the dog can be allowed to sniff the baby closely if it has had a great deal of experience with it and has shown no signs of becoming exited or agitated. There is no hard and fast rule for when this should take place – owners must use their own judgment here.

8. During the days, weeks, and months which follow, make a deliberate effort to pay more attention to the dog (i.e. talking to it more, petting it and playing with it more, rewarding it for following commands, etc.) when the infant is present than when it is sleeping in its room. *(This will help ensure that the baby continues to be closely associated with all of the "good things in life" rather than a sign to the dog that less attention will now be available from parents because they are busy attending to the baby. Essentially, if parents get the feeling that the dog may feel left out, the time to make it up to it is when the baby is awake and nearby not when it is sleeping.)*

9. As a general rule, never leave the dog and baby alone in the same room together. Fixing a screen door or gate across the doorway to the baby's room may be helpful for times when the mother must step outside for a moment or go to the bathroom and therefore cannot keep a close watch on the two at all times.

10. Keeping the dog muzzled in the presence of the baby is a reasonable option in some cases. However, care should be taken not to directly associate the muzzling process itself with the appearance of the baby. The dog should also sometimes wear the muzzle at times when the baby is absent so as to avoid any association at all between wearing the muzzle and the baby.

concerning such dogs closely resemble dominance-related aggression patterns. The aggressive behavior is generally directed toward family members and is precipitated by petting or by ordering the animal to do something" (p. 235). She also suggests that the behavior is more commonly reported in Bernese mountain dogs, English cocker spaniels, springer spaniels, and St. Bernards. Hart and Hart (1985) add Doberman pinschers and German shepherds to this list.

Hart and Hart (1985) state that autopsies of dogs with this aggression syndrome usually reveal "no pronounced pathology of the nervous system or other organ systems". However, they also point out that a "mild degree of encephalitis has been observed upon careful microscopic examination of parts of the brain in some dogs" (p.48). These authors suspect that a "painstaking neuropathological examination" might turn up other evidence of brain pathology.

At present, it is difficult to know what to think about this problem which, while uncommon, is apparently common enough and different enough from the typical dominance aggression pattern to be provisionally regarded as distinct syndrome in its own right – as all of the above authors do. Basically, more information required. Both more detailed case history information and more results of the kinds of painstaking neuropathological examinations which Hart and Hart suspect would provide additional evidence of central nervous system pathology.

For now, however, the counselor should simply be aware that such a syndrome exists and take special precautions to protect the safety of family members when these problems are reported to him/her. In this connection, Hart and Hart (1985) suggest that although some specialists report that anticonvulsant drugs such as *primidone, phenobarbital*, and *diphenylhydantoin* are sometimes "useful in controlling the attacks", it is best to advise clients to euthanize such dogs given the unpredictable, explosive, and extraordinarily dangerous nature of the attacks. O'Farrell (1992) essentially agrees, pointing out that while administering *primidone* or treating the problem as dominance aggression usually produces some improvement, the attacks are so ferocious that even if the treatment improves the problem, the dog "may still not be tolerable to live with". In short, extreme caution by placing the safety of family members above all else is called for and not experimentation with types of drugs or behavioral treatments which *might* help improve the problem or control the attacks.

Pathophysiological causes of aggression problems

The list of pathophysiological conditions which are known to sometimes cause aggressive behavior is long: neurological impairment, cardiovascular disease, cerebral and hippocampal neuronal degeneration, psychomotor epilepsy, viral, bacterial, or fungal infection, trauma, infestations of parasites, chemical abnormalities, metabolic diseases, toxicoses, malformations, and others (Voith, 1989; Reisner, 1991).

The history of such problems often differs in some obvious ways from the problems which have been discussed throughout this and the last three chapters. But this is not always the case as when, for example, an animal which is in pain begins reacting with self-protective aggression when approached or touched by family members. Here, suspicion of a pathophysiological problem is aroused not by the form and environmental context of the problem, but by the fact that there has been a noticeable change in the animal's behavior.

In general, behavior specialists should always recommend a thorough veterinary examination – and inform the family veterinarian that they suspect that the behavior problem is somehow associated with some pathophysiological condition – whenever (1) the problem does not fit one of the usual behavior problem patterns, (2) there is any kind of odd or puzzling feature of the animal's behavior which cannot be explained, or (3) there has been a fairly sudden and/or dramatic change in the animal's behavior which is not the obvious consequence of some change in its environment.

The following quote from Reisner (1991) describes what is required from the veterinarian in such cases:

"If the primary complaint is behavioral, physical causes must be excluded from the diagnosis. Patient data should include a thorough history and results of physical and neurologic examinations. An extended office visit may be required to obtain sufficient information. Ancillary tests, including serum chemistry analysis, urinalysis, plain and contrast radiography, electroencephalography, cerebrospinal fluid analysis, and more specialized diagnostic tests also may be indicated." (p. 207)

References

Borchelt, P.L, Lockwood, R., Beck, A. M., and Voith, V.L. (1983): Attacks by packs of dogs involving predation on human beings. *Public Health Reports* **98**, 57–66.

Borchelt, P.L., and Voith, V.L. (1982): Classification of animal behavior problems. *Veterinary Clinics of North America: Small Animal Practice* **12**, 571–585.

Campbell, W.E. (1992): *Behavior Problems in Dogs.* Goleta, California, American Veterinary Publications, Inc.

O'Farrell V. (1992): *Manual of Canine Behaviour.* British Small Animal Veterinary Association. Shurdington, Cheltenham, Gloucestershire, UK.

Reisner, I (1991): The pathophysiologic basis of behavior problems. *Veterinary Clinics of North America: Small Animal Practice* **21**, 207-224.

Voith, V.L. (1984): Procedures for introducing a baby to a dog. *Modern Veterinary Practice* **July**, 539–541

Voith, V.L. (1989): Chapter 43: Behavioral Disorders. In Ettinger, J.S. (ed.) *Textbook of Veterinary Internal Medicine.* Philadelphia, W.B. Saunders Company, pp. 227–240

Wright, J. C. (1991): Canine aggression toward people: Bite scenarios and prevention. *Veterinary Clinics of North America: Small Animal Practice* **21**, 299–314.

14   Aggression Towards Other Dogs

The present chapter makes use of the functional scheme for classifying aggression problems towards human beings discussed in Chapter 9 to classify and attempt to understand problems involving aggression towards other dogs. The fact that the same basic types of aggression problems occur when other dogs are targets of aggression should not be surprising, for dogs which have had a great deal of exposure to humans early in life behave towards them as if they were conspecifics rather than members of an alien species. And conversely, dogs with little or no experience with other dogs early in life may be unable to interact with them normally later. In extreme cases, they may behave as if other dogs are not recognized as conspecifics at all.

Except for the omission of an intragroup play aggression problem category, the scheme presented in Table 14.1 is identical to that presented for aggression towards human beings in Chapter 9. Here again, viewing the problems within the framework of the *intraspecific vs. interspecific* and *intragroup vs. extragroup* dimensions proves to be of considerable value in terms of classifying and understanding the similarities and differences between the various common and less common types of interdog aggression problems.

The problem of intragroup defense of young will not be discussed below because it usually does not represent the kind of problem for owners which lead them to seek expert advice. Other problems will be discussed only in combined form (e.g. *extragroup* self-protective, group-defensive, and competitive aggression considered together under the general heading of "aggression towards dogs in the neighbor-

Table 14.1: Functional scheme for classifying interdog aggression problems

Intraspecific aggression *(dog responding to other dog as conspecific)*		Interspecific aggression *(other dog responded to as member of alien species)*
Intragroup aggression *(between fellow group members)*	**Extragroup aggression** *(towards dogs outside of the family)*	
Competitive aggression *(dominance-related or possessive)*	Competitive aggression *(dominance-related or possessive)*	Competitive aggression *(interspecies competition)*
Self-protective aggression	Self-protective aggression	Self-protective aggression
Defense of young	Group-defensive aggression	Group-defensive aggression
		Predatory behavior

hood"). While the distinction between them is clear in the theoretical or functional sense, in specific problem cases it is often not at all clear whether one or some combination of the various implied types of motivations is involved.

Figure 14.1 presents a breakdown of cases involving interdog aggression as either a major problem (main or major secondary problem in 40 cases) or minor problem (9 cases) in 49 of a series of 147 dog cases (33%). As can be seen, aggression towards dogs outside the family by a dog which otherwise shows no special problem interacting with other dogs – and presumably perceives them and responds to them as conspecifics – is by far the most common type of problem which accounts for almost three-quarters of all cases.

One preliminary note: the fact that dogs show similar general types of aggression towards other dogs as they do towards human beings does not, of course, imply that a dog which shows a particular type of problem towards human beings will also show that same problem towards other dogs. Indeed the opposite is usually the case. Dogs can be aggressive to humans under a variety of circumstances but never have the slightest problem with other dogs, and vice versa.

Competitive aggression between dogs in the same home

The intragroup competitive aggression category subsumes what are commonly referred to in the literature as intermale or interfemale dominance aggression as well as the more specific, resource-related possessive aggression where, for example, the more submissive of a pair of animals may sometimes be able to aggressively defend a particularly valued resource like food against a more dominant packmate.

Only dominance aggression between males or females in the same home will, however, be discussed in this section. Most problems which are brought to the behavior counselor involve the nature of the general, dominance-related relationship between two animals rather than highly situation-specific problems like aggression which only occurs, for example, in the vicinity of food bowls. Owners may be able to easily cope with these latter problems by doing something like feeding the dogs separately.

In the 6 out of 49 interdog aggression cases from Figure 14.1 involving dogs in the same home (i.e. intragroup), three exhibited the intermale and three the interfemale pattern.

Possible causal factors

Lack of stable dominance-submission relationship

One common scenario is the development of mutual threatening and fighting several or more days following the taking in of a second adult or near-adult dog into the home. Another is the case in which threatening/fighting develops between an adult dog that has been in the family for some time and a younger, now-larger dog

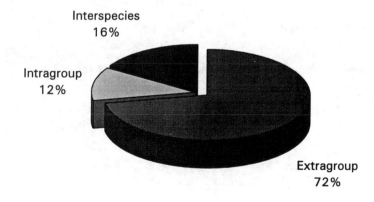

Interspecies
16%

Intragroup
12%

Extragroup
72%

Figure 14.1: Relative frequency of the major types of interdog aggression problems

POSSIBLE CAUSAL FACTORS

Lack of stable dominance-submission relationship
(e.g. new dog in family; younger dog maturing and challenging previously dominant dog's position)

Effects of experience
(e.g. aggressiveness can greatly increase after serious fighting)

Erroneous owner beliefs
(aggression is always aberrant, undesirable, and calls for immediate human intervention)

Lack of appropriate training
(e.g. difficult for owner to prevent/suppress aggression when dogs not well-trained to obey commands)

Hormonal influence
(problem more common in males)

Unintentional owner fostering
(owner favors/supports less dominant of two dogs in competitive/confrontation situations)

Unintentional owner reinforcement
(e.g. attempting to end aggression by petting aggressive dog, distracting it with tidbits, toys, playing, etc.)

Lack of owner dominance
(lack of owner dominance implies lack of "authority" to intervene to stop or prevent fighting)

COMPETITIVE AGGRESSION BETWEEN DOGS IN THE SAME HOME

- Fighting between dogs in the same home in situations involving dominance-related interactions and/or direct competition over valued objects, locations, etc.

POSSIBLE TREATMENT ELEMENTS

Increase owner understanding
(e.g. nature of dominance hierarchies; function of stable dominance-submission relationships in preventing fighting)

Change maintenance conditions
(e.g. keep dogs separated when alone)

Castration
(of more submissive male or both males; only when problem directly connected with estrus in bitches)

Cessation of ineffective treatment methods
(e.g. scolding aggressor; always intervening to suppress aggression)

Increase owner dominance
(to increase owner control capability)

Avoid problem situations
(e.g. feed dogs separately; avoid other competitive situations)

Physical aids
(e.g. leash/muzzle)

Correct owner mistakes
(e.g. supporting/favoring less dominant of two dogs in confrontation/competition situations)

Conventional obedience training
(to increase owner control capability)

Behavior therapy methods
(e.g. counterconditioning of non-aggressive behavior; desensitization; habituation)

Medicaments
(e.g. progestin therapy)

of 6-12 months of age that has matured sufficiently to begin challenging the older dog's dominant status. Basically, serious fighting may
occur where (1) a stable dominance-submission relationship has not yet formed between
pairs of males or females or (2) a reversal of the
present dominance-submission relationship is
inevitable and just beginning.

Hormonal influence

Problems of this type are much more common
between males. In general, males seem on average to be more intensely concerned than females with dominance-submission relationships
and all of the "rights and privileges" to which
more dominant animals have first or sole access. Females in families form dominance hierarchies as well, but often the development of
such relationships involves little or no serious
fighting. Owners can often state clearly which
of the two is dominant by, for example, observing which takes the lead in certain situations,
gets the toy or bone when there is only one, or
pushes in front to be greeted or petted first. But
when questioned, owners often report that
there has never been any kind of serious aggressive confrontation between the two. This is,
however, not always the case. Sometimes females fight viciously with one another and
must be separated to prevent serious injuries.
Unlike males, where a stable dominance-submission relationship finally develops which
drastically reduces problems between the two,
some females may persist in fighting with each
other and their fights become more vicious and
bloody as time goes on.

Such interfemale aggression is therefore regarded by some authors (e.g. Neville 1991) as
being potentially more dangerous than intermale aggression. In some cases, owners have
indeed reported that one female's surrendering
and turning over and lying submissively on its
back did not inhibit the aggressor's attack as
usually happens in fights between males. It is
not at all clear why this should be so. Perhaps it
is some kind of domestication-produced aber-
ration. More interestingly, perhaps the function
of aggression in females under some circum-

stances is less of a "test of strength" to settle
the matter of the dominance-submission relationship between the two but rather an attempt
to expel a rival from the group. A further possibility is suggested by the observation that in
some serious fights between wolves over dominance when, for example, the previous alpha
male is finally beaten by a challenger, submissive behavior may be insufficient to inhibit the
attacker's aggression and thus the beaten animal has no choice other than to flee or keep aggressively defending itself to avoid being more
seriously injured (Feddersen-Petersen, 1993).
Perhaps under some circumstances, therefore,
dominance-related fighting between two particularly highly-motivated combatants – male or
female – simply does not follow the same rules
as in confrontations where the stakes are not so
high.

Effects of experience

In the most severe cases of intermale or interfemale fighting between family dogs, owners often report that after the first serious fight, the
animals' level of aggressiveness towards one
another is increased to such an extent that they
begin fighting almost the instant they see each
other after having been separated for awhile.
Another experience-related causal factor suggested by O'Farrell (1992) is where "either dog
has an early history of poor socialization to
other dogs, which might make it less able to
understand the other's body language". Presumably, this would somehow prevent the
formation of an aggression-preventing dominance hierarchy.

Unintentional owner fostering

Most owners make the mistake of favoring or
supporting the less dominant dog by scolding
or otherwise punishing the aggressor or making
sure that the subdominant dog is petted first,
gets the only bone or toy available, gets more
frequent and positive owner attention, or is
awarded privileges like lying on the furniture or
sleeping in the owner's bedroom which the
other does not have. This is often particularly

true in cases where the "top dog" status of one dog which has been in the family for years comes under serious challenge by some aggressive newcomer. This kind of owner favoring naturally intensifies competitive interactions between the dogs and works against the formation of a stabile hierarchy because either the owner is in the position to partially suppress the more dominant dog's aggression or he/she is perceived by both dogs as being an ally of the less dominant dog. Another possibility is that the owner's preferential treatment of the less aggressive of the two dogs acts to delay its perception and acceptance of its new subdominant status.

There are several reasons why owners react this way. As discussed at length in Chapter 2, owner behavior is basically human parental behavior, the result of the operation of a behavioral system which evolved to care for and successfully raise a maximum number of healthy children. When children are involved, this kind of democratic, fairness-based treatment may well be adaptive in a sense that it would result in the smaller and weaker children being given the preferential treatment (e.g. more intensive care, better protection) needed to develop into healthy adults. But instinctively behaving in this way towards the family dog can be inappropriate and represent a fundamental misunderstanding of the peace-keeping function of stable dominance-submission relationships.

Another psychological element may be the owners' tendency to unthinkingly perceive dog aggression in human aggression terms, which leads them to dislike, disapprove of, and scold the aggressive dog as one might do with an overtly aggressive member of any small human social group. This too is potentially adaptive in human social groups in which the "social pressure" that would result when all group members reacted this way is a force that would, in the long run, discourage and counteract disruptive aggressive behavior by group members. However, it can have an adverse effect on the interdog aggression problem for obvious reasons.

And finally, an additional reason for such counterproductive owner intervention is purely practical. What could be a more logical and natural way to stop aggression than to scold and punish the aggressor? Although this type of owner reaction might be called for in some cases of persistent and potentially dangerous aggression, when problems are not so dangerous or are just beginning to develop within the family, it is counterproductive and only makes the problem worse.

Erroneous owner beliefs

Not understanding the positive role aggression between dogs can play in establishing a clear-cut, stable, and therefore peaceful dominance-submission relationship between dogs in the family, many owners regard it as aberrant, undesirable in any form, and totally inexplicable in dogs which are given everything they need or want and otherwise seem to be quite fond of each other. Another erroneous belief is that such fighting must necessarily be dangerous to one or both dogs and should be prevented at all costs.

Unintentional owner reinforcement

As with other forms of aggression, owners often unintentionally reinforce and thereby contribute to the progressive worsening of the problem when they attempt to stop aggression or prevent growling from developing into fighting by trying to calm the aggressive dog by, for example, petting it or trying to distract it with a toy, tidbit, or invitation to play.

Lack of appropriate training

Aggression between dogs whose fighting is too vicious to be allowed to occur can sometimes be completely prevented or suppressed by the owner when both dogs are firmly under his/her control. The lack of basic obedience training – which also includes training animals to stop misbehavior on command – can therefore be regarded as a major contributing factor in some interdog aggression cases.

Lack of owner dominance

A related factor which affects the owner's capability to suppress aggression in cases where this is called for can be the nature of the relationship between the owner and one or both dogs. If there is some kind of dominance problem between the owner and one or both dogs, they tend to be disobedient and slow to obey, and they tend to ignore owner commands and other attempts at control in situations where they are highly motivated to do something the owner wishes to suppress. Particularly in potentially dangerous cases where owner suppression of fighting is especially critical, owners should be questioned closely about the way both dogs respond to them in the various kinds of situations in which dominance problems between owner and dog are revealed (see Chapter 10).

Starting from the observation that aggression tends to be more common among higher ranking members of a wolf pack, O'Farrell (1992) suggests that the dogs' aggressiveness towards one another may partially reflect the lack of sufficient owner dominance, which results in the dogs perceiving themselves as occupying relatively higher ranks in the family than otherwise would be the case.

Possible treatment elements

Increase general owner understanding

The first step in helping owners deal with this problem is to explain to them the nature of dominance hierarchies in dog packs, the role of aggressive behavior and postures and gestures signaling dominance and submission in their formation and maintenance, and the function of such hierarchies in determining the access of individual dogs to limited food, resting place, mate, etc. resources in a way which avoids most potentially dangerous aggressive confrontations. Basically, owners must understand that such problems between dogs in the same family are normal under certain circumstances, that serious fighting indicates that a stable dominance-submission relationship has not yet developed between the two animals, and that solving the problem therefore involves taking steps to promote its formation.

Avoid problem situations

If the problem is highly situation-specific as in cases of so-called possessive aggression where fighting is limited to contesting some specific type of resource (e.g. food), having the owner arrange things so as to avoid such situations completely (e.g. feeding dogs separately) can represent a sensible and fully satisfactory solution to the problem. In cases where problems occur in many types of competitive situations, arranging things so as to temporarily avoid some of them (e.g. feed dogs separately, play with dogs separately, remove all toys from the home) may be helpful in preventing fighting while other remedial measures are taking effect.

Change maintenance conditions

If the aggression is potentially dangerous, it is often a wise precaution to keep the two dogs separated from one another whenever they are left alone.

Physical aids

As is always the case when aggression is potentially dangerous and difficult to control, physical aids such as keeping one or both dogs on leashes or muzzling them in certain situations may be called for.

Castration

One retrospective survey of the effects of castration on intermale aggression reported that it was effective in reducing or eliminating the aggression in 5 out of 8 dogs (Hopkins et al. 1976). Most workers in the field apparently agree that this approx. 60% level of effectiveness seems consistent with their clinical experience; for in spite of the small-scale, uncontrolled nature of this study, its results are widely cited in the literature as a guideline.

The related advice given to owners of males is to identify the more dominant of the two – or the one which will surely end up to be dominant in the long run – and then have the other dog castrated to try and amplify the difference in aggressiveness between the two and thereby facilitate the rapid formation of a stable domin-ance-submission relationship. In cases where fighting between two very similar males (e.g. brothers from the same litter) is intense and neither of the two is able to establish itself as dominant over the other, castration of both males is often recommended. This can help if the effects of the castration differ between the two, giving one a competitive advantage over the other, or if the operation lowers the aggres-siveness of both dogs to an equal extent.

Spaying is only recommended for bitches if the interfemale aggression is directly associated with estrus (Voith 1989).

While O'Farrell (1992) suggests that *del-madinone* should be given prior to castration to judge whether or not it will be effective, Hart and Hart (1985) state that it is difficult and perhaps impossible to predict in which animals the operation is going to be the most success-ful.

Given that male dominance aggression to-wards other male dogs is often effectively treat-ed with castration, it is interesting to ask why castration apparently doesn't help nearly as of-ten or to nearly as great an extent in reducing what is supposedly the same kind of domin-ance aggression towards human family mem-bers? One possibility is that humans do not re-act to the change in the castrated dog's odor the way another dog might. In this connection, Hart and Hart (1985) suggest that the effects castration have on intermale aggression are due both to a lowering of competitive motivation and to a change in the castrated dog's odor, which makes it less likely to provoke aggres-sion in other dogs. A second possibility is that dominance aggression towards human beings differs in some crucial ways from dominance aggression towards other dogs. Perhaps it is its defensive rather than offensively competitive element which is more pronounced here. And finally, it is surely also the case that behavior di-rected towards human beings is never precisely the same as similar behavior directed towards other dogs. Indeed, in spite of strong resem-blances between the behavior of domestic dogs towards humans and conspecifics, it is prob-ably a mistake to assume that the behavior is

identical – in effect, that the dog doesn't per-ceive the difference between dogs and human beings.

Correct owner mistakes

A potentially serious mistake in all cases of competitive aggression between dogs in the same home is supporting the less dominant dog in competitive or confrontation situations by, for example, scolding the more dominant dog or making sure that the submissive dog gets the disputed resource (bone, toy, resting place) or privilege (best place on sofa, greeted/petted first by owner). Indeed, owners must learn to do the opposite and always favor the more dominant dog by petting, greeting, and feeding it first, perhaps allowing it privileges which the other doesn't have, and siding with it by scold-ing the other animal whenever there is an ag-gressive confrontation between the two no matter which dog appears to have started it.

Owners usually know which of the two dogs is dominant or will soon become dominant as soon as the younger dog becomes a little older. But sometimes this is not so obvious. Here, owners should be advised to observe the two more closely to see which goes through door-ways first, gets in and out of cars first, greets family members first, appropriates the resting places which both seem to prefer, or gets the bone or toy when only one is available.

Cessation of ineffective treatment methods

As discussed above, scolding the aggressor can make the problem worse in cases where the ag-gression is not so dangerous that it must be suppressed at all costs. A second method which is counterproductive in all but the most serious cases is to always intervene and sup-press aggressive behavior when one or both dogs start growling. Although it may be diffi-cult for the owner to decide whether or not to intervene in specific situations, it is sometimes best with dogs which do not seem to be danger-ously aggressive towards one another – or which have fought previously without injuring each other – to simply stand back and let the two settle things in their own way.

Conventional obedience training

In the case of potentially dangerous aggression and in situations where aggression is continuously recurring because neither of the two dogs can seem to gain the upper hand, owner intervention and control of both dogs may be imperative. Where such control possibilities are limited because of a simple lack of training, conventional obedience training using the methods described in Chapter 8 or by attending an obedience training class should be recommended.

Increase owner dominance

One or both dogs may ignore owner commands, scolding, and other required control measures because of the kind of "lack of respect" indicative of a dominance problem between dog and owner. If no such problems exist, owners are usually in a position to exercise the necessary authority to stop or prevent aggression between dogs if this is required. But if there are problems in this area, some of the recommendations for increasing owner dominance discussed in Chapter 10 may be called for.

Systematic behavior therapy methods

In some cases, it may be desirable and feasible to extend the obedience training process into the various potential problem situations in which fighting often breaks out to counter-condition non-aggressive behavior like sitting, lying down, and staying sitting or lying on command. One look at how well-trained dogs in dog sport clubs have learned to essentially ignore the presence of other dogs when told to lie down and stay until released is enough to demonstrate the possibilities for control through persistent, long-term training which are available to the highly-motivated owner.

Sometimes, the interdog aggression problem between family dogs is so severe that the dogs begin viciously fighting with one another on sight. In this case, some type of desensitization/counterconditioning or habituation behavior therapy method can be applied like, for example, keeping the dogs entirely separated from one another except for several hours a day

when they are confined by leashes to opposite sides of a room. They are then fed and often rewarded with tidbits for following commands in this situation, and over the course of several days, the distance between the two is progressively reduced as they learn to remain relaxed and non-aggressive in each other's presence.

Medicaments

Progestin therapy can be effective in reducing intermale aggression in both intact and castrated males. Hart and Hart (1985) recommend a 0.5 mg/kg/day oral treatment with *megestrol acetate* or a single dose of 5 mg per kg *medroxyprogesterone acetate* injected SQ or IM. The effects are only temporary, however, and such treatment is therefore best regarded as supplementary for cases in which a temporary reduction in aggressiveness may be helpful to a behaviorally-oriented treatment method. (See the "drug therapy" subsection in Chapter 8 for side effects and other important drug-related information.)

Self-protective aggression towards another dog in the home

It is difficult to assess the extent to which fighting between two dogs in the family may sometimes also involve self-protective aggression (i.e. either pain-elicited or fear-related). At least some of the types of fights described in the last section may well involve this element on the part of the dog which is attacked. Here is another case where observational research is needed. Certainly an experienced canine ethologist analyzing filmed confrontations from a number of problem cases could take us much farther in differentiating and characterizing the various forms of the interdog aggression problems than one can go on the basis of owner reports alone.

Aggression towards other dogs in the neighborhood

Many dogs become involved in aggressive confrontations with other dogs during walks. Often this involves intermale aggression. There

SAMPLE RECOMMENDATIONS

Competitive aggression between dogs in the same home

Between males:

- There is a good chance that castration of the dog which is least dominant – or which will almost certainly end up being the least dominant – will reduce or eliminate the problem.
- Drug therapy with a hormone preparation may help to temporarily reduce the aggression to a level which allows you to successfully apply the other treatment recommendations (*i.e. those listed below under scenarios A or B*).

Between females:

- Spaying is only helpful in cases where the aggression problem only occurs when one of the dogs is in heat.

Scenario A: *the aggression does not seem particularly dangerous and is a sign that a stable dominance hierarchy between the two males or females has not yet developed.*

- Never give the more submissive of the two dogs special privileges (e.g. being allowed up on the furniture) which the other dog doesn't have.
- Always support the dominance relationship between the two by letting out, greeting, feeding, petting, etc. the most dominant of the two first, by making sure that it is given the toy, bone, etc. when only one is available, and by making sure that it has exclusive access to the most desirable feeding/resting places.
- Stop punishing the wrong dog. Whenever one or both dogs growl, immediately scold the more submissive dog even though it appears to you that the other dog started the trouble.

Where it is not clear which dog is dominant:

- Watch the dogs closely over the next few days to determine which one goes through doors and gets in and out of cars first, pushes in front to be greeted and petted first when you return home, gets the toy or bone when only one is available, and so on.

Where an overprotective owner has been too quick in the past to interfere in minor aggression confrontations between the two dogs:

- Only intervene in fights between the two when it is clear that one or both dogs might be injured. Basically, an occasional fight is normal and may be beneficial in establishing the kind of relationship between the dogs which will prevent future fighting.

Scenario B: *the aggression is especially vicious and dangerous.*

- Never leave the two dogs alone together.
- The dogs should be well-trained over a period of weeks and months to come on command when called, and to sit, lie down, and stay sitting or lying when told to do so even in situations when they are highly excited or obviously want to do something else.
- Scold any growling with enough authority to immediately stop the behavior. When the growling has ended, call the dog, ask it to sit, and immediately reward compliance.

- Avoid unintentionally rewarding aggressive behavior by petting or talking to the aggressor to calm it down, or by distracting it with playing, food rewards, etc.
- Temporarily avoid placing the dogs together in competitive situations like feeding where aggression is commonly elicited.

Special behavior therapy method for dogs which immediately begin fighting on sight:

- Keep the dogs tied up on opposite sides of a room for several hours a day. Feed them and reward them with food tidbits for following commands often in this situation. As the dogs learn to remain more relaxed and non-aggressive in each other's presence, gradually reduce the distance apart over several days. At other times, keep the dogs entirely separated from one another.

(Additional recommendations from Chapter 10 to strengthen owner dominance are often required in all of the above types of cases.)

---

are, however, several other common scenarios as well. Females may be aggressive to other females. And both males and females may be especially aggressive to all other dogs, only to dogs of a certain type, or only to known individuals with which they have had problems in the past. Such aggression may vary greatly from displaying a decidedly self-protective/fearful quality on the one hand, to being bolder, more purely offensive on the other. And finally, some dogs which seem neither particularly fearful of nor aggressive towards other dogs seem nevertheless to have a way of provoking aggression in dogs they approach and greet in what appears to the owner to be a basically friendly, non-aggressive way.

As in the case of aggression towards unfamiliar humans, several categories are commonly used by pet problem counselors to classify aggression problems between dogs in the neighborhood such as *intermale, interfemale, fear, predatory, territorial,* and *protective* aggression. This is basically an empirical system – a reflection of the fact that if anyone who has seen a large number of interdog aggression cases were to sort the various problem scenarios into categories on the basis of common characteristics without any kind of preconceptions about the number of categories or characteristics of each, he/she would probably arrive at something similar: A category for ag-

gression between males, one for aggression between females, one where the dog shows obvious fear and reacts only when approached, cornered, etc., one for animals which viciously attack and perhaps kill other dogs as if they were members of an alien species, and two for other remaining cases depending on whether or not the intensity or probability of aggressive behavior is correlated with how near or far away the dog is from its home.

Classifying problems is this way is therefore an objective reflection of reality. It is also useful in a practical sense: the terms intermale, fear, etc. aggression do indeed refer in a fairly straightforward way to common scenarios, and as such there is no reason why they need to be abandoned. But to increase our understanding of these various types of interdog aggression problems, one must go farther than this. Is intermale aggression in this context the same as intermale aggression in the home? Does it have the same function? And does it have the same function as interfemale aggression in this context? Is it only dogs showing what anyone would describe as fear aggression that are in some sense "reacting out of fear"? Or are territorial and protective aggression sometimes also a reflection of the animal's fear of other dogs or types of dogs as appears to be the case with similar forms of aggression towards human beings? Is predatory aggression really predatory? Or is it a form of interspecies competition or perhaps even another form of intraspecific behavior where dogs are viciously attacked in spite of being recognized as conspecifics? And how do all of these various forms of aggression towards other dogs during walks relate to forms of aggression towards other dogs in the family on the one hand, and towards human beings who do not belong to the dog's family on the other?

Excluding until later the interspecific aggression case where dogs do not seem to respond to other dogs as conspecifics because of insufficient experience with them during the first three months of life, the classification system presented at the beginning of the chapter suggests that from a biological point of view, aggression towards dogs outside of the family can be profitably categorized as *self-protective*, *group-defensive*, or *competitive* aggression depending on whether the primary biological function of the aggressive behavior is for the dog to (1) defend itself against some immediate threat to its physical safety, (2) join with other group members to defend against outsiders who may represent a similar kind of immediate threat or threaten the group's existence more indirectly by exploiting the group's critical food, shelter, etc. resources, or (3) establish or maintain clear dominance over individuals encountered which, in a social group, would translate itself into a variety of advantages related to have exclusive or prior access to resources like food, mates, and resting places without having to fight for them.

Although this functional scheme neatly subsumes fear aggression as self-protective aggression and territorial and protective aggression as forms of group-defensive aggression, intermale (or interfemale) aggression between strange dogs is a form of competitive aggression which is more difficult to understand from a functional perspective than intermale aggression between dogs in the same family. Why should a male risk life and limb to establish its dominance over a strange male when there is nothing in the immediate situation they are competing over and it is likely or possible that they will never encounter one another again in the future?

There are several possible answers to this intriguing question. The first is that intermale aggression between strange males is basically intragroup behavior which is being performed outside of its normal social group context. A common observation made by ethologists in birds, fish, and other species is that when deprived of the opportunity to perform various types of species-typical behavior like, for example, hunting, sexual behavior, and aggressive behavior in their normal context, animals display increasingly heightened motivation to perform such sequences to the extent that finally minimally adequate and sometimes normally completely inadequate stimuli may elicit them. Thus, much of the intense interest, excitement, play, *and* aggression elicited by strange dogs during walks may be symptomatic of the state of partial deprivation of contacts with conspecifics in which most of our pet dogs are forced to live. Deprived of contacts with conspecifics for all but a short period of time every day, dogs leave their homes highly motivated to engage not in only extragroup behavior with the dogs they meet on the streets, but also types of intragroup play and dominance-related social behavior for which their human packmates are inadequate elicitors.

A second possibility is that intermale aggression between strange dogs may be best regarded as competitive not in the sense of the establishment or maintenance of a certain position in a social group dominance hierarchy, but rather as a means of settling the matter of "rights" to use certain territorial resources between members of different groups – therefore reflecting a fundamentally *group-defensive* function. While such encounters also seem entirely functionless in this regard in the sense that the males may encounter one another often and continue to share a common territory, one must consider how this kind of extragroup behavior might function in a natural environment setting. In theory at least, dominance-related threats and skirmishes in areas adjoining both groups could affect movement and territory use patterns of neighboring packs in ways (e.g. through future avoidance by the more submissive animals of places in which such confrontations took place) which are precluded among urban and suburban dogs that are members of human families whose territorial behavior takes an entirely different form. From this perspective, intermale aggression between strange males would be essentially a form of group-defensive aggression whose aim is to communicate to an intruder that the resident of this territory is a tough customer whom it would be advisable to avoid in future. In effect, its primary function is to settle what amounts to a kind of potential territorial dispute with a minimum of potentially dangerous fighting and in a way which precludes the need for further confrontations in the future.

A final possibility for accounting for intermale aggression between strange dogs is that such behavior is profitably looked at as a form of competitive or dominance aggression which has little or nothing to do with defense of the group or its territory. Rather, the behavior may be aimed at quickly settling the dominance question so that future aggressive competition between two individuals which are now essentially beginning the process of establishing some kind of new social relationship with one another will be avoided. Indeed, the initial aggressive interactions which occur between strange males can sometimes turn out to be a prelude to more positive behavioral interactions between the two animals – particularly if the one has no difficulty asserting its dominance over the other. For example, if the less aggressive dog reacts submissively to the other's dominant behavior, the tone of the social interactions may change dramatically and the two may soon end up playing together. Thus, even though the two individuals may be strangers to one another, the function of such behavior would not be to encourage the submissive animal to depart and keep out of area in the future, but rather to establish or confirm a certain kind of relationship between individuals which allows them to engage in various types of positive behavior like playing without fighting in competitive situations as when, for example, the two dogs are trying to play with one stick or one human being.

Essentially this view postulates that for our domestic dogs, the distinction between intragroup and extragroup behavior is not always as clear as in would be if the dogs were living wild in stable packs which defend group territories and regularly drive intruders away. In effect, it is being suggested here that this type of extragroup competitive aggression might lead naturally and quickly to intragroup behavior – that perhaps it is the first step in the *group formation process* which might be expected to occur when, for example, strays which eventually band together initially encounter one another, or when a new individual is allowed to join an existing group. This type of intermale aggression along with play between strange dogs and indeed the tendency for most family-owned dogs to be strongly drawn to one another other during walks may therefore be another indication of how highly our pet dogs are motivated to form groups with real conspecifics in spite of our belief that they have all that they need. Essentially, the state of partial social deprivation inherent in the domestics dog's life isolated from true conspecifics for all but a small proportion of every day would be in evidence here as well.

The remainder of the present section consists of a discussion of possible causal factors and treatment elements for all of the various forms of aggression towards dogs encountered during walks which do not reflect early experience effects which are severe enough to make dogs incapable of normal social behavior with conspecifics. Although diverse forms of aggression and related problem scenarios are involved, the many similarities in the approach to treatment makes it easy to consider them together in a single section while, at the same time, pointing out where differences in causal and treatment elements exist for the various types of problems.

Possible causal factors

Genetic predisposition

A genetic predisposition is often suspected for some of these problems. For example, some

POSSIBLE CAUSAL FACTORS

Genetic predisposition
(e.g. intermale/interfemale aggression)

Hormonal influence
(e.g. intermale aggression often reduced by castration)

Insufficient early experience with conspecifics
(possible source of fear of all dogs; behavior of socially inexperienced dog may provoke aggression)

Aversive past experiences
(e.g. conditioned fear to known individuals or dogs of certain type due to past attacks)

Lack of basic obedience training
(low owner control capability)

Insufficient owner dominance
(low owner control capability)

Unintentional owner reinforcement
(e.g. petting/distracting dog to reduce fear/aggression)

AGGRESSION TOWARDS OTHER DOGS IN THE NEIGHBORHOOD

POSSIBLE TREATMENT ELEMENTS

Avoid problem situations
(e.g. alter walk schedule/route to avoid known enemies, choose off-leash times/ places more carefully)

Castration
(for intermale aggression)

Training in problem situations
(combination of reward and punishment to improve behavior in presence of other dogs)

Conventional obedience training
(increase owner control capability)

Increase owner dominance
(increase owner control capability)

Correct owner mistakes
(e.g. stop unintentional rewards/ineffective scolding; don't always intervene in fights)

Systematic behavior therapy methods
(e.g. countercondition non-aggressive behavior in series of situations involving increasingly close proximity to other dogs)

Medicaments
(progestin therapy as adjunct to retraining measures in intermale aggression cases)

Change care/maintenance ground rules
(e.g. keep dog on leash in potential problem situations; provide more experience with other dogs)

Physical aids
(muzzle, head collar)

males are highly aggressive to other males during walks while others rarely if ever get involved in any kind of aggressive interaction. And in most cases, there is no viable explanation of why these individual differences exist in terms of the dogs' past experiences with other dogs, home environment, treatment by owners, lack of contact with conspecifics, and so on – which seems to point to genetic differences between the animals.

Hormonal influences

While so-called fear, territorial, and protective aggression are unaffected by castration, intermale aggression towards dogs in the neighborhood can often be reduced or eliminated in this way, which obviously implies that some sort of hormonal influence is involved.

Insufficient early experience with conspecifics

Some dogs have difficulties getting along peaceably with other dogs. In some cases, owners report that the dogs were taken away from their littermates at a relatively young age and had little contact with conspecifics during the following months. Although this kind of early experience-related effect may not be severe enough to make the dogs completely incapable of normal social behavior with other dogs, it may nevertheless produce lasting effects on the dog's behavior towards conspecifics. Such dogs may be mildly fearful of other dogs or act somewhat uncertain as to how to behave towards them. Perhaps they tend therefore to perform odd or partially incorrect versions of species-typical behavior or tend to incorrectly interpret the communicative behavior of conspecifics. And even if they are not unusually aggressive to other dogs, their behavior may tend to provoke aggression in others. Indeed, many owners describe just such a scenario: their dog approaches other dogs in a basically friendly and non-aggressive way, but even the most gregarious neighborhood dogs will have little to do with it, and may growl and snap if it persists in trying to engage them in social interactions.

Aversive past experiences

So-called fear aggression towards other dogs is common. For example, owners may report that the dog is noticeably fearful and therefore aggressive towards certain dogs or types of dogs (e.g. large dogs, small dogs) with which it has had problems with in the past. But the conditioning effects of aversive past experiences can produce a somewhat different outcome as well. Rather than behaving overtly fearfully, some dogs act like they simply don't "like" certain kinds of dogs or individuals and are, therefore, inclined to be offensively aggressive towards them under any and all circumstances. In response to the question of why think this might be so, owners often point to specific incidents in their dog's past where such problems began. Commonly, the dog was attacked by a certain individual and later is especially aggressive towards this individual and perhaps other dogs which resemble it. Additionally, owners frequently report that dog was in fact noticeably fearful during the weeks and months following the incident, but the behavior towards the type of dogs it often attacks has become increasingly less fearful and more purely offensive over time.

Interestingly, it is not always the larger dogs which are most feared. Sometimes large dogs are especially fearful of and hence aggressive towards small dogs ever since they were suddenly and viciously attacked by an especially aggressive dog of this size. One must be careful here, however, for it is theoretically possible that attacks on smaller dogs could also be a case of a dog which tends to be aggressive to all dogs but is essentially too fearful to take on someone its own size.

Lack of basic obedience training

Often dogs which make the most problems in the presence of other dogs are those which have not been trained by their owners to respond to commands and inhibit misbehavior when ordered to do so.

Insufficient owner dominance

Naturally, owners of dogs that are often disobedient or slow to obey are particularly helpless when in comes to preventing and ending fighting with other dogs. As always, the dominance-related relationship between owner and dog is an extremely important area to explore during the consultation.

Unintentional owner reinforcement

Owners should always be questioned closely about what exactly they do when their dog starts, for example, growling at another dog. If the answer is that they try to distract the dog with something it likes like an invitation to play, a tidbit, ball, etc., or if they assume the dog is fearful and pet and talk reassuringly to it to try and reduce the fear, they should be warned that they may be contributing to the problem by reinforcing the problem behavior.

Possible treatment elements

Avoid problem situations

In some cases, it may be possible for owners simply avoid problem situations. For example, animals which have run free in the past can be kept on a leash during walks, walk schedules or routes can be changed to avoid known enemies, or off-leash times and places can be chosen more carefully. Many owners of dogs which frequently become involved in aggressive confrontations with other dogs learn to satisfactorily cope with the problem simply by making adjustments of this sort.

Castration

As discussed earlier, castration can sometimes produce a dramatic reduction in intermale aggression. It does not, however, appear to have a beneficial effect on the other forms of aggression towards strange dogs.

Conventional obedience training

The first step in increasing the control capability of owners who have little or no control over their dogs in problem situations – or potential problem situations – is conventional obedience training either using the methods discussed in Chapter 8 or by joining an dog obedience training class.

Training in problem situations

In cases where a conventional retraining approach is indicated, the general training principles are the same as in the case of group-defensive aggression towards strange human beings. Namely, the consistent application of some combination of (1) promptly-administered food or and/or social *rewards* for desirable behavior in potential problem situations (e.g. coming to the owner, sitting and staying quietly sitting instead of threatening potential targets) with (2) *punishment* which is intense enough to immediately suppress problem behavior.

However, specifying precisely how owners should behave under any and all circumstances can be even more difficult here than in the case of aggression towards human strangers, for it is unrealistic and counterproductive to train dogs to stay away from other dogs entirely. Should a dog be trained to stay away from known enemies with which it has had problems in the past? Or should the two be allowed to work out the matter of dominance between them even if this means standing back and watching them fight until one or the other submits? Theoretically, this may seem like the most reasonable solution. But fights between dogs can sometimes result in serious injuries or even cause the death of one of the combatants. And what about the case of the first encounter with a strange dog? How should the owner of a dog which is sometimes, but not always aggressive to strange dogs behave in this situation? Intervene immediately to prevent problems? Or allow the two approach and interact with one another at least until problems begin to develop? Many of the interactions dogs have with other dogs in the neighborhood (presented for interdog aggression problems) are in fact peaceable and in the long run extremely beneficial to the dogs, and more positive experiences interacting with other dogs is one of the best medicines for some dog-aggressive dogs. But how then is one to decide which encounters to prevent and which to allow, when to intervene during the early stages of an aggressive confrontation and when to stand back and do nothing, and when to stop fighting or let it run its full course?

Obviously, these are often difficult decisions for owners to make. But make them they must, for these questions reflect the complexities and uncertainties inherent in the situations within which these interdog aggression problems occur. Owners must essentially learn to adjust their behavior to the many kinds of dogs, owners, and situations encountered. Experience teaches them which of the dogs in the neighborhood are best avoided and which need not be avoided either because no aggressive confrontations occur or because confrontations are usually tolerably mild. Experience also teaches them to assess strange dogs from a distance and during the early stages of the close contact between dogs. Warnings and information elicited from other owners are helpful here too. For example, some owners of males which are aggressive to other males routinely call out ahead to approaching owners if their dog is a male, and if it is, immediately attach the leash to their own male's collar. When interactions between dogs do turn aggressive, owners must do their best by closely observing both dogs to judge how serious the confrontation will turn out to be. And finally, the sometimes irrational wishes of other owners to prevent minor skirmishes must often be respected in the interests of avoiding making neighborhood enemies oneself. Although it is easy for "dog people" who know better to ridicule overprotective owners who are frightened when their dog becomes embroiled in any kind of aggressive confrontation with another dog, these anxious owners too are a fact of life with which the owner who seeks to maintain friendly relations with the other dog owners encountered daily must diplomatically deal.

Particularly with a dog that is predictably aggressive towards certain types of dogs or certain individuals in the neighborhood with which the dog has had a number of problems in the past, the use of the *early intervention method* which is often useful to train the dog

to come to its owner and follow commands in the presence of potential targets like joggers and bicyclists may be profitably applied here as well. The dog is called as soon as one of its arch enemies or one of the types of dogs towards which it is invariably aggressive is sighted and then rewarded with its favorite tidbits for approaching the owner instead of the other dog. However, to be effective and to avoid the danger of inadvertently rewarding aggressive behavior, the dog must be called *before* it begins showing any kind of aggression. (See Chapter 12 for a more detailed discussion of this method).

Finally, some owners are able to essentially accomplish the same early-intervention objective by simply exercising more authority at this time by calling the dog and firmly commanding it to come if it doesn't come immediately as soon as they spot another dog with which there is likely to be problems. When combined with rewarding the dog with a tidbit or petting and praise for compliance, this method can sometimes be highly effective in avoiding problems, increasing owner control, and counterconditioning desirable behavior (e.g. immediately coming to the owner) in potential problem situations.

Increasing owner dominance

In a great many interdog aggression cases, the difficulty owners have in controlling and retraining dog-aggressive dogs reflects some kind of owner-dog relationship problem which also must be addressed by the counselor's recommendations. Often, substantial progress must first be made using either the direct or indirect methods described in Chapter 10 for increasing owner dominance if the owner is going to stand a chance of improving the dogs behavior towards other dogs.

Correct owner mistakes

Overprotective owners who always intervene before their dog's threatening of other dogs provokes fighting may be making a mistake. Most fights are short-lived and not dangerous to either party. And it usually doesn't take the small dog which has picked a fight with a much larger one long to realize that it's time to give up, roll over, and admit defeat – which is just the kind of lesson from which some dogs benefit.

Another common mistake is when owners unintentionally reward threatening by petting and talking to their dog as if trying to calm it down or convince it that there is no reason it should be aggressive. Even if the reinforcing effect per se is minor, such positive reactions may signal owner approval and support to the dog, which in turn may act to increase the aggression.

Finally, owners which scold or scream at other dogs or their owners, scream at their own dog, or scold it too mildly to have any effect may simply be making the problem worse. Such owner behavior may be misinterpreted by the dog as the owner's having joined in the fray on its side and so increases the aggression via the kind of social facilitation effect which produces coordinated aggressive displays in pairs or groups of dogs. However, scolding can be indicated for some problems and when it is effective enough to end the threatening *immediately* and *every time* it occurs. If punishment is indicated but scolding is ineffective – as is often the case with mild-mannered clients – the owner must employ some other punishment method like, for example, leash correction or the production of some sound (e.g. from a compressed air device) which the dog finds aversive.

Systematic behavior therapy methods

The use of tidbits or social rewards (i.e. petting and praise) to countercondition obedience to basic commands like come, sit, stay, etc. in the presence of other dogs is a necessary adjunct to punishment-produced suppression of aggression in cases where this is indicated. Although rewarding obedient, non-aggressive behavior is normally carried out on an informal basis in whatever naturally occurring situations it seems appropriate, there are cases in which this approach can be incorporated into a more systematic behavior therapy procedure. Obedience training can, for example, be first carried

out on the edge of a large field where dogs are playing or being trained. Over the course of time, the distance away from other dogs can then be gradually reduced as the dog learns to ignore the other dogs and continue following owner commands during these practice sessions.

However, even a relatively simple behavior therapy procedure such as this requires a dedicated owner who understands the long-term nature of the training program and is patient, highly-motivated, and self-disciplined enough to see it through. Unfortunately, all too few clients are interested in such an option. In general, they are extremely fond of their pet and would dearly love to solve the burdensome problem. But they are busy people with many other demands on the time, and they tend therefore to be unwilling to invest as much time and effort as this kind of long-term retraining effort would require.

Medicaments

Many behavior specialists recommend the use of progestins, *megestrol acetate* or *medroxyprogesterone acetate*, as an adjunct to retraining measures in some serious cases of intermale aggression. Hart and Hart (1985) report that clinical experience leads one to expect a 75 % improvement rate with castrated males. However, it is widely recognized that the beneficial, aggression-reducing effects of these medicaments are only temporary, the long-term administration of these drugs sometimes have serious side effects, and it is therefore only by placing the primary emphasis on retraining or problem management measures that a satisfactory solution to the problem can be achieved. (See the "drug therapy" subsection in Chapter 8 for side effects and other important drug-related information.)

Change care/maintenance conditions

Deciding to routinely keep the dog on a leash in potential problem situations is one helpful change which owners who have previously always let their dog run free can make. Another

SAMPLE RECOMMENDATIONS

Aggression towards other dogs in the neighborhood

- Use the dog's favorite tidbits as rewards for quiet, obedient, non-aggressive behavior in the presence of other dogs. Don't give the dog any tidbits at all at other times.
- In the beginning, it is to be expected that this approach may only be successful in situations where the dog is not so excited or aggressive (or when other dogs are not so nearby).
- Avoid unintentionally rewarding aggression by using petting, food rewards, playing, or other distraction measures to try and end the dog's threatening of other dogs.

In cases where punitive measures to suppress aggression are also appropriate:
- Every time the dog barks or growls at another dog, scold or otherwise punish it severely enough to stop the aggression immediately.
- As soon as the dog has quieted down in this situation, tell it to sit or lie down and give it a tidbit and/or pet and praise it when it obeys.
- Screaming at the dog or scolding it to stop it from being aggressive is only to be recommended if it really does stop the aggression. If not, you are not reacting with enough authority and you may be actually stimulating the dog to become even more aggressive.

In cases where the aggression is mild and simply spending more time interacting with other dogs might help to reduce the seriousness of the problem:
- Frequent playtimes with other dogs is the best medicine against this kind of problem.
- Do not intervene in every aggressive confrontation. Sometimes it is better to let the dogs settle such matters for themselves.

In cases where the dog represents a serious danger to other dogs:
- If possible, avoid aggressive confrontations with the dog's arch enemies by changing walk schedule/routes.
- The dog should be kept on the leash during walks until its behavior towards other dogs has improved.
- If the dog is impossible to keep under control even when kept on a leash, some kind of head collar which makes it easier to physically control is to be recommended. Muzzling the dog is another option.

Example of early intervention method which is useful in some types of cases:
- If the dog is off leash, call it and reward it with a tidbit for coming as soon as you see another dog coming but *before* your dog starts being aggressive. Then tell it to sit or lie down, reward it for obeying, and then reward it several times again for not being aggressive when the other dog is nearby.

Additional recommendations in some cases of intermale aggression:
- There is a good chance that castration will reduce or eliminate the problem of fighting with other males.
- Temporary drug therapy with a hormone preparation may help to reduce the aggression to a level which allows you to carry out the behavioral training program.

(Additional recommendations from Chapter 10 to strengthen owner dominance are often required in all of the above types of cases.)

is to alter walk schedules or routes to increase the amount of daily contact which their dogs have with other dogs. This is certainly not necessary or helpful in all cases, but for some dogs which have had too little contact with other dogs in the past and therefore often provoke aggression in other dogs with their awkward, uncertain, mildly fearful, or otherwise peculiar behavior, this may provide beneficial experiences which may help reduce the frequency and severity of interdog aggression problems.

Physical aids

In some particularly serious cases, having the dog wear a muzzle or head collar during walks may be called for. Neville (1991) sometimes recommends both to eliminate the danger to other dogs posed by some particularly vicious animals and to provide the owner with a more effective means of physically controlling the dog during confrontations with other dogs.

Interspecific aggression towards other dogs

Interspecific group-defensive/self-protective aggression

Dogs which are taken away from their litter and deprived of all contact with other dogs before 6 weeks of age may have difficulties interacting with conspecifics later in life. And dogs which are taken away much earlier than this are likely to be aggressive to other dogs or otherwise socially inept in interacting with them (Hart and Hart, 1985; O'Farrell 1992). They may direct virtually all of their later social behavior towards human beings and either ignore other dogs entirely or treat them as undesirable intruders which must be avoided or driven away. As is the case with other similar imprinting-like phenomena in the animal world, this early experience effect is largely irreversible and there is usually no way to train or teach such a dog to interact normally with or "like" other dogs.

Do dogs which completely ignore or are aggressive to all other dogs really fail to perceive

them as conspecifics? It is difficult to say with certainty. Many examples of imprinting in other species where later *intra*specific sexual behavior, for example, is directed towards the members of another species often involve animals which do not seem able to interact normally with members of their own species. This has led some animal behaviorists to hypothesize that some kind of species misidentification may be involved (e.g. Grier and Burk, 1992). Indeed, if it is granted that dogs are flexible enough to respond to and perhaps also perceive human beings as conspecifics, then perhaps it is not so unreasonable to suspect that failure to perceive true conspecifics as fellow species members is also possible.

However, there is a second possibility for accounting for the aggressive behavior of such dogs. Namely, that in spite of the fact that they perceive other dogs as conspecifics, they lack the critical early experiences required for the development of a normal social behavioral capability. They therefore turn out to be somewhat incompetent in carrying out and reacting properly to (i.e. correctly interpreting) species-typical social behavior, and this in turn provokes aggressive reactions in other dogs so often that they finally become conditioned aversive stimuli which elicit defensive aggression in the socially inept animals.

Without careful research into the question, there is no way to be sure whether dogs that are aggressive to all other dogs or otherwise do not interact normally with them are displaying true interspecific behavior. As a result, the use of this term in Figure 14.1 should be regarded as tentative. Such behavior may also represent some combination of *intra-* and *inter*specific behavioral elements, or it may resemble only in certain limited ways the self-protective/group-defensive behavior directed towards the members of other species.

Predatory "aggression"/interspecies competition

In cases where large dogs immediately and viciously attack smaller dogs (and all other smaller animals like cats, rabbits, etc.) on sight – grabbing them by the neck and viciously shaking them without showing the slightest trace of the species-typical behavior normally seen when strange dogs first encounter one another – true *interspecific* predatory or interspecies competitive behavior may be involved. However, this problem seems to be relatively rare. For example, from eight of my interdog aggression cases (out of a total of 49) in which the dogs never interacted with other dogs and were invariably aggressive towards them, only one fitted this pattern.

References

Borchelt, P.L., and Voith, V.L. (1982): Classification of animal behavior problems. *Veterinary Clinics of North America: Small Animal Practice* **12**, 571–585.

Feddersen-Petersen, D. (1993): Verhaltensprobleme älterer Hunde. *Der praktische Tierarzt* **74**, 46–49.

Grier, J.W., and Burk, T. (1992): *Biology of Animal Behavior*. St. Louis. Mosby-Year Book Inc.

Hart, B.L., and Hart, L.A. (1985): *Canine and Feline Behavioral Therapy*. Philadelphia: Lea & Febiger.

Hopkins, S.G., Schubert, T.A., and Hart, B.L. (1976): Castration of adult male dogs: Effects on roaming, aggression, urine marking, and mounting. *Journal of the American Veterinary Medical Association* **168**, 1108

Mech, L.D. (1970): *The Wolf: The Ecology and Behavior of an Endangered Species*. New York, The Natural History Press.

Neville, P. (1991): *Do Dogs Need Shrinks?* London, Sidgwick & Jackson Ltd.

Nott, H.M.R. (1992): Social behaviour of the dog. In Thorne, C. (ed) *The Waltham Book of Dog and Cat Behaviour*. Oxford, Pergamon Press.

O'Farrell V. (1992): *Manual of Canine Behaviour*. British Small Animal Veterinary Association. Shurdington, Cheltenham, Gloucestershire, UK.

15   Fear Problems

Pet behavior counselors are frequently confronted with fear problems in dogs. Dogs may try to run away, hide under a table or behind their owner, tremble, whine, bark, pant, and perhaps become aggressive in response to fear-eliciting stimuli.

Excluding problems related to separation anxiety (Chapter 16) and the various forms of self-protective aggression discussed in Chapters 11-14, owners in 31 out of 154 consecutive dog problem cases (i.e. approx. 20%) reported that fearful behavior was one of their dog's major behavior problems. A total of 54 different fear problems was mentioned for these 31 dogs. Figure 15.1 summarizes the nature of the fear-eliciting stimuli for the various fear problems reported.

While the specific percentages shown in the figure differ from those reported by the several articles referred to by Tuber et al. (1982), for the most part these studies agree with the present statistics that fear of sudden loud noises, traffic and street noises, human strangers, and other dogs are the most commonly reported problems involving fearful behavior in response to specific stimuli.

Fear problems can sometimes be quite bizarre. In a recent case, an owner contacted me to make an appointment because his dog was terrified of airplane vapor trails. During the house call, it became apparent after seeing the dog hardly react to the trail left by a jetliner passing overhead that it was not the vapor trails per se, but the empty blue sky itself which was eliciting the fear: the dog continuously starred into the vacant sky, shivered, and kept trying to press up against the owners' legs when it was walking down the relatively open residential streets. The husband and wife assured me that on cloudy days the animal was an entirely different dog – not exhibiting the slightest trace of fear. The dog's "blue sky phobia" was also in evidence indoors. Whereas on cloudy days the dog normally lies next to the large sliding glass door that leads out onto the terrace, on blue-sky days the dog always lies under the coffee table well away from the door which provides a vantage point from which the dog can constantly scrutinize a wide strip of the blue sky through the top of the door.

Figure 15.2 presents additional statistical information on the prevalence of fearful be-

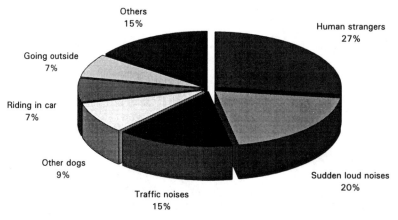

Figure 15.1: Relative frequency of various stimuli eliciting fearful behavior in 54 fear problems (n=31 dogs)

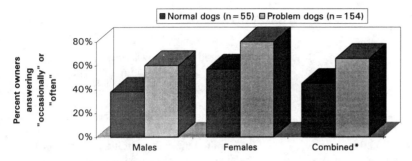

■ Normal dogs (n = 55) ▨ Problem dogs (n = 154)

Figure 15.2: Relative frequency of "occasionally" or "often" answers by owners of problem dogs vs. normal dogs to the question "How often does your dog show excessive fear reactions?" (* Excluding 31 dogs specifically presented for fear problems)

havior in both problem dogs and those from the normal, non-problem dog population. Using the client information form described in Chapter 6, the owners of 154 problem dogs and 55 non-problem dogs were asked to indicate how often (i.e. "often", "occasionally", or "never") their dog displayed "excessive fear reactions".

The following three aspects of the results presented in the figure are worth mentioning:

- Excessive fear reactions seem to be more prevalent among females in both populations.

- Excessive fear reactions are more commonly reported in problem animals then in those from the normal population. Even excluding the previously-mentioned 31 dogs specifically presented for fear problems, a modest difference between the two samples is still apparent (i.e. difference between the two "combined" bars). This still leaves, however, some dogs in the problem dog sample which show fear responses in connection with aggression and separation anxiety problems. It is likely therefore that the fearful behavior associated with these problems accounts for much of the difference between the two groups.

- Of particular interest is the relatively high frequency (45%) in the "combined" sample with which owners from the normal dog population checked the "often" (twice) or "occasionally" (23 times) columns. Apparently, it is entirely normal for dogs to show "excessive fear reactions" in response to loud noises, strangers, other dogs, etc. from time to time.

Possible causal factors

Genetic factors

Four types of evidence suggest that the predisposition to react extremely fearfully to environmental stimuli may be in part genetically determined in some animals. First: in contrast to other problems like dominance aggression, the tendency to react fearfully to stimuli later in life is partially predictable from the assessment of fear reactions of puppies from about 8 weeks of age onwards (Goddard and Beilharz, 1985). Second: the histories of some fearful dogs do not indicate any kind of early deprivation or later traumatic experience effects. Sometimes one dog out of a litter may turn out to display severe fear problems whereas other dogs from the same litter which had essentially the same early and later experiences turn out to be normal in this regard. Third: using selective breeding, Murphree and colleagues (Murphree et al., 1967, Murphree 1972, Dykman et al., 1979) bred two strains of German shorthaired pointers – one which is essentially normal and the other which develops extreme fear reactions to noise, novel stimuli, and even familiar human beings at about 3 months of age. And fourth: it is well-known that wolves tend to be "neophobic" in that they tend to react fearfully to novel stimuli – one of the characteristics which has been obviously selected against during the domestication process.

These types of evidence do not, however, indicate that fear problems are due to genetic factors in most dogs. Probably the opposite is the case; most problems reflect either early experience deficits, later aversive experiences, or a

POSSIBLE CAUSAL FACTORS

Genetic factors
(suspected where fear not result of past experiences)

Effect of traumatic/aversive events
(e.g. punishment, traffic accident, attack by other dog, teasing by children, loud noises in neighborhood, etc.)

Restricted early experience
(e.g. with strangers, children, traffic noises, etc. during first 3 months of life)

Unintentional owner reinforcement/ fostering
(e.g. unintentional rewarding of fearful behavior; owner's emotional/avoidance behavior may intensify animal's fearful response to situations/stimuli)

FEAR PROBLEMS
• Fear of strangers, loud noises, traffic, other dogs, etc.

POSSIBLE TREATMENT ELEMENTS

Avoid problem situations
(especially when fear very intense)

Correct owner mistakes
(e.g. stop unintentional rewards)

Systematic behavior therapy methods
(systematic densensitization/counter-conditioning; flooding)

Conventional obedience training
(to increase owner control in problem situations)

Increase owner dominance
(when lack of owner dominance relevant to problem)

Cessation of counterproductive treatment methods
(e.g. stop exposing animal to situations evoking great fear)

Medicaments
(e.g. anxiolytics indicated in some cases)

Training in problem situations
(ignore fearful behavior and elicit/reward non-fearful behavior in problem situations)

Increased owner authority
(to increase owner control in problem situations)

combination of the two. But in some cases, the apparent absence of such experiential effects in some dogs' histories coupled with information that dogs were abnormally fearful even as young puppies suggest that a genetic predisposition may be involved – a suspicion which can be of great practical importance in terms of determining treatment methods and setting treatment goals.

Restricted early experience

Many studies have provided evidence that dogs which have had restricted experience with humans or novel environments during the first three months of life – the 3rd to 12th week is commonly regarded as the critical time period for this effect – react fearfully to such stimuli later in life. In reviewing some of these studies,

Borchelt and Voith (1985) make a point of emphasizing that such fears are not rigidly irreversible as is commonly believed and, therefore, some instances of fearful behavior reflecting a lack of early experiences with certain stimuli are at least partially reversible through later experiences. However, this result is the exception. For most of the dogs in these studies, treatment procedures designed to reduce the level of fear had little or no effect. It is not surprising therefore that in many cases that come to the attention of behavior problem counselors, dogs whose later fear of human strangers, children, city environments, etc. seem causally related to impoverished early environments have remained extremely fearful in spite of having had a great deal of later experience with the feared stimuli. For these dogs, the tendency to react fearfully to certain specific stimuli may indeed be irreversible, and the therapeutic aim therefore becomes more focused on helping clients cope with rather than eliminate the problem.

Effect of traumatic/aversive events

Fear of a certain type of stimulus can be acquired as the result of a single traumatic event. For example, an animal can become extremely fearful of riding in cars after being involved in a traffic accident or it may react fearfully towards all big black dogs after having been attacked and seriously injured by one. However, the fear acquisition process can also be more gradual, involving a series of negative experiences with types of stimuli which it eventually fears. Frequent punishment by the owner, teasing by children, and being startled by loud noises in a certain place in the neighborhood can all lead to fear problems which increase in intensity with every additional experience.

Unintentional owner reinforcement/fostering

What could be more natural for the human parent than to pick up, hug, distract, or speak reassuringly to a frightened young child? All owners are naturally inclined to unthinkingly react this way to a frightened pet. These owner reactions can have two interrelated effects. Firstly, they may function as rewards and thereby strengthen if not the underlying fear itself, at least some of the overtly fearful behaviors like running to owners for protection, cowering behind their legs, and whining and trembling. Secondly, the owner's concerned and perhaps even alarmed behavior may inadvertently communicate an erroneous message to the dog that this is indeed a potentially dangerous situation or stimulus which even the owner fears. Indeed, some owners actually do learn to fear these situations or stimuli and therefore do they what they can to avoid them simply because they find it so disturbing to see their dog apparently suffering in this way.

Possible treatment elements

Avoid problem situations

With extremely fearful animals, recommendations for preventing a worsening of the problem and increasing basic owner control capabilities may be required along with those for reducing the animal's fear. The first is to temporarily avoid problem situations (e.g. changing walk routes to avoid feared stimuli, avoiding contact with strangers, avoiding taking the dog in the car or on public transportation) especially with animals which are extremely fearful. When animals become intensely fearful in the presence of a feared stimulus, this tends to maintain the animal's fearfulness and perhaps make it react even more fearfully the next time the stimulus is encountered. Like pain, fear is an intensely aversive state which has great power to affect animals' reactions to situations in which it is elicited.

Often this strategy of avoiding problem situations is recommended as a temporary measure which remains in effect until the animal has learned – via the various training measures discussed below – to be exposed to less threatening approximations to the feared stimulus/situation without becoming fearful.

Cessation of counterproductive treatment methods

Owners sometimes think that simply exposing animals to a feared situation is enough; sooner or later the animal will learn that nothing bad is going to happen to it and relax. This is theoretically true in the sense that an animal which is left in a fear-eliciting situation long enough may eventually relax to some extent. However, the time-scale on which this might be expected to happen is more on the order of several hours rather than the few minutes which the owner assumes will be sufficient to start this habituation process. As discussed above, exposing the animal to feared stimuli for periods of time which are too brief for it to learn to relax will probably make the problem worse and not better.

Correct owner mistakes

A mistake which all owners make is to respond to the fearful dog as one would respond to a fearful young child. Namely, to try to reduce the fear by calming, reassuring, or distracting the animal by petting it, picking it up, trying to get it to play, or giving it a food reward. Although these kinds of owner reactions may work in the short-term sense that an animal's trembling and crouching do indeed decrease at the time, in the long run they may (1) reinforce components of the fear response like trembling, hiding behind the owner, etc., and (2) be interpreted by the animal as a sign that the owner too finds the situation in some way threatening or more significant than it really is. As considered above, this inadvertent message is sometimes not entirely erroneous. Owners do in fact tend to become sensitized to and perhaps even learn to fear these kinds of situations because of their dog's strong negative reactions to them. Consequently, they too may try to avoid them or escape from them as soon as possible as much for their own sake as for that of their dog.

Medicaments

For the treatment of fear problems, medicaments are sometimes useful in the following types of cases:
- As the sole treatment when recent trauma is the source of the problem (e.g. dog is very

fearful when riding in a car a few days after being in a traffic accident).
- If it is not practically feasible to carry out the systematic behavior therapy which would be needed to reduce the fear.
- As a temporary adjunct to training or behavior therapy methods when the animal is initially too fearful to respond appropriately to the counterconditioning procedure.
- To protect the animal from becoming intensely fearful in situations where exposure to a fear-eliciting stimulus is inevitable (e.g. at the first sign of approaching thunderstorm).

The following drugs have been reported to be sometimes effective with fear problems in dogs:

Diazepam at the following doses:
- 0.1-0.5 mg/kg po (Shull-Selcer and Stagg, 1991; Voith and Borchelt, 1885)
- 0.55 to 2.2 mg/kg po as needed (Marder 1991)
- 1 to 2 mg/kg po bid – tid (Hart and Hart, 1985)

Paradoxical excitability or hyperactivity is a common side effect (Voith and Borchelt, 1985) which can sometimes be overcome by increasing the dose (Shull-Selcer and Stagg, 1991). All authors emphasize that owners should stay at home to observe the dog's reaction to the drug the first time it is administered.

Voith (1989) warns that diazepam may increase aggression in fearful dogs and recommends that it should not be given to dogs which are fearful of people, particularly those which have been aggressive in the past.

A longer-acting benzodiazepine, *clorazepate dipotassium*, has also been used effectively for the treatment of noise or thunder phobias at doses of 5.6 mg/dog po for small dogs, 11.25 mg/dog po for medium-sized dogs, and 22.5 mg/dog po for large dogs (Shull-Selcer and Stagg, 1991).

According to Marder (1991) and Shull-Selcer and Stagg (1991), *buspirone* and the beta-blocker, *propranolol*, have been occasionally used with some success. Marder recommends dosing buspirone at 2.5-10 mg/dog po bid-tid.

Voith and Borchelt (1985) and Marder (1991) suggest that the *phenothiazines* (e.g.

acetylpromazine dosed at 0.5-1 mg/kg po, according to Marder) are only useful for managing extremely fearful dogs, but not for helping to reduce or eliminate fear problems themselves. Voith and Borchelt (1985) and Shull-Selcer and Stagg (1991) suggest that the same is true of *phenobarbital*. Marder (1991) only uses phenothiazines to treat, for example, "dogs with loud-noise phobias or separation anxiety that are extremely destructive or jumping through windows".

The following quotation from Shull-Selcer and Stagg (1991) sums up the general views expressed above and presents sensible guidelines for the prescription of drugs in cases where they are required:

"Acetylpromazine maleate and phenobarbital are used commonly in veterinary medicine to aid in the management of fearful dogs. In the treatment of noise phobias, sedation to the point of disorientation and ataxia frequently is required before the behavioral component of the fear response is adequately attenuated. In some dogs with high-intensity fear responses, heavy sedation may be the only effective treatment...When the phobic fear response is less intense, however, the less sedating anxiolytics may be effective ... (and therefore) ... are recommended as the initial drugs of choice for dogs with low to moderate intensity fear responses." (p. 364)

Before prescribing medicaments, the reader is advised to refer to the "drug therapy" subsection in Chapter 8 for side effects and other important drug-related information.

Systematic behavior therapy methods

The classical desensitization/counterconditioning behavior therapy approach which can sometimes be employed to reduce an animal's fear of specific persons or specific stimuli is analogous to a similar procedure which the several sources cited by Shull-Selcer and Stagg (1991) claim is "widely accepted as the most reliable treatment for phobic disorders in humans". Interestingly, the procedure was originally developed as an experimental treatment for phobic fears in animals – to reduce cats' fear

of cages in which they were subjected to intense electrical shock (Wolpe, 1958).

The behavior therapy approach is based on the following principles:

- The procedure is only useful for (1) reducing fears of *specific stimuli* – a certain individual, specific type of person, or certain type of noise rather than all persons or all loud noises – which can be (2) presented to the animal in a *graded intensity* ranging from very mild in the beginning (e.g. person far away, noise at low intensity) to progressively more and more intense (e.g. person closer, noise louder) as the animal becomes desensitized to each intensity level.

- The animal must not be exposed to the feared stimulus except during the behavior therapy sessions. Where exposure is inevitable (e.g. to a thunderstorm), keeping the animal's fear response low with medication may prevent the loss of progress which has been achieved during the behavior therapy sessions.

- At each stage, the animal is rewarded with food tidbits for performing some competing behavior in the presence of the feared stimulus which is incompatible with fearful behavior like following a command and/or waiting for another food reward in a "relaxed" manner (i.e. without noticeable signs of fear like lowered head and tail). This eliciting and strengthening of a competing behavior incompatible with the fearful behavior is referred to as *counterconditioning*.

- The cardinal rule of the procedure is that the animal must never be exposed to a version of the feared stimulus which evokes a noticeable fear response. It is acceptable if the animal becomes only very slightly uneasy, for this soon habituates with repeated presentations and rewards. But if the animal reacts very fearfully at any time, this is a sign that the procedure is being improperly applied (e.g. intensity has been increased too quickly), and the stimulus intensity must again be reduced down to a level which doesn't elicit fear. Ideally, the whole procedure should be carried out in such a way that the animal never shows more that the slightest trace of uneasiness when exposed to the various versions of the feared stimulus.

Tuber et. al (1982) presents a detailed and excellent account of how these general treatment principles can be applied to the treatment of separation anxiety (see Chapter 16) and fear of thunderstorms, loud noises, and unfamiliar persons and places. In all of these cases, the principles are always the same. First expose the animal to only mild versions of the feared stimulus or situations and reward it with food tidbits, petting, etc. for following commands while remaining non-fearful in this situation. Then later, systematically and gradually extend such training to a graded series of stimuli or situations to which the animal used to react somewhat more – but not too much more – fearfully, while making sure that the whole procedure is carried out in such a way that the animal never becomes fearful.

Fear of thunderstorms is an interesting example which is discussed at length by Voith and Borchelt (1985), Tuber et. al (1982), and Hart and Hart (1985). After acquiring a commercial recording of thunder and testing it at high volume to make sure that it does indeed elicit an intense fear response, training is begun by playing the recording at a volume which is low enough not to disturb the dog while rewarding it for sitting, lying down, and staying when it shows no signs of fear. Over the course of many sessions, the volume of the recording is gradually increased until the dog shows no fear when it is played at real thunderstorm intensity. In the final step, owners are instructed to carry out this kind of training session at home when a real thunderstorm is taking place.

Although this procedure can indeed train dogs to remain unafraid while hearing a thunderstorm recording which formerly elicited great fear, all authors who have worked extensively with this procedure (e.g. Tuber et. al, 1982; Voith and Borchelt, 1985; Shull-Selcer and Stagg, 1991) admit that the apparently successful therapy often does not transfer to the real storm situation. Presumably, the problem is that the recording duplicates only a limited portion of the combined auditory (thunder +

sounds of wind and rain), visual (lightning flashes), and possible electromagnetic stimulus complex which the dog is exposed to during a real thunderstorm. Even the auditory component itself may be problematic, for it may lack the high-energy percussive sound wave characteristics of real thunder (Shull-Selcer and Stagg, 1991). Another related problem is that storms may even differ from one another in terms of their precise auditory characteristics due to, for example, interactions with atmospheric conditions like wind velocity and direction, relative humidity, and temperature.

In general, therapeutic success with systematic desensitization/counterconditioning behavior therapy procedures is much higher where feared stimuli are more faithfully reproducible during training sessions (e.g. fear of gun shots, fear of a specific person).

Another human behavior therapy procedure which can sometimes be applied to treat dog fear problems is *flooding*. Here, the animal is exposed to the fear-eliciting stimulus at full intensity for as long as necessary for the fear response to wane considerably, which can take several hours. The procedure generally calls for one of these lengthy sessions per day on many different days. The primary rule here is that this method can only be successful if the animal is much less fearful at the end of the session than it was at the beginning. If the animal is taken out of the situation too soon, when it is still just as fearful as it was at the beginning, the problem is likely to get worse rather than better.

While not widely used to treat fear problems in companion animals, there are situations in which the flooding approach can be appropriate and helpful. Dogs which fear crowds, for example, can be taken to a busy shopping center two or three times a week and kept for several hours in an area like a main passageway in which there is constant heavy flow of pedestrian traffic. This ensures continuous exposure to the fear-eliciting situation. One obvious disadvantage is time-consuming nature of this approach: only the most committed owner would consider it given that it might entail spending 4, 5, or more hours a day, a few days a week, for at least several weeks in an environment which can be stressful for the owner as well. Another potential disadvantage of the procedure is that when initially exposed to this situation, the animal's fear may increase dramatically to the point where it becomes panicky and perhaps dangerously aggressive to anyone who comes too near. Initially, owners must therefore be cautious in this regard even though their dog is never aggressive in other situations. Muzzling it, for example, might be a wise precaution where close contact with strangers cannot be avoided.

Training in problem situations

The formal behavior therapy methods described above are often not practically feasible for many of the kinds of fear problems which dogs display (e.g. fear of traffic noises or strangers on the street). Then too, fear problems may not be so intense as to necessitate a time-consuming systematic behavior therapy approach given that considerable improvements can often be achieved in the real-world problem situations themselves by applying less elaborate treatment measures. The following paragraphs discuss some of these alternative measures which can be beneficial in many kinds of cases.

• *Totally ignore the dog's fearful behavior:*
When the dog begins acting fearfully on the street, the owner should simply walk on as if nothing has happened. He/she shouldn't look at or talk to the dog, slow down, speed up, change directions, or wait for it if it stops. Unless the fear is very intense, the dog will overcome it and catch up as soon as it sees that the owner is not going to stop and wait or come back to it this time. If the dog is on the leash, the owner should pull it onwards, perhaps with the help of a sharp tug on the leash, when it plants its feet and refuses to move. In other situations like in the home, owners should simply pretend not to see the dog's fearful behavior and perhaps do something else that requires them to get up, move around, or leave the room without looking at the dog, talking to it, or paying any kind of attention to it.

• *Early intervention method:*
If the owner spots the feared stimulus (e.g. an approaching person or bicycle) outside when it is still some distance away, before the dog becomes fearful, it may be appropriate to call the dog, reward it with a tidbit for coming, and give it commands and reward it several times for performing correctly as the feared stimulus passes by – provided, that is, the animal can be induced to pay more attention to the owner while more or less ignoring the feared stimulus or becoming only mildly uneasy when it passes by. If on the other hand, the animal's fear response cannot be prevented by eliciting the alternative behaviors *before* it starts acting fearfully, this technique should only be used in situations where the animal's fear is much less intense (e.g. where the feared stimulus passes by at a greater distance). Basically, no food rewards should be given after the animal has already become very fearful, for they may reinforce the fearful behavior and make the problem worse. In such cases, it is better to simply ignore all fearful behavior and reserve this early intervention method for other, more favorable situations.

• *Campbell's "jolly routine":*
Campbell (1992) describes a similar early intervention method which he recommends to owners to combat a variety of behavior problems. Basically, instead of calling the dog (before it begins behaving fearfully) and rewarding it for coming and following commands with food tidbits after a person, bicycle, etc. the dog fears is spotted approaching, the owner is instructed to apply the "jolly routine". What specifically the owner does depends on what "turns the dog on" in the sense of making its tail wag and arousing its playfulness or enthusiastic interest. The owner might, for example, clap his/her hands, bounce a ball, laugh and act happy, or say something the dog always responds positively to like "you want to go out?", uttered in the same provocative way in which it is uttered at home before taking the dog out for a walk.

Like the early intervention method using particularly desirable food rewards, applying the jolly routine just before problem behavior begins is also a means of eliciting and then rewarding behavior which is incompatible with the problem behavior and, therefore, basically a counterconditioning procedure. It also has the additional advantage of ensuring that owners are communicating an entirely positive emotional message to the dog about their own reaction, which may also contribute to changing a dog's general perception of the feared situation.

Most behavior counselors recommend using food rewards because these have a powerful effect on the behavior of all problem dogs, are easy for any owner to administer, and if anything their effect increases in strength with repetition rather than waning as may happen if the dog begins to habituate to the owner's repeated attempts to elicit play and other positive behavior. But for dogs for which the sight of a ball or stick in the owner's hand has an immediate and powerful energizing effect, the Campbell method can be ideal.

• *Controlled exposure to feared stimulus analogously to the desensitization behavior therapy method:*

If the dog's fear response to approaching cars, bicycles, dogs etc. is so intense that showing it a ball or offering it a tidbit fails to elicit the desired competing behavior (and thereby prevent fearful behavior), it may be necessary for the owner to apply this method in stages: it is first carried out at a place which is relatively distant from passing cars, bicycles, or dogs, and then it is later applied progressively closer to the stimuli the dog fears over the course of several days or weeks. With stimuli which are physically constrained in their movements like cars driving on roads and bicycles on bicycle paths, it is easy for the owner to control this distance aspect. However, with a problem like fear of other dogs, the owner must seize opportunities whenever they spontaneously arise by applying the early intervention method only when, for example, an approaching dog is between 50 and 100 yards away for the first few days, between 30 and 60 yards for the next few days, then 20 and 40 yards, and so on. This minimum distance requirement basically rules out using the method at times when the owner knows from experience it won't elicit the desired behavior and, therefore, might even be detrimental.

Conventional obedience training

Teaching the dog to respond correctly to come, sit, down, and stay commands is an important preliminary step in most of above procedures for reducing an animal's fear. The above description of the early intervention method, for example, assumes that the dog has already been well-trained to come, sit, and stay on command. There is another aspect of most fear problems, however, that make conventional obedience training imperative. Excessively fearful dogs often tend to pull strongly on the leash, try to run away, stop and refuse to walk onwards, refuse to walk in certain directions, and try to pull the owner back home – behavior problems which many owners are powerless to combat. In extreme cases, walks are full of these kinds of owner-dog confrontations, and owners must either do what the dog wants or spend five minutes convincing, coaxing, or bribing it to walk where and how they wish at every street corner. When the dog is small, the only way some owners can cope with the dog's fear-motivated stubbornness and unruliness is to pick it up and carry it for awhile every time they come to one of these problem spots. From the owner's viewpoint, these accompanying control problems can be far more bothersome than the animal's fearfulness itself.

Increased owner authority

Another characteristic feature of many fear problem cases is the reluctance of some owners to "get tough" with their dogs and thereby end disobedience as soon as it starts. Either they feel sorry for the dog when they see or assume that it is reacting out of fear, or they think that their scolding or firm commanding of the dog will only make it more fearful. For some owners, it is therefore enormously helpful to simply be told that they should no longer tolerate the dog's disobedience no matter how fearful it is. In this connection, the specific advice given depends on the details of the problem situation. Along with such measures as ignoring the dogs attempts to stop or change directions, and inducing a reluctant dog to start walking again with a sharp tug (or series of sharp tugs) on the leash, it is sometimes recommended for situations in which scolding is appropriate that the dog should be sharply reprimanded just as one would do with any normal dog in this situation. In general, it should be explained to owners that fear or no fear, the dog must be trained to understand and obey commands and other leadership behavior just like any other dog. This can mean "getting a little tougher" with it particularly when the more gentle, understanding approach is obviously creating more problems than it solves.

Increase owner dominance

Of course, the above description of a dog which is unruly, tries to pull the owner in another direction, ignores commands, and must be picked up and carried arouses the suspicion that a dominance problem between owner and dog may also be involved in some cases. Indeed, some fearful animals do show a mild dominance problem or even dominance aggression. Thus, owners should be questioned closely concerning how the dog reacts to commands in other situations, whether it ever growls at family members, is generally slow to obey commands, or is often pushy and demanding. And when called for, some of the recommendations from Chapter 10 for improving owner dominance can be given.

References

Campbell, W. E. (1992): *Behavior Problems in Dogs.* Goleta, California, American Veterinary Publications, Inc.

Dykman, R.A., Murphree, O.D., and Reese, W.G. (1979): Familial anthropophobia in pointer dogs? *Arch. Gen. Psychiatry* **36**, 988–993

Goddard, M.E., and Beilharz, R.G. (1985): Early prediction of adult behaviour in potential guide dogs. *Applied Animal Behavioural Science* **15**, 247–260.

Hart, B.L., and Hart, L.A. (1985): *Canine and Feline Behavioral Therapy.* Philadelphia: Lea & Febiger.

Marder, A.R. (1991): Psychtropic drugs and behavioral therapy. *Veterinary Clinics of North America: Small Animal Practice* **21**, 329–342

Murphree, O.D., Dykman, R.A., and Peters, J.E. (1967): Genetically determined abnormal behavior in dogs: results of behavioral tests. *Conditioned Reflex* **2**, 199–205.

Murphree, O.D. (1972): Reduction of anxiety in genetically timid dogs: Drug-induced schizokinesis and autokinesis. *Conditioned Reflex* **7**, 170–176

O'Farrell V. (1992): *Manual of Canine Behaviour.* British Small Animal Veterinary Association. Schurdington, Cheltenham, Gloucestershire, England

Shull-Selcer, E.A., and Stagg, W. (1991): Advances in the understanding and treatment of noise phobias. *Veterinary Clinics of North America: Small Animal Practice* **21**, 353–367.

Tuber, D.S., Hothersall, D., and Peters, M.F. (1982): Treatment of fears and phobias in dogs. *Veterinary Clinics of North America: Small Animal Practice* **12**, 607–623.

Voith, V.L., and Borchelt, P.L. (1985): Fears and phobias in companion animals. *Compendium on Continuing Education for the Practicing Veterinarian* **7**, 209–221.

Wolpe, J. (1958): *Psychotherapy by Reciprocal Inhibition.* Palo Alto, California, Stanford University Press.

SAMPLE RECOMMENDATIONS

Fear problems

Some basic recommendations applicable in many types of cases:

- For the present, avoid exposing the animal to situations in which it becomes very fearful.
- Fearful behavior (e.g. trembling, cowering) should always be completely ignored; that is, you should never pet the dog, talk to or look at it, try to distract it, or pick it up when it shows signs of fear.
- When the dog makes problems during walks by, for example, refusing to go on, ignore this completely and continue onwards without pausing or paying any attention to the dog no matter what it does to try and stop you. A series of sharp tugs on the leash is appropriate if the animal plants its feet and tries to resist being pulled onwards.
- As far as training, control, disciplining, etc. are concerned, consider the dog to be completely normal and treat it accordingly.
- If the dog ignores your command to stop engaging in especially undesirable behavior like pulling strongly on the leash or barking at passersby, exercise more authority and scold it severely enough so that it stops immediately every time this happens.
- The dog should always be rewarded in some way when it exhibits no fear in situations in which it usually reacts fearfully.

Scenario A: *example early intervention methods for reducing dog's fear of bicyclists*

- If the dog is off leash, call it and reward it with a food tidbit for coming as soon as you see a bicyclist coming but *before* it starts showing noticeable signs of fear. As soon as it comes, ask it to sit or lie down, reward it for obeying, and then reward it again for not paying much attention to the bicyclist as he/she passes by.

OR

- Cheerfully call the dog at the moment it spots an approaching bicyclist but *before* it starts acting fearfully and try to engage it in whatever game (e.g. chasing a ball) it likes the most. Act enthusiastic about the game and unconcerned or unaware of the passing bicyclist. Don't play the dog's favorite game with it at any other time.
- If its fear is too great for these methods work as envisioned, arrange to be somewhat farther away from the path when bicyclists pass by. After the dog has learned to ignore them in this situation, move the whole routine progressively closer to sidewalks or bicycle paths over the coming days and weeks.

Scenario B: *dog is mildly fearful of but not aggressive to children*

- Daily contact with selected, understanding, and patient children who wait for the dog to approach them – rather than try and force close contact with it – could help to gradually reduce its fear of children.
- After the dog has practiced the basic sit, come, etc. commands with you for a few days, the children should take over conducting the daily sessions and thereafter they should be the only ones to give the dog tidbits, play with it, and so on.

Scenario C: *example systematic behavior therapy method to reduce fearfulness in a dog which becomes fearful during car rides (e.g. trembling, whining, salivating, panting)*

- **Critically important:** Every one of these steps must be thoroughly practiced until the dog has learned to remain fully relaxed without showing the *slightest trace of fear* in this situation before it is time to move on to the next step:
  (1) During the course of 2-3 brief practice sessions daily, use food rewards to train the dog to come, sit, lie down, and stay sitting or lying on command first in the home and then outside in the yard. Don't give it tidbits at any other time.
  (2) Practice the basic come, sit, down, and stay commands next to the car with the car doors closed.
  (3) Carry out the same training with the car doors open.
  (4) Reward the dog with food tidbits for getting into the parked car and following commands there.
  (5) Reward it for following the basic commands in the parked car with the doors closed.
  (6) Reward it for following the basic commands in the car with the motor running (but without driving).
  (7) Reward it when it stays sitting or lying and shows no fearful behavior when the car is first simply put in gear.
  (8) Reward it for remaining non-fearful when the car is driven just a meter or two.
  (9) Gradually increase the length of these little trips (stopping after 5 meters, then 10, 20, 50, etc. and giving the dog a food reward for patiently remaining sitting without showing signs of fear).
  (10) Gradually increase the length of these short trips.

- If the animal becomes fearful at any stage during this procedure, you have tried to move from one stage to the next too quickly. Go back to one of the previous stages where the dog shows absolutely no fear and try again, but this time progress much more slowly from stage to stage than you did before.
- During the whole of the behavior therapy procedure, the dog should never be taken for a normal ride in the car. Even occasional trips of this sort would wipe out any gains made during the special training exercises.
- Given that the animal's fear is quite intense, it will probably take several weeks of daily practice sessions such as these to eliminate it.

Scenario D: *using drug therapy to treat a dog which becomes extremely fearful during occasional car rides when the car is driven very fast.*

- The dog should be medicated with an effective tranquilizer before every trip when the car will be driven fast.
- Medicate the dog prior to the next 20 trips when the car will be driven fast. Then administer only half this dose for the next 20 trips, then half the dosage again for the 20 next trips, and so on until the drug is no longer needed.
- The dog should *never* be taken for fast rides without first receiving the appropriate dosage.

16   Separation Anxiety

Dogs that make serious problems when left alone in the home show three common symptoms which may occur singly or in combination.

- *Excessive vocalization:* many dogs bark, whine, or howl so loud and long that they create a severe disturbance for neighbors in apartment buildings. In many cases, neighbors have become hostile to the owners who are basically forced to do something about the problem if they wish to go on living in the building.
- *Destructive behavior:* dogs may cause damage by scratching on doors or the floor or walls around doors or windows, or they may destroy mattresses, sofas, etc.
- *Elimination behavior:* either defecation, urination, or both.

This problem is relatively common. Between 10 and 30% of the cases of behavior counselors involve dogs of this type. This might be just the tip of the iceberg, for many people who have this kind of problem with their dog simply accept the fact that their dog cannot be left alone. They either take it everywhere or leave it with a friend or neighbor when a separation is inevitable. Leaving the dog in the car, sometimes for hours, is another common strategy for coping with this problem. Some dogs find this much more acceptable to being left alone at home.

Even though the symptoms of excessive vocalization, destructiveness, and elimination are often associated with other problems as well, the separation anxiety problem is easy to diagnose in most cases. Owners are aware that their dog finds it aversive to be alone. It's clear from the damage and nature of the dog's destructiveness that it is not just being playful. The vocalization is too persistent to be an immediate response to external stimuli. And the dog may even eliminate in the home after it was taken outside and had eliminated there a half-hour earlier.

As the name of this syndrome implies, the assumption has always be made in the pet problem literature that since these animals apparently become extremely anxious when left alone, the problem is most appropriately treated as a type of fear problem.

According to this theory, being alone is unnatural for highly social animal like dogs. They must therefore learn to tolerate being alone without becoming afraid by simply being left alone often, as most wise owners make a point of doing. However, some dogs which were not accustomed to being left alone when they were young react fearfully when left alone for the first time later in life – a kind of "phobic" reaction or fearful response to a situation that is, objectively speaking, harmless which tends to increase steadily as a result of the every experience the animal has being left alone and becoming fearful at this time.

The following facts are given in support of this fear hypothesis:

- The presence in some cases of elimination and escape-oriented destructive behavior (e.g. scratching on doors) are consistent with the hypothesis that fear is the underlying problem.
- Sometimes the problem first appears in an animal which was badly frightened by a thunderstorm when alone.
- Animals often apparently become fearful even before owners leave home and show signs like shivering, head lowered, and ears flattened that are indicative of fear.
- Animals often show the most frequent/intense symptoms during the first half hour or so of the owner's absence, presumably because the fear is maximally intense at this time.

- The dog greets owners when they return home with an excessive outpouring of affection and enthusiasm, which gives one the impression that the dog must feel like it has been rescued from an intensely distressing or frightening situation.
- Such dogs usually follow owners around continuously, refusing to accept a closed door separating them from family members and protesting loudly until it is opened. This too is interpreted as being a sign that they become distressed or fearful as soon as there is any sort of separation.
- A desensitization/counterconditioning treatment procedure which is conceptualized as being basically a method of gradually reducing the underlying fear is often successful.

O'Farrell (1992) departs somewhat from this classical view in the course of making some specific suggestions of how the three major types of symptoms should be interpreted. Being pack animals, dogs become uneasy or agitated or anxious when left alone – reactions which relate as much to what she refers to as excitement or over-excitement problems as to phobias. This state of uneasy or anxious agitation then leads to the symptomatic behaviors for various reasons: "chewing and digging are displacement activities produced by the increase in anxiety, which can also result in uncontrolled urination and defecation", scratching on the door is interpreted as "an attempt to follow the rest of the pack", and barking and howling "as attempts to attract its attention". Theoretically interesting here is O'Farrell's raising of the possibility of interpreting some symptoms as *displacement activities* (i.e. out-of-context behavior in response to some sort of conflict or stress situation) and the explicit recognition of some symptoms as *instrumental behavioral strategies* that are biologically understandable given the dog's agitated, distressed state and environmental situation.

Taking O'Farrell's suggestions as a starting point, the following discussion will consider these and other features of the separation anxiety syndrome from a combined ethological and experimental psychological perspective with the aim of developing a more detailed and comprehensive view of the nature and causes of this intriguing behavior problem.

Like O'Farrell, this broader, more comprehensive theoretical approach starts from the assumption that although animals may not become extremely fearful when left alone as earlier investigators assumed, they are reacting to what is for them and indeed probably for all dogs an inherently stressful or aversive environmental situation. Differences between dogs in how stressful or aversive they find the situation – and how specifically they are predisposed to react to it – presumably reflect a variety of factors such as genetic predispositions (e.g. in gregariousness, activity needs, vocalization thresholds), the dog's age, and previous experience coping with various types of aversive environmental situations. Age is obviously an important factor, for puppies are easily accustomed to being alone whereas with older dogs, several weeks of training using special methods may be required.

Although training puppies to tolerate being alone is simply a matter of leaving them alone often from the first day onwards, understanding why this should be the case involves more than positing some simple habituation process. Most importantly as far as the nature of the separation anxiety problem is concerned, being left alone exposes puppies to this mildly or intensely aversive situation at a time in their lives in which they have a natural tendency to develop acceptable (to owners) behavioral strategies for coping with this temporarily impoverished environment. Barking, whining, and howling when the bitch goes away for a time to eat, drink, or eliminate would surely be maladaptive for puppies in a natural setting: it could attract predators, signal nearby predators that they are now alone, or interrupt or delay the bitch's food-acquisition behavior. In human homes, puppies that are left alone are usually confined in a place where they can't damage anything other than their toys by biting and chewing – and it is likely therefore that any displacement or frustration-related aggressive behavior would be directed towards them. Puppies readily play with or chew on small objects left within their reach at times when they are motivated to be active and there is nothing interesting or compelling in the environment to respond to. And of course puppies sleep a lot and perhaps tend to sleep more or sooner when the surrounding environment is monotonous. Taking all of these factors together, the behavioral reactions that are elicited in the puppy in what for it too might be the stressful, impoverished, or aversive situation of being alone tend to be those like playing, chewing on appropriate objects, or sleeping which remain acceptable to owners when it matures into an adult dog.

This story is, however, quite different for an older dog that is confronted with the situation of being left entirely alone for the first time in its life. Barking and howling are natural forms of calling which can function to bring separated members back to the pack, or vice versa. Destructive behavior directed towards points of escape in the home can be easily interpreted as attempts to escape and rejoin the pack. Destructive behavior directed towards sofas, mattresses, etc. could be a type of displacement activity or redirected aggression related to the frustration-producing situation of having all avenues of escape blocked. As any dog owner can confirm, adult dogs are indeed highly motivated to remain in close contact with family members at all times – and quickly become uneasy, agitated, and disturbed when they cannot. It is rare that dogs which are not on a leash stray farther than a certain relatively fixed distance away from owners. Accordingly, most dogs can be easily trained to come more quickly and reliably when called by convincing the owner to always call only once and then turn and walk directly away.

Thus, the picture of an animal which engages in problem behavior when alone is not necessarily one of a highly fearful animal, but rather of an animal which finds its present situation aversive and has become agitated, anxious, and/or frustrated by its failure to solve its present problem by vocalizing or trying to escape. And unlike the young puppy, the more mature dog's natural reactions to this situation – to call louder and longer, to scratch harder on the door to get out, and then to become

even more agitated, anxious, or aggressive when these problem-solving behaviors do not succeed – are those which develop naturally into the separation anxiety problems of destructiveness and excessive vocalization. Although elimination behavior has no such instrumental behavioral element, it is probably reasonable to assume that it is a response to the increased levels of stress, excitement, or anxiety which are inherent in this situation.

This portrait of a distressed, anxious, agitated, frustrated animal reacting with ineffective problem-solving behaviors to an impoverished/inadequate environmental situation is only the starting point for understanding the problem. For at first glance, animal learning theory would seem to predict that while the older animal being left alone for the first time might react this way initially, in the long run these behaviors would wane if they did not turn out to be effective means of solving its problem. They don't, however, and the separation anxiety tends to worsen rather than improve over the course of time.

Several factors are probably involved here. Firstly, while many dogs with the separation anxiety problem may not actually become fearful (or as fearful) as is commonly believed, it seems fair to assume that the animal experiences great distress and discomfort at this time. Like fear itself, such aversive states add to the aversiveness of the situation and, in effect, may therefore be self-perpetuating or self-strengthening.

A second factor which may help to account for the progressive worsening of the problem is that many dogs exhibiting this problem are rather demanding, pushy types of pets not only when a door is closed in their faces, but under any and all circumstances when they want something from owners. Their owners reactions to the closed-door situation is an example of why the dogs are this way: these tend to be owners who give in easily and give the dog what it wants when it protests long and loudly enough. Essentially, a dog which has learned in whatever context that it pays off to be persistent with its begging and demanding will not give up nearly as quickly as an animal which is rarely allowed to get its way with such behavior. Interestingly, this can help to create conditions where the persistent vocalizing or scratching on the door of the dog which is left alone is more likely to be rewarded by, for example, the owner's return than might otherwise be the case. In particular, the dog's whining/barking/scratching may be reinforced every time it hears signs of the owner's return (e.g. the owner's car driving in the driveway, footsteps in the hall) or signs that *might* indicate his/her return (e.g. any car driving in the driveway, any footsteps in the hall) when it is engaging in the problem behavior. Animal experiments in which rewards were given to animals randomly – without any connection whatsoever to what animals were doing at the time – showed that even these have powerful effects on animals' behavior, causing, for example, the development of elaborate "superstitious behavioral rituals" in pigeons like whirling in circles, pacing figure 8's in the cage, and repetitive head-bobbing. Under these circumstances, each pigeon tends to develop its own distinctive, sometimes rather bizarre ritual which it repeats faithfully and precisely over and over again as if believing that this is the way one goes about gaining access to grain. The coincidental reinforcement of different behaviors in different pigeons during the initial sessions are thought to be the reason why each pigeon develops its own idiosyncratic ritual: whatever behavior is coincidentally reinforced is more likely to be repeated. This in turn further increases the probability that it will be in the act of being performed when the next "reinforcement" is delivered.

The separation anxiety situation bears a resemblance to these experiments in the sense that in reality, nothing the animal can do will produce the reward (i.e. the owner's return) which the dog is highly motivated to obtain. However, animals don't behave this way. To the contrary, their whining/barking/scratching is often extremely persistent, being exhibited off and on for many hours a day. This can in part be accounted for by assuming that when they persistently bark, whine, or scratch on the door, such behaviors are likely to be coincidentally rewarded – particularly after

short owner absences – strengthening the dog's tendency to repeat them and thereby increasing the percentage of the animal's time is spent barking and whining. This in turn increases the chances that the owner's return or outdoor noises that are in any way similar to stimuli which signal the owner's return may act as a rewards and strengthen the behavior further. From this point of view, the greater intensity/frequency of symptoms during the first half hour may also reflect higher owner return probabilities at this time and not, as commonly thought, merely the fact that aversiveness is greatest during this time.

A third factor contributing to the progressive development of the problem in some cases is that neighbors in apartment buildings may reward the dog's incessant vocalization or scratching by going up to the door, talking through it to the dog, trying to calm or scold it, etc. – a natural reaction of a neighbor who is being driven crazy and, like the dog itself, trying to do something to solve his/her own problem. Owners too make similar mistakes. As an attempt to solve the problem, they may wait outside of the door for awhile and then come back in when the dog starts to make noise to quiet it down either with quiet reassurance that "Mummy won't be gone long", or by scolding it, which may not be aversive enough to outweigh the rewarding effects of the owner's return.

Incidentally, this rather complex view of the dynamics of the development and maintenance of the separation anxiety problem may also help account for the destructiveness. Animal experiments indicate that aggression towards conspecifics or objects may be elicited when an expected reward does not occur – a type of situation which anyone who has deposited coins in a vending machine that is out of order knows all too well can elicit both frustration and aggression. Perhaps the howling animal is not only frustrated because the howling is producing no effect, but hearing a car door slam in front of the house and therefore expecting the owner will soon walk in through the door, the failure of the owner to appear might be sufficient to trigger off this kind of reactive aggression. Such false alarms may be common particularly in apartment houses where many people come and go during the day.

That intense fear can be involved in some cases of separation anxiety seems clear: the dog which shows the problem after being frightened by a storm is an example. Cases where the owners have hidden outside and stormed in and severely punished the dog for barking might be another. However, it seems likely that rather than being *the* underlying cause of the separation anxiety problem, fear is at most accurately regarded as a contributing factor which increases the aversiveness of a situation and, hence, the animal's reaction to it in cases where the problem has developed to this severe extent.

The observation that these animals often show apparent signs of fear like shivering, head lowered, ears flattened, or looking "depressed" when they see owners preparing to leave the home may often involve attention-getting behavior rather than genuine fear. Such behaviors immediately alarm and arouse the sympathies of many owners, causing them to delay their departure and lavish attention on their pet to reassure it or plead with it not to make problems this time. And this, in turn, accounts for why these types of behavior are common components of the attention-getting behavior of animals which have essentially been inadvertently trained by their well-meaning owners to use these kinds of behaviors instrumentally – a means to an end. "Oh, you poor baby! Is it as bad as all that?" And presto, the shivering, crouching, pathetic-looking creature is petted and talked to and fussed over and picked up more or less whenever it feels like it.

If separation anxiety is not really primarily a fear problem, then why does the classical systematic desensitization/counterconditioning approach to accustoming the animal to being alone without becoming fearful (e.g. Voith and Borchelt, 1985) work as well as it does? The answer may be that along with reducing the aversiveness of the situation (and related fear, anxiety, agitation, frustration, etc.) via desensitization, the procedure also functions to countercondition acceptable behavioral responses on the part of the dog to the aversive

situation of being left alone. In short, one conclusion which might be drawn from this speculative discussion of the nature of the separation anxiety problem is that it is the counterconditioning and not the desensitization aspect of the traditional behavior therapy procedure which may well be most critical. And this has important practical implications; for the traditional approach to treatment can be easily modified to optimize counterconditioning effects while, at the same time, de-emphasizing fear-reduction as an explicit treatment goal.

Possible causal factors

Aversive environmental circumstances

In general, it seems fair to assume that for a highly social animal like a dog, being left alone is inherently aversive. Most dogs learn to cope with these periods of isolation early in life by, for example, sleeping, chewing on acceptable objects, or doing something else which causes owners no problems. Others, however, react with ineffective instrumental behavior, displacement activities, frustration or nonreinforcement-elicited aggressive behavior, and symptoms of intense emotional arousal like elimination in the home which indicate that they find the situation especially aversive and/or have failed to learn to respond to it with behavior acceptable to owners.

Inherited predispositions

Part of the answer to the question of why only some dogs become a problem in this regard may be that variations in how aversive such circumstances are for individual animals reflect inherited genetic differences between dogs with respect to such characteristics as gregariousness, vocalization/chewing/playfulness tendencies, and activity levels and related needs for physical exercise. A dog that sleeps a lot, is not particularly active, has a relatively high bark-eliciting threshold in the situations in which these dogs often bark, likes to chew on things, often plays with objects, and is not as highly motivated as many other dogs to remain

POSSIBLE CAUSAL FACTORS

Aversive environmental circumstances
(i.e. highly gregarious animal left alone
for long periods of time)

Lack of early experience
(being left alone during first few months
of life)

Traumatic experience
(e.g. dog badly frightened by thunderstorm
when alone)

Reinforcement effects
(e.g. owner returns when dog in process
of barking/howling; neighbor tries to quiet
from outside of door)

Owner-dog relationship problem
(e.g. dog pushy/demanding in other situations)

Inherited predispositions
(e.g. gregariousness, activity levels,
playfulness, vocalization tendencies)

Sudden change in family circumstances
(e.g. adult dog left alone for first time in
life after death of owner/other dog in family)

Conditioned emotional effects
(e.g. fear/emotional distress self-
strengthening; punishment increases
aversiveness of dog's situation)

Outside eliciting stimuli
(e.g. stimuli from outside home can trigger
off bouts of howling, destruction)

SEPARATION ANXIETY

• Destructive behavior, elimination, and/or persistent vocalization
when left alone in home

POSSIBLE TREATMENT ELEMENTS

Avoid problem situations
(don't leave dog alone except during
short training absences)

Systematic behavior therapy procedures
(special counterconditioning/desensitization
method)

**Change owner-dog interactive ground
rules**
(recommendations to decrease dog's
pestering, pushy, demanding behavioral
tendencies)

Care/maintenance condition changes
(e.g. acquiring a second dog may be
helpful in certain types of cases)

**Cessation of ineffective treatment
methods**
(punishment contraindicated)

Correct owner mistakes
(e.g. reentering room/home when dog
barking/howling)

Physical aids
(crate/cage if dog destructive or eliminates
in home)

Drug therapy
(anxiolytic medicaments reportedly effective
in a small minority of mild cases)

in close physical proximity to family members or conspecifics is probably far less likely to develop the separation anxiety problem than dogs which display the opposite characteristics.

Lack of early experience

Another relevant factor is the experiences dogs have had being left alone very early in their lives. Most dogs are left alone often during the first weeks and months in the home. They must learn from the first night onwards to sleep alone in the kitchen. Their whining and barking protests are ignored and soon cease. And from that time onwards, they are left alone for lengths of time varying from a few minutes to a few hours every day. However, dogs exhibiting the separation anxiety problem tend to have a rather different kind of history. They may have slept in the owner's bedroom from the first night on. And their family situation may have been such that there was always someone at home with them – most commonly an elderly person – or they were always allowed to accompany family members on trips away from home and so were never once left at home alone during the first few months of life.

Sudden change in family circumstances

Often the separation anxiety problem appears suddenly in response to some change in family circumstances which results in the dog being left alone for the first time in its life (e.g. following the death of an elderly person or another animal which has always kept the dog company in the owner's absence). Another common scenario is when a dog which has stayed alone for hours practically every day for years makes problems when left alone again after it was exposed to a period of several weeks or months where someone in the family was always there (e.g. due to temporary unemployment or an extended illness).

Traumatic experience

The classic example is when the separation anxiety problem appears suddenly after a dog which fears thunderstorms was left alone in the home during such a storm. In this case, it can probably be assumed that a genuine phobic fear reaction is involved which parallels, for example, the suddenly acquired fear of riding in cars exhibited by a dog that has been involved in a traffic accident.

Conditioned emotional effects

Theoretically speaking, it can be assumed that once the problem develops to the point where being alone is highly aversive – that is, the animal is experiencing severe emotional distress rather than becoming just mildly uneasy – conditions are produced which lead to a vicious circle of the animal's distress adding to the aversiveness of the situation and leading, in the long run, to steadily increasing levels of distress under similar situations: an effect which directly parallels the development of phobic fear reactions in animals and man. Indeed, this is what makes the treatment of human phobias so difficult. To be successful, the required behavior therapy must control exposure to fear-eliciting stimuli in such a way that any fear elicited is mild enough to permit the habituation which must occur before the intensity of the fear-eliciting stimulus is raised to its next, slightly-more-intense level. In comparison, exposure to fear-eliciting stimuli which are more intense than this can destroy the effectiveness of the procedure, increasing rather than decreasing the level of fear elicited by the situation. Something similar is assumed to occur in the case of separation anxiety in dogs: if the aversiveness of the situation remains below a certain threshold, simple habituation (i.e. leaving the animal repeatedly alone) may result in the animal becoming accustomed to the situation. But if the situation is more aversive that this, each new separation leaves a lasting negative impression on the animal which adds to rather than reduces aversiveness on future occasions. In effect, such emotional reactions turn out to not only be self-perpetuating, but self-strengthening as well.

From this perspective, it is also understandable why owner punishment for vocalization, destructive behavior, or elimination is contra-indicated. Although waiting outside the door and then rushing in and punishing the dog when it starts barking may reduce barking temporarily – or at least cause the dog to wait longer after the owner has left before starting to bark – such owner tactics are likely to add considerably to the aversiveness of the dog's situation. The same can be said for punishment long after the act when, for example, a dog that has eliminated in the home or destroyed something is punished when the owner returns home hours later. In short, punishment is likely to increase the aversiveness of the situation and hence fuel the vicious circle, self-strengthening character of the problem.

Reinforcement effects

One frequent scenario is when the owner leaves the apartment, waits outside the door for awhile to see if the dog makes problems, and then reenters the home and tries to quiet or reassure the dog if it starts whining or barking. Even scolding the dog at this time could be rewarding if the scolding is mild enough not to outweigh the dog's relief at seeing the owner reappear. Another source of unintentional reinforcement is neighbors. Being bothered by the dog's whining, barking, or howling – or reacting out of sympathy for the dog – neighbors may try to quiet or reassure the dog by talking to it through the door. And finally, simply the sound of a car turning into the driveway, the elevator operating, or any unusual outside sound which might at first suggest to the dog that the owner is returning has the potential of reinforcing problem behavior.

There is another interesting possibility here too. Animal experiments have shown that an apparently neutral stimulus change of any sort such as a light going on or off can reinforce and strengthen behavior, particularly where animals are being kept for long periods of time under isolated, monotonous environmental conditions. Obviously, such a reinforcement effect might occur in the separation anxiety situation as well where the "understimulated" dog might welcome most any kind of change (e.g. an outdoor sound) in its monotonous surroundings.

In summary, a variety of types of events related or entirely unrelated to the dog's problem behavior have the potential of reinforcing and strengthening it if they occur when the behavior is in progress. Furthermore, as the problem becomes increasingly severe and the dog spends a greater and greater percentage of its time vocalizing, scratching on the door, or tearing up paper, these types of reinforcement events are likely to become correspondingly more frequent and contribute to the progressive worsening of the problem.

Contributory role of outside stimuli

Some owners report having been informed by neighbors that the dog often begins one of its minutes-long bouts of barking or howling in response to some outdoor noise like the ringing of the doorbell or the postman delivering mail. This effect could be due to a combination of increased general arousal with the interruption of sleeping or some acceptable competing behavior which the dog might have been performing at the time. A further possibility with sounds like a car door slamming or footsteps approaching the front door which often signal owner return is that the dog may become agitated and perhaps even aggressive when the sound is not followed by the return of the owners (i.e. expected reinforcement fails to occur).

Owner-dog relationship problem

In many cases, dogs are not only demanding and pushy when they are separated from the owner by a closed door in the home, but they are demanding and pushy in other situations as well. Often, separation anxiety symptoms like vocalizing or scratching on the door seem to be a reflection of the dog's general approach to getting whatever it wants from owners – and the owner's past tendency of allowing him/herself to be manipulated in this way.

Possible treatment elements

The treatment method outlined in the sample recommendations box is a modified version of the approach recommended by O'Farrell (1992). The main difference is a reduced emphasis on desensitization in favor of more exclusive concentration on training the dog to engage in acceptable behavior like sitting or lying quietly in its bed or chewing on a nylon chew.

Avoid problem situations

The cardinal rule for all therapeutic approaches to the separation anxiety problem is that the dog must not be left alone at any time except during the short owner absences required by the behavior therapy procedure. Leaving the dog alone for a period of time much longer than this is likely to cause a major setback which requires essentially returning to very short absences and starting the retraining process of slowly increasing absence time all over again.

Cessation of ineffective treatment methods

Punishment for undesirable behavior long after it has occurred – for example, when the dog has eliminated during the owner's absence and is punished when the owner returns home – is contraindicated for two reasons. First: to be effective, punishment must be delivered either during or immediately following (within a second or two) the punished behavior. And second: conditioned fear resulting from overly harsh owner punishment at the time of his/her arrival may increase the aversiveness of being left alone and thus make the problem worse instead of better.

Systematic behavior therapy procedure

The behavior therapy procedure outlined in the sample recommendations box has two beneficial effects on the dogs behavior. The duration of absences is strictly controlled so that the dog is only left alone for lengths of time which it can tolerate without becoming distressed. This in turn facilitates habituation to the aversive situation of being left alone – the *desensitization* element. Additionally, the procedure is designed to train the dog to engage in some kind of acceptable behavior during owner absences like, for example, lying or sitting quietly and purposefully waiting in its bed or chewing on a nylon bone – the *counterconditioning* element.

All behavior therapy approaches to the separation anxiety problem share these two desensitization and counterconditioning features. However, the present procedure differs from classical approach (e.g. Voith and Borchelt, 1985) in that the main emphasis is on arranging the situation to encourage the dog to develop specific alternative behavioral strategies to cope with what is assumed to be the inherently aversive situation of being left alone. In comparison, the classical approach regards the counterconditioning feature of the procedure as being primarily a supplementary measure whose main function is to accelerate the reduction of the aversiveness of being left alone produced by habituation.

Correct owner mistakes

If the dog starts barking when it is being trained to remain quiet when alone in another room in the home, or if owners hear the dog vocalizing when they return after being absent from the home, they should not enter the room or home respectively until the dog has remained completely quiet for at least 2 or 3 minutes. To be avoided at all costs is returning when the dog is vocalizing or shortly thereafter, for this could function as a powerful reinforcement of the dog's barking or howling behavior.

Change owner-dog interactive ground rules

To the extent that a dog's vocalizing or destructive behavior when left alone may be in part an expression of pushy or demanding behavioral tendencies that are in evidence in other contexts as well, advising the owner to never reward begging or pushy behavior, and ignore the dog whenever it comes for attention, may provide a helpful supplement to the behavior therapy procedure.

Physical aids

Particularly when the dog is destructive or eliminates in the home, training it to enter and remain in a large crate or cage when alone – after pretraining it over the course of several days to go into and stay in it without experiencing problems by (1) putting its bedding there and (2) using food tidbits to reward it for entering and remaining some time in the crate, first with the door open and then with the door closed – can be a highly effective way of preventing problem behavior. Ideally, this approach should be recommended as a supplement to rather than in place of the behavior therapy procedure. Essentially, the behavior therapy procedure can be the same except that the dog is sent into the cage instead of its bed before the owner leaves the room.

Care/maintenance condition changes

Obtaining a second dog generally does not solve the problem (Voith and Borchelt, 1985). However, O'Farrell (1992) suggests that it may be successful with dogs "which have a history of close bonding with other dogs" or those whose problem began after the death of another dog in the household.

Anxiolytic medication

Some American specialists have reported successful treatment of mild cases of separation anxiety using *amitriptyline HCl, imipramine hydrochloride,* or *megestrol acetate* (Voith and Borchelt, 1985). Voith and Borchelt (1985) recommend *amitriptyline HCl* dosed at 1–2 mg/kg or *megestrol acetate* at 1–2 mg/kg for 10 to 14 owner absences, half this dose for the next 10 to 14 absences, and then a further 10 to 14 absences at a quarter of the initial dose before discontinuing the medicament. (See the "drug therapy" subsection in Chapter 8 for side effects and other important drug-related information.)

Although the effectiveness of this drug therapy approach has not been systematically compared with that of behavior therapy, most authors are of the opinion that while the behavior therapy approach can be highly effective even in the most severe and long-standing cases, drug therapy alone works only occasionally and only in mild cases where barking is the only symptom.

Cautionary note

It is critical for the counselor to bear in mind that the major practical problem with a behavior therapy approach such as this one is that some owners have great difficulties training their dogs to stay in one place for an extended period of time. In general, obedience training should always be physically demonstrated to owners who have never done it before. After the dog has initially been taught to come, sit, down, and stay on command by the counselor, the owner should be given the plate of small rewards and asked to take over while the counselor watches and offers advice. In separation anxiety cases, it may be wise to recommend a second consultation a few days later during which the owner's basic training procedure and the dog's responses to it can be observed. In short, without considerable help with the basics, owners may well become discouraged and frustrated and give up without even getting past the preliminary stage of training the dog to stay in one place for more than a few seconds.

References

Borchelt, P. L. and Voith, V. L. (1982): Diagnosis and treatment of separation-related behavior problems in dogs. *Veterinary Clinics of North America: Small Animal Practice* **12**, 625–635.

O'Farrell (1992): *Manual of Canine Behavior.* Shurdington, Cheltenham, Gloucestershire, England, British Small Animal Veterinary Association.

Voith, V. L. and Borchelt, P. L. (1985): Separation anxiety in dogs. *Compendium on Continuing Education for the Practicing Veterinarian* **7**, 42–53.

SAMPLE RECOMMENDATIONS

Separation anxiety

To reduce dog's pushy, demanding behavioral tendencies:

• The dog should *never* be allowed to get what it wants (e.g. food, petting, playing, attention, going outside) when it begs or shows pestering, pushy, demanding behavior of any kind such as barking, whining, jumping up on you, nudging, licking, or scratching to get something. It should simply be ignored at such times or sent away if it becomes too bothersome.

• You should determine the times and duration of all social and physical contact with the dog. Whenever it comes to you for attention, to play, or to be petted without having been called, it should be totally ignored. After it gives up and goes away, it can then be called and petted and played with as normal.

Example behavior therapy approach to train the dog to wait quietly or chew on a nylon chew in its bed or on a special rug instead of barking/howling in front of the door:

• In 2-4 brief daily practice sessions, use the dog's favorite food tidbits to train it to come and sit, lie down, and stay either in its bed or on a small scatter rug in a room well away from the main door of the home. If a rug is used, it should be laid down at the beginning of the training session and put away out of sight when the session is over.

• Except for these special sessions, the dog should not be left alone in the home at any time during the whole behavior therapy process.

• A few chews or toys should always be placed in or directly in front of the bed or on the rug, and they too should always be put away after the session is over. The dog should not have access to toys or chews at other times.

• Staying and quietly waiting in its bed or on the rug is rewarded with petting, praise, and tidbits during the training sessions. By starting with very short time requirements (i.e. a few seconds) and gradually increasing them, the dog should be trained to do this for:
  – up to 3 min. when owner remains in the same room.
  – up to 3 min. when owner often goes in and out of room with the door open.
  – up to 3 min. when owner often goes in and out of room and closes the door each time.
  – up to 10 min. with door continuously closed but where owner remains in the home.
  – up to 10 min. with door open but with the owner out of the home.

• The rule is to never leave the dog alone longer than it has learned to remain quietly waiting in its bed or on the rug without showing signs of being disturbed by being left alone. If it leaves the rug and is waiting for you in front of the door when you reenter the room, or if it shows any signs of distress, it is being left alone for too long a time, and the training should concentrate only on much shorter absences for a few days.

• The length of the absences from the room or home should always be varied so irregularly that the dog never knows whether you will be gone for 5 sec. or 5 min.

• Should it happen for any reason that the dog begins barking or howling while you are out of the room or home, make no sound and simply wait until it has remained completely quiet for at least 3 full minutes before you open the door and come in.

- Never scold or otherwise punish the dog in this situation even if you are in a position to catch it in the act of barking.
- Once the dog has been well trained to stay in its bed or on the rug for 10 min. even when you leave the home, absences can be gradually prolonged further (i.e. 15 min., 20 min., 30 min., 45 min., 1 hour, etc. irregularly interspersed with much shorter absences of 1, 3, 5, or 10 min.).
- Providing the dog with more opportunities for vigorous exercise immediately before training sessions can greatly help to accelerate progress. Even after the problem is solved, the dog should always be given a long period of strenuous exercise before being left alone.

17   Elimination Behavior Problems

Twenty-three out of a sample of 149 consecutive dog cases (approx. 15 %) involved the problems of urination and/or defecation in the home. This is close to the 20% figure given by Voith and Borchelt (1985). These authors also cite a survey of 800 owners of dogs who brought their dogs to a university clinic for medical treatment which indicated that 5.5% of the animals in this sample from the normal dog population sometimes eliminated in the home.

The major dog elimination-related problems are *inappropriate urination/defecation, urine marking, submissive urination, excitement-related urination,* and urination and/or defecation related to *separation anxiety* or *fear responses*. In the latter case, the elimination may either be a direct response to fear-eliciting stimuli like thunderstorms or other loud noises, or it may be an indirect consequence of such reactions as when a dog fears traffic noises and therefore avoids going outside to a degree which overrides its inhibition against eliminating in the home (Voith and Borchelt, 1982).

Inappropriate urination/defecation (i.e. dog not fully housebroken)

Distinguishing between inappropriate urination/defecation and urination and/or defecation caused by separation anxiety can sometimes be problematic (e.g. when the problem occurs during the night when the animal is confined to the kitchen away from the rest of the family). Voith and Borchelt (1985) list the following symptoms which suggest separation anxiety rather than loss of housebreaking habits is involved:

- Dog well-housebroken when it has access to owner.
- Dog may sometimes vocalize or become destructive as well as eliminate when alone.
- Elimination usually occurs not long after the owner leaves the dog alone (i.e. often within a few minutes). With housebreaking problems, the dog usually eliminates several hours after the owner's departure (Voith and Borchelt, 1982).
- Dog shows signs of anxiety or distress prior to owner's departure.

Obviously, the mere fact that the dog only eliminates in the home in the owner's absence does not in itself settle the matter of whether separation anxiety or loss of housebreaking habits is involved. Elimination that only occurs in the owner's absence may simply indicate that the dog has been punished when caught in the act of eliminating in the home and therefore learned to inhibit the behavior when someone is present. Then too, the problem may not occur when the owner is home simply because the dog is let out more frequently (Voith and Borchelt, 1982, 1985).

Possible causal factors

Pathophysiological conditions

The onset of urination or defecation in the home in a dog which is well-housebroken is often a sign of some pathophysiological condition. Based on Reisner (1991) and Parker (1989), the following are some of the organic disorders which can lead to inappropriate urination or defecation: inflammatory diseases such as cystitis, urethritis, prostatitis, vaginitis, enteritis, and colitis, diarrheal diseases, irritable bowel syndrome, hypoglycemia, hypocalcemia, diabetes mellitus, diabetes insipidus, medullary washout, and any cause of polyuria such as hyper- or hypothyroidism or hyper- or hypoadrenocorticism.

POSSIBLE CAUSAL FACTORS

Pathophysiological conditions
(can be symptomatic of various medical conditions or residual consequence of past pathophysiological conditions)

Inadequate care/maintenance conditions
(e.g. dog not taken outside often enough)

Lack of appropriate training
(in puppies or in older dogs which were never fully housebroken)

Consequence of other behavior problems
(e.g. can develop as result of elimination in home related to separation anxiety or fear problem)

INAPPROPRIATE URINATION OR DEFECATION
• Dog not fully housebroken

POSSIBLE TREATMENT ELEMENTS

Cessation of ineffective methods
(e.g. punishment long after elimination)

Change of care/maintenance conditions
(e.g. dietary changes; feeding schedule changes; confine dog under special conditions when left alone; keep outside for long periods)

Application of effective housebreaking methods
(follow basic rules for housebreaking puppies or older dogs)

Medicaments
(laxative or diuretic in rare cases where dog completely inhibits urination and/or defecation outside)

Reisner (1991) points out that if both urination and defecation are involved, the problem is unlikely to be organic unless spinal or other neurological disease is involved. She also provides an extensive account of various causes of urinary incontinence. This medical problem is, however, easily distinguished from the urination behavior problems discussed in this section which involve normal canine elimination behavior that is being performed in the home rather than outside.

As Voith and Borchelt (1985) point out, a housebreaking problem may follow an illness in which the dog could not help eliminating in the home. After the medical problem is remedied, the new elimination habit persists for the same learning-related reason which causes a dog to become housebroken in the first place: namely, after having eliminated in a particular place or on a particular surface a few times, the animal develops a preference for (or loses its inhibition against) eliminating there.

Lack of appropriate training

Voith and Borchelt (1985) point out that dogs with housebreaking problems "generally have a history of never having been well housebroken". Often owners admit that the dog has always had occasional accidents after it has sometimes appeared for weeks or months at a time that such problems were finally past.

Of course, the owner's failure to carry out effective training is a common cause in cases where puppies and juvenile dogs are taking abnormally long to become housebroken. Often the pattern here again is a series of apparent improvements followed by relapses before the owner seeks professional help.

Inadequate care/maintenance conditions

Not taking or letting a dog out as often as it requires can be the primary cause of the problem in an older dog or the reason why a puppy never becomes fully housebroken. With some illnesses, the animal needs to urinate or defecate much more frequently than normal – a fact which owners must adjust to. Factors like diet, number of feedings, timing of daily feedings, or availability of drinking water can influence the problem too. In a recent case, simply stopping feeding a 5 month-old Labrador in the evening – its third meal of the day – was enough to stop occasional nightly defecation in the hall.

Consequence of other behavior problems

It is also possible that a dog which initially eliminated in the home as a result of separation anxiety or a fear-related problem may lose its desirable housebreaking habit of inhibiting elimination until it is outside.

Possible treatment elements

Cessation of ineffective methods

From the standpoint of the basic principles of animal learning, it is easy to understand why the usual method applied by owners of taking the dog back to the scene of the crime and punishing it hours after it has eliminated there never solves the problem. To be effective, punishment must be delivered during or immediately following (i.e. within a second or two) the punished behavior. This should be explained to owners and they should be advised to entirely abandon this punishment method in favor of exclusive concentration on other genuinely effective methods. The fact that most dogs that are punished in this way eventually become housebroken does not mean that the method works. Obviously, these owners have done other things right like, for example, closely supervising the dog when it is inside and making sure to take it out and remain outside long enough at times when it usually urinates or defecates.

One reason owners persist in applying this futile delayed-punishment method is that the dog's apparent "guilty" look when they return home convinces them that the punishment has at least taught the dog to know that "he has done something wrong" – which seems to be a step in the right direction. However, as is briefly explained in the following quote from Voith and Borchelt (1982), the supposed "guilty" look implies nothing of the sort:

"Some dogs ... learn to associate the presence of urine and/or feces in the home, the return of the owner, and the likelihood of punishment. These dogs are reported as 'looking guilty' only 'when they have done something wrong'. What owners interpret as 'guilt' are canid submissive and avoidance behaviors. The dog only displays these postures when there are elimination products in the home because this is the only time the dog is punished." (p. 641)

Application of effective housebreaking methods

Effective housebreaking involves arranging conditions so that the animal only eliminates outside in places acceptable to the owner. If this is achieved, the dog's preference for eliminating at these sites, and its related tendency to inhibit elimination at others, develops without having to train the dog to do anything in the normal sense of the term. From puppy age onwards, dogs display a natural tendency to select and repeatedly use particular locations for elimination. Essentially, all owners must do is steer the development of this location preference in the desired direction by doing whatever is necessary to ensure that elimination takes place only at the desired locations for a few weeks. To do this, the following rules should be applied with young dogs:

- The dog should be taken outside to the place the owner wishes it to eliminate at times when it is likely that it will soon need to urinate or defecate. These are:
  - As soon as the owner returns after being away from home for some time.
  - Shortly after the dog wakes up.
  - Shortly after eating.
  - Whenever the owner notices that the dog is engaging in pre-elimination behaviors such as circling, sniffing, or some other behavior (e.g. restlessness in the area of front door) which might indicate that the dog needs to eliminate.
  - After a certain specific period of time has passed since it last eliminated. This varies from dog to dog, and owners must therefore adjust their tactics to their dog's particular rhythm.
- The dog should be closely supervised when the owner is home particularly when considerable time has passed since the last elimination or when the dog goes to the room or corner where it has eliminated previously.
- Mild punishment like startling the dog with a hand clap or other loud noise is appropriate, but only if it is actually caught in the act of eliminating or squatting. This interrupts the elimination sequence so that the dog can be immediately taken outside to eliminate there instead. It also trains the dog to inhibit elimination in the owner's presence, which is helpful if the dog can be closely supervised when the time of its next elimination is drawing near.
- When left in the home alone, the dog should be kept under conditions in which it is likely to inhibit elimination until the owner returns. For example, it can be confined to a room where it has never eliminated in the past, or a barrier can be used to confine it to a small area (e.g. a corner of the kitchen) close to its bed or blanket. Areas preferred by puppies for elimination are always some distance away from their usual sleeping/resting sites.
- If the owner is going to be gone too long for the puppy to inhibit its elimination, newspapers can be laid down over the area where the dog is likely to eliminate. This prevents the formation of other surface preferences (e.g. on carpets), and the size and location of areas covered by newspapers can be easily manipulated later to help in the housebreaking process if a strong preference for eliminating on them does indeed develop.

The same basic approach to preventing elimination inside the home and arranging things so that the dog is always outside when it needs to eliminate is used to housebreak adult dogs which have never been well housebroken or have lost their inhibition against eliminating inside for some reason. One or more of the following methods may also be helpful depending on the specifics of the case:

- When alone, the dog can be kept close to its bed by keeping it on a leash or by confining it in a large crate or cage along with its bedding. The dog should be gradually accustomed to being in the cage by placing its normal bedding materials inside and using food rewards to first entice it inside and then train it over the course of several days to remain inside with the door left open for increasingly long periods of time. Finally, closing the cage door first briefly and then for progressively longer periods of time is incorporated into the training procedure. O'Farrell (1992) suggests that adult dogs can probably be left in such a cage for 2–3 hours at a time during the day and for the whole night.
- If the dog is strongly accustomed to defecating at particular time in the night and there is no underlying gastrointestinal disorder, Hart and Hart (1985) recommend "training its intestinal system" by first getting up at say 12.00 midnight to take the dog outside and then, over a period of several weeks, getting up progressively later and later (i.e. 1.00, 2.00, 3.00, 4.00 a.m. etc.) until the dog learns to go all night without defecating.
- A similar method is recommended by O'Farrell (1992): the dog sleeps next to the owner's bed tied by a leash which is connected to the owner's wrist so that he/she will awaken when the dog gets restless and gets up and starts to wander around looking for

SAMPLE RECOMMENDATIONS

Inappropriate urination and defecation in the home

Basic rules for housebreaking puppies:

- Urination and defecation in the home must be completely prevented either by carefully supervising the dog or confining it to a small area close to its bed where it is unlikely to urinate or defecate when it must be left alone.
- Take the dog outside as often as possible. Pay close attention to when during the day the dog needs to urinate or defecate, and adjust your schedule for taking it out accordingly.
- Make sure to take the dog out immediately after you come home, shortly after it eats, shortly after it wakes up, or when you see it sniffing, circling, or getting restless in the way it usually does (or at the particular location it usually soils) before urinating or defecating.
- Stay outside long enough each time until the dog has urinated and/or defecated.
- Startle the puppy by loudly clapping your hands if you actually catch it in the act of defecating or urinating, or if it squats with that intention. This interrupts the behavior and allows you time to take it outside so that it can finish its business there.
- Don't punish the dog when you discover later that it has urinated or defecated somewhere in the home. If you don't catch it in the act, it won't know what it is being punished for even when you show it the spot. Basically, there is nothing you can or should do to the dog when you discover a spot later.
- If you are going to be gone long and know, therefore, that it is inevitable that the dog will urinate or defecate inside, cover the area in which it is confined with newspapers so that at least it will later prefer to go on these rather than on your carpets, kitchen tiles, etc.

A selection of alternative recommendations for different types of cases involving older dogs:

- House-train the dog as if it were a puppy. That is, it must be taken out when urination or defecation is very likely (e.g. after eating, after waking up, just after you return home after a long absence, when it shows by becoming restless, sniffing the floor, or circling that it will soon have to urinate or defecate). In addition, it must be watched very closely in the home so as to prevent elimination there as much as possible.
- The dog should be taken outside more often and rewarded for urinating and defecating there. As soon as it squats outside, praise it. And as soon as it stands up after eliminating, give a particularly good food reward. Don't give it tidbits at any other time.
- It is appropriate to mildly punish the dog (e.g. by scolding it or startling it by loudly clapping your hands) for urinating or defecating in the house, but only if it is actually caught in the act. Punishment more than a few *seconds* after the dog has eliminated is completely ineffective.
- Stop feeding the dog in the late afternoon. A single large meal in the morning is enough.
- Do not allow the dog access to water after 6 p.m.
- By (1) confining the dog to another room at night, (2) keeping it in a small room with another kind of floor surface, (3) gradually accustoming it to spend the night in a large cage containing its bed and water bowl, or (4) allowing it to temporarily sleep in your bedroom, find some new nightly arrangement so that defecation in the night is fully prevented.
- When none of the recommended methods prevent the urination or defecation between 3 and 6 a.m., you should get up at 3 o'clock to take it outside. If this helps, you can then get up later and later over the course of the next few weeks (3.30, 4.00, 4.30, 5.00, etc.).

a place to urinate. The owner then makes the dog lie down again, waits until it is calm, and then takes it outside to urinate. "On subsequent occasions the lengths of time the dog is required to wait should be gradually extended until eventually the dog lasts all night" (p. 112).

- The dog should be rewarded with praise, petting, and food tidbits (which it doesn't receive at any other time) as soon as it eliminates outside. It is difficult to say with certainty if and how much this measure really facilitates the development of acceptable elimination habits. With puppies, it is unnecessary. But with older dogs whose problem may be much more difficult to correct, one tries to maximize all potentially or possibly helpful factors.

- This also applies to cleaning the sites. It is important to do this with puppies as well in order to prevent residual odors from triggering off elimination. But in difficult cases with older dogs it may pay to make doubly sure in this regard. O'Farrell (1992) recommends diluted bleach, a biological detergent, or a commercial odor eliminator.

Change of care/maintenance conditions

Changing the dog's diet, water intake, or feeding schedule can often be very helpful. A diet with a lowered fiber content may reduce the frequency of defecation (O'Farrell, 1992). Not feeding or allowing the dog unlimited access to water from the late afternoon onwards may be very effective in helping to reduce or eliminate defecation or urination in the night respectively.

Naturally, a change as simple as shifting the dog's nightly location from one room to another can sometimes be helpful when it exhibits a strong preference for eliminating at one particular location or on one particular floor surface.

As Voith and Borchelt (1982) point out, with dogs whose location and substrate preferences for sites inside the home are so well-entrenched that they completely inhibit elimination outside, keeping them continuously outside until they do eventually eliminate there

may be required in cases where this is feasible. Manipulating food and water access can be used to support this method. An example given by these authors is to withhold water for 12 to 24 hours and then allow the dog to drink as much as it wishes before immediately taking it outside and keeping it there until it urinates.

Medicaments

In some cases, administration of a diuretic or laxative may also be helpful in arranging conditions so that the animal has no other choice but to repeatedly eliminate outside in spite of strong inhibitions against doing so (Voith and Borchelt, 1982, 1985).

Urine marking

According to statistics presented by Voith and Borchelt (1985), 40% of dogs presented for urine marking in the home began showing the behavior by one year of age and 90% before the age of two. Urine marking is almost exclusively a problem involving males which regularly expel small amounts of urine in a few specific locations in the home. The marked locations are usually the vertical surfaces or corners of objects (e.g. chair and table legs), and the objects are marked using the typical male raised-leg posture. In most urine marking cases, no clear-cut eliciting stimuli are obvious to owners. But in other cases, dogs are reported to mark in response to visiting dogs, an estrous bitch in the neighborhood, or visitors or new objects in the home.

It is difficult to account for why particular dogs urine mark in the home. Although the behavior is assumed by most workers in the field to be a territorial behavior, Voith and Borchelt (1985) point out that domestic dogs mark both inside and outside of what might be considered to be their territory, scent marking does not keep other dogs out of territories, and dogs typically enter the territories of other dogs to mark. These authors also discuss the possibility that urine marking may function to identify the residents of an area to a strange dog by allowing it to compare the odors of the scent marks with those of the individuals it encounters there – a theory which would help account for the fact that dogs often mark within sight of each other and then investigate each other's marks. Finally, these authors mention possible sexual attractant, courtship, orientation, dominance communication, alarm signal, and population density related functions. They also refer to a study which indicated that dogs are twice as likely to mark over the urine of familiar dogs and four times as likely to mark over that of strange dogs than over their own urine. The resulting portrait of urine marking is of an important *communicative* behavior which is somehow associated with relations between neighboring groups and individuals. However, none of this information helps account for why a small minority of dogs mark in the home where they never encounter other dogs and/or the urine of other dogs.

Given that urine marking in the home is certainly "out-of-context" in the sense that dogs do not normally mark near to their den area (Hart and Hart, 1985), one possibility is that the behavior is either a *displacement activity* (i.e. an "irrelevant" activity which is triggered off by some sort of conflict situation) or a *vacuum activity* reflecting high marking motivation combined with the absence of normal eliciting stimuli (e.g. urine marks of other dogs, sight of other dogs marking). Even though this line of speculation still does not answer the question of why certain dogs mark and not others, it may be a more productive approach to putting the behavior problem in some kind of intelligible ethological perspective than is, for example, the approach taken by Neville (1991). He suggests that dogs mark in the home because they feel nervous, excited, insecure, or vulnerable – and accordingly, that a dog might be marking to try to "boost his own sense of security by surrounding himself more with his own smell" (p. 248). This is a version of the explanation recently given by O'Farrell and Neville (1994) for urine marking in cats, and the reader is referred to Chapter 20 for a detailed critique of such approaches to explaining animal behavior problems.

One popular belief is that urine marking by male dogs is often correlated with dominant behaviors or with dominant personalities and, therefore, increasing an owner's dominance over the dog will solve the problem (e.g. Neville, 1991; O'Farrell, 1992; Campbell, 1992). However, there seems to be no evidence to support this view. Voith and Borchelt (1982) express the following view on this subject:

"In our experience, urine marking has not been correlated with dominance-related problems in companion dogs. Moreover, the research literature does not indicate a clear relationship between urine marking and dominance in many canid species. In wolves, submissive individuals urine mark, although less frequently than dominant wolves. The function of urine marking involves more than simply a signal of dominance." (p. 640)

My case statistics support this view. Not one of the 54 dogs in my most recent cases of dominance aggression or other dominance-related behavior were spontaneously reported by owners to show even occasional urine marking. And in the five cases of urine marking males seen during this time period, not one showed any kind of dominance problem or had what might be described as a "dominant personality". Suggestive evidence was also yielded by the behavioral problem checklist section of the client information form described in Chapter 6. Excluding animals specifically presented for elimination problems, 11% of 64 males with mild or severe dominance problems had shown occasional urination in the home at some time in the past whereas this figure was 15% for 48 males not exhibiting any type of dominance problem. Although these figures are not easily interpreted in the sense that the question asked did not discriminate between urine marking and other types of urination problems, one might reasonably expect the difference between the two groups of dogs to be in the opposite direction if indeed urine marking in the home was more prevalent among dominant animals.

Given that many problem dogs show more than one serious behavioral problems, it is not surprising that one might be occasionally confronted with dogs which show both dominance-aggression and urine marking problems. But in such cases, the two problems obviously need not be directly associated with one another. While reducing a dog's abnormally high dominance is usually a good idea under any circumstances, given our present state of knowledge there appears to be no justification for routinely recommending this as a treatment for urine marking.

Possible causal factors

Genetic predisposition

This is one possible answer to the question of why particular dogs mark in the home. This is not to say that it is possible to definitely establish this in individual cases, but rather that the urine marking problem need not reflect any of the other causal factors mentioned below. It is theoretically possible, for example, that the genetic makeup of the dog could be such that marking motivation is abnormally high or the marking behavior threshold, or effect of mechanisms normally functioning to inhibit all forms of urination in the home, are abnormally low. A genetic predisposition cannot be ruled out as a contributing factor even in cases where there are clear-cut eliciting stimuli like a bitch in heat next door or a visiting dog in the home, for here too the question remains of why some dogs mark under these circumstances whereas most others don't.

Social eliciting stimuli

In two of my last five cases there were two and five other dogs respectively living and marking in the home. In a third case, a Yorkshire terrier only marked when visiting a dachshund owned by the client's mother. Certainly this last case is a clear-cut example of the effect of social eliciting stimuli on the urine marking problem. As far as the first two cases are concerned, it is interesting to speculate whether all of these dogs would have started marking if they lived in separate homes and did not encounter other dogs in the home, observe other dogs marking in the

home, or smell the urine marks of other dogs in the home. Probably not.

Urine-elicited marking

A very special type of social eliciting stimulus is the olfactory stimuli emanating from old marks. Both in wolves (e.g. Mech and Peters, 1977) and in dogs, urine marks elicit interest and overmarking – more so for strange dogs than familiar ones, and more so for familiar dogs than for the dog's own urine (Dunbar and Carmichael, 1981). But dogs still investigate their own urine marks and mark over them. In the home, it can therefore be assumed that the eliciting effects of the lingering odor from previous urine marks can play a role in the persistence or progressive worsening of the problem.

Hormonal factors

Urine marking in the home is much more common in males than females, and castration can often help to reduce or eliminate the behavior in males (e.g. Hopkins et al., 1976). These facts indicate that hormonal influences can also play a major role.

Two other kinds of findings indicate the possible importance of hormonal influences on urine marking in dogs. During estrus, the frequency of urination in females is greatly increased, which may be a form of hormone-influenced urine marking functioning to provide information concerning the female's reproductive condition to males in the surrounding area. And Fox (1963) cites experimental evidence that leg-raising behavior prior to urination can be induced by testosterone injections in both young males and females – an example of a direct effect of hormones on urination behavior.

Possible treatment elements

Castration

Castration of intact males is often helpful. One uncontrolled retrospective survey of 10 dogs castrated for urine marking in the home reported a rapid decline in the problem in three dogs

---

POSSIBLE CAUSAL FACTORS

Genetic predisposition
(as possible contributing factor in some
cases)

Social eliciting stimuli
(e.g. visiting dog in home, estrous bitch
nearby, other dog marking in home)

Urine-elicited marking
(old marks often investigated and
marked over)

Hormonal factors
(problem much more common in males;
castration often helpful)

URINE MARKING

- Male raises hind leg and deposits small amounts of urine on vertical
  surfaces or corners of objects in the home

POSSIBLE TREATMENT ELEMENTS

Castration
(often effective with intact males)

Cessation of ineffective methods
(e.g. punishment long after the marking took
place)

Training in problem situations
(e.g. punishment when caught in act;
countercondition competing behavior
in some cases where specific eliciting
stimulus identified)

Changes in care/maintenance conditions
(keep away from marked rooms/sites; put
dog's bed at marked site; clean marked
sites thoroughly)

Medicaments
(progestin therapy)

---

and a gradual decline in two additional ones
(Hopkins et al., 1976).

According to Hart and Hart (1985), urine
marking outside of the home is unaffected by
castration which is "...probably related to the
fact that olfactory stimuli from the urine of
other dogs, which are the most important stimuli in evoking urine marking, are strongest outside the home." (p. 239)

Cessation of ineffective methods

All owners try to eliminate urine marking in the
home by punishing their dogs as soon as spots
have been discovered. Typically, the dog is tak-
en back and shown the marked spot and then
punished by being scolded or hit with its nose
held close to the spot in hopes that it will un-

derstand why it is being punished. Experimental research on the effect of punishment which
occurs more than a few seconds after a behavior is performed clearly indicates, however, that
this method cannot possibly exert a direct suppressive effective on the future probability of
the behavior (Borchelt and Voith, 1985). If it
sometimes seems to be effective, it could be
that this form of punishment produces a general avoidance of the site and, hence, might
exert an indirect effect on problems where site-
stimuli are crucial in eliciting the behavior.
There are, however, other methods for training
dogs to stay away from marked sites, and
owners should therefore be firmly advised to
give up entirely the idea that this delayed punishment method will solve the problem.

SAMPLE RECOMMENDATIONS

Urine marking

- Clean the marked sites thoroughly because the lingering urine odor may elicit further urine marking.
- The dog should be scolded or otherwise punished (e.g. by making a sudden loud noise) if it is actually caught in the act of urine marking in the home. Such punishment should be strong enough to immediately suppress the behavior.
- Stop punishing the dog at times when you don't actually catch it in the act of urinating. This is a completely ineffective method for solving the problem because the dog cannot associate the punishment with the act of urinating itself.
- Placing the dog's food bowl, water bowl, or bed at the marked location(s) often helps prevent urination at these sites.
- If the dog always marks in response to some very specific event like a new dog coming into the home or the mailman bringing mail, watch the dog especially closely at these times, call it the instant it starts heading for the place it usually marks, and give it a few great food rewards (which it never gets otherwise) for coming and staying beside you until the critical time has past. However, if it has already started urinating, don't reward it. Scold or startle it severely enough to stop the behavior immediately.
- The chances are about 50:50 that a castration will help reduce or eliminate the problem.
- Drug therapy using a hormone preparation is sometimes helpful in controlling this problem.

Training in problem situations

Mild punishment by scolding or startling a dog that is actually caught in the act of marking, however, is to be recommended. While this usually only trains the dog to refrain from marking when the owner is present, this can be a step in the right direction by helping to reduce the overall frequency of marking in the home and creating conditions where close owner supervision in certain key situations can prevent the problem entirely.

When marking occurs in response to a very specific stimulus like, for example, the entrance of dog or visitor into the home, it may be possible to countercondition some alternative behavior such as lying down or coming to fetch a food reward in response to the stimuli that often elicit marking. Here, the early intervention method of calling the dog as soon as it perceives the eliciting stimulus but *before* it starts marking (or pre-marking sniffing, going to the site, etc.), and then rewarding it with an especially attractive tidbit which occupies it until the critical eliciting time period is past, is

one possible approach. However, application must be 100% consistent over a considerable time period to completely and permanently change the dog's reaction to the eliciting situation.

Changes in care/maintenance conditions or home environment

Some potentially helpful measures involving changes in the dog's care/maintenance conditions or home environment are the following:

- Denying the animal access to marked areas in the home.
- Temporarily housing the family's second dog with a relative to attempt to assess whether or not the removal of the other pet has an impact on the frequency of urine marking.
- Placing and keeping the dog's bed, food bowl, or water bowl at marked sites.
- Cleaning each site thoroughly after a mark has been discovered to reduce the residual urine odor which may elicit further marking.

Medicaments

Hart and Hart (1985) recommend the administration of the long-acting progestin, *medroxy-progesterone*, when castration is not effective or the male has been previously castrated. The recommended dose is a single injection of 5 to 10 mg/kg which may need to be repeated once or twice at 1 or 2-month intervals. *Megestrol acetate* is also often recommended for various male behavior problems. Marder (1991) recommends a dose of 2.2 to 4.4 mg/kg/day po with a progressive reduction of dosage by half every two weeks. Burghardt (1991) recommends 2 to 4 mg/day but with a more quickly tapering dose of once a day for 3–4 days, once every second day for 4–8 days, twice a week for 2–4 weeks, and then once a week indefinitely. (See the "drug therapy" subsection in Chapter 8 for side effects and other important drug-related information.)

Submissive urination

Most commonly puppies but also unusually fearful or submissive older dogs sometimes urinate as part of a submissive behavioral display towards human beings in the greeting situation or when a person scolds the animal, punishes it some other way, or displays some kind of dominant behavior like picking it up, bending over and petting it, or staring directly at it. Other behavioral components of the submissive display may involve lowering of the head and neck, flattening of the ears against the head, retracting the lips to form the so-called "submissive grin", evading eye contact, and crouching down in a semi-squat position or rolling over onto its back with one hind leg raised (Voith and Borchelt, 1985).

In a series of 71 cases in which there was no serious elimination problem, 5 out of the 54 owners of males (approx. 9 %) and 3 out of 17 owners of females (approx. 17 %) indicated in one of the questions in a behavior checklist that submissive urination sometimes occurred. This is consistent with Hart and Hart's (1985) contention that the behavior is more common in females. The fact that the urination was most commonly elicited in these eight cases in response to the owner's punishment in an effort to correct other behavior problems is also consistent with the ethological view that the biological function of submissive urination and other forms of submissive behavior is to inhibit further aggression by another dog.

In one additional case in which submissive urination was the primary behavior problem, two Shih Tzu bitches, a 4-year-old mother and one of her 1-year-old female offspring, were involved. The older dog urinated in response to being picked up prior to being brushed and during the brushing itself (which the dog hated) and the younger dog urinated when being greeted both by strangers and family members. According to the owner, some of the other puppies from the same litter as the younger female had also shown the problem to differing degrees, which suggests a genetic predisposition towards submissive urination was involved.

Possible causal factors

Genetic predisposition

In the above case example, a genetic predisposition towards submissive urination or reacting unusually submissively to situations which normally do not elicit this kind of extreme reaction in other dogs seems clear.

History of punishment

Sometimes the problem develops in a dog with no previous history of being excessively submissive or fearful as a direct result of the owner's application of punitive measures first to control another behavior problem and then later, to control the submissive urination itself. When this kind of conditioned reaction to owner behavior is involved, treatment measures, goals, and prognosis can be somewhat different than in cases involving dogs that were extremely submissive from the start.

Restricted early experience

Submissive urination may also occur in a dog which reacts fearfully to human beings or hu-

POSSIBLE CAUSAL FACTORS

Genetic predisposition
(suspected in cases where no obvious environmental cause)

Early experience deficit
(e.g. submissive urination associated with fear of certain types of human beings because of lack of experience with them early in life)

History of punishment
(problem can result from the owner's application of punishment measures)

Unintentional owner eliciting/fostering
(problem can be response to dominant/ aggressive owner behavior)

Unintentional owner reinforcement
(e.g. owner stops doing something to the dog or comforts/reassures it in response to urination)

SUBMISSIVE URINATION

- Puppy or submissive older dog urinates and shows other submissive behavior when approached, punished, picked up, greeted, etc.

POSSIBLE TREATMENT ELEMENTS

Avoid problem situations
(avoid behaving towards dog in ways which elicit urination)

Cessation of unintentional reinforcement
(e.g. giving dog attention when it shows problem behavior)

Cessation of counterproductive treatment methods
(e.g. stop punishment of urination)

Systematic behavior therapy methods
(e.g. desensitize dog to being picked up; countercondition sitting/standing in greeting situations)

man beings of a certain type because of insufficient experience with them during the first three months of life. The often irreversible nature of such early experience deficits implies that treatment must be based on the assumption that the problem behavior must somehow be eliminated or controlled even though there is little one can do about the underlying fear.

Unintentional owner elicitation

Owners may approach and bend over, pick up, pet, groom, or gaze lovingly at their overly submissive dog completely unaware that these be-

haviors may be perceived by it as being dominant behavior which tends naturally to elicit a submissive behavioral response. Given that owner punishment is essentially a form of aggressive behavior, it is not surprising that it too is a potent elicitor of submissive behavior. Such an effect can also operate on a more general, relationship level in the sense that being overly strict, punitive, and perhaps bullying towards the dog in a variety of circumstances can encourage the development of extreme submissiveness which, in turn, increases the probably of submissive urination in the various problem situations.

SAMPLE RECOMMENDATIONS

Submissive urination

- Whenever the dog urinates, it should be completely ignored; that is, no scolding and no positive kinds of attention like talking to or petting it which might reward the behavior.
- Stop severely scolding and otherwise punishing the dog for urination or any other problem behavior. Use the recommended reward-based methods instead.

Urination occurs in the greeting situation: *(3 treatment alternatives)*

- Greeting of guests and family members should be kept briefer and calmer.
- Arrange greetings so that they always take place outside of the home.
- Do not greet the dog after you return home until you have been home long enough for the dog to have calmed down completely.

Example behavior therapy method to reduce submissive urination when being picked up to be brushed and when being brushed:

- At times when the dog must be brushed thoroughly, only do so outside until it has been trained to accept brushing without urinating.
- Frequently give the dog food tidbits as a reward during the following types of practice sessions. Over a period of several weeks, practice each stage several times a day until the desired goal has been achieved before going on to the next stage. Reward the dog in the home:
  - for sitting, lying down, and coming on command
  - for not showing fear or insecurity when being picked up (at first just slightly above the floor and then later, increasingly higher)
  - for not showing fear or insecurity during brushing (at first only when brushed very lightly with one or two brush strokes, and then after brushing for progressively longer periods of time).
- Do not give the dog tidbits except during these practice sessions.

Unintentional owner reinforcement

Stopping whatever one is doing as soon as it elicits the urination whether it be punishment or petting, picking up, or bending over the dog is a natural and indeed advisable owner response which nevertheless reinforces the submissive behavior and therefore may make it more probable in the future. This is an understandable aspect of the dynamics of the situation considering that the function of submissive behavior performed in direct response to threatening forms of dominant or aggressive behavior is to inhibit further threatening or more severe aggression.

Of course, another possible type of reinforcement which can affect the behavior is reacting sympathetically by reassuring or petting the dog when it urinates as part of a display of extreme submission.

Possible treatment elements

Avoid problem situations

Simply not picking up a dog which shows submissive urination in response to being physically handled in this way, for example, might be the most sensible way to deal with certain types of problem situations. In the above-described Shih Tzu case, the owner had learned to avoid picking the dog up after approaching it from the front or side. By approaching it and picking it up from the back, however, urination was usually prevented. Making sure that the greeting or brushing occurs outside, where urination is not a problem, could also be classified as a means of avoiding problem situations. Another would be for the owner to stop punishing the dog for other behavioral problems if this kind of punishment elicits submissive urination.

Cessation of counterproductive treatment methods

Punishment of the submissive urination is strictly contraindicated for obvious reasons. Most owners discover this on their own after seeing the problem rapidly worsen as a result of punishing the dog for urination.

Cessation of unintentional reinforcement

Although the rewarding effect of submissive urination that occurs when the owner stops doing whatever has elicited the behavior is unavoidable, other possible forms of reinforcement like giving the dog a lot of attention and sympathy when it reacts submissively can be easily avoidable. Dogs should neither being punished nor rewarded for the behavior. Instead, they should simply be totally ignored and therefore not approached, talked to, or even looked at.

Systematic behavior therapy methods

Sometimes dogs can be gradually *desensitized* to and/or *counterconditioned* to perform alternative behaviors (i.e. other than urination) in problem situations using behavior therapy methods. The method of training the dog to be picked up without urinating described in the sample recommendation box below is an example of one such procedure. The dog was to be frequently picked up by the owner without being brushed (desensitization element) and rewarded with tidbits for not urinating and for remaining relaxed/non-fearful when picked up (counterconditioning element). Using instrumental learning techniques to gradually train a dog to remain sitting or standing when greeting owners is another example of a countercondi-

tioning procedure. It could be used to correct the problem in an animal that has the tendency to submissively roll over onto its back and urinate when being greeted.

Excitement-related urination

In the behavior problem checklist mentioned in the last section, 5 out of 71 (7%) owners of dogs without serious elimination problems indicated that the dog sometimes urinated when playing or greeting owners after an extended absence. Voith and Borchelt (1985) point out that this kind of problem is especially common in puppies and that they usually outgrow it within a few months.

Given the nature of the situation in which the urination occurs, the fact that the dog may urinate while standing or walking, and the experiences most people have had at some time in their lives with involuntary urination, most owners understand from the start that no conventional housebreaking problem is involved. Consequently, most refrain from punishing the dog and instead try to cope with the problem by in some way arranging things so that the dog doesn't get so excited at certain key times.

Possible causal factors

Genetic predisposition

Why do some dogs exhibit this problem and others don't? The answer is more likely to involve differences in the dogs' genetic makeup rather than past experience. Although learning can be involved in the sense that a series of rewarding experiences in a particular type of situation may increase the dog's level of arousal when exposed to it again, even here the question still remains as to why some of these extremely excited dogs urinate whereas most others don't.

Unintentional owner fostering

To the extent that owners behave in ways which elicit vigorous play or excited greetings, they may be contributing to the problem.

POSSIBLE CAUSAL FACTORS

Genetic predisposition
(possible explanation of why some dogs are incontinent in excitement-eliciting situations)

Unintentional owner fostering
(owner behavior during greeting/playing may increase dog's excitement)

Inadequate care/maintenance conditions
(e.g. excitement greater after period of social isolation/lack of activity)

Physiological factors
(e.g. low bladder/bladder sphincter tone)

EXCITEMENT-RELATED URINATION

• Dog urinates while standing or walking when highly excited during greeting, playing, etc.

POSSIBLE TREATMENT ELEMENTS

Avoid problem situations
(e.g. greet outside; avoid greeting/overstimulating dog at certain times)

Cessation of ineffective/undesirable treatment methods
(punishment contraindicated)

Drug therapy
(e.g. to increase tone of bladder sphincter)

Change of care/maintenance conditions
(e.g. don't leave animal alone so long; take outside more often; provide it with more opportunities for play/exercise)

Training in problem situations
(elicit or countercondition behavior not associated with excitement-related urination in problem situations)

Inadequate care/maintenance conditions

A common scenario is when a young active dog which is left alone for long periods of time becomes overly excited when the owner returns home. Essentially, some kind of social or activity deprivation effect would be involved. Of course, the animal's increased need to urinate after hours alone in the home is relevant here as well. Perhaps it is the excitement combined with a full bladder that is the problem.

Physiological factors

Basically, the excitement-related urination problem is a situation-specific form of incontinence. Voith's (1989) suggestion that drugs which increase the tone of the bladder sphinc-

ter or decrease the tone of the bladder may be helpful in some cases implies that the primary cause may be some physiological disorder.

Possible treatment elements

Avoid problem situations

Usually dogs do not show the problem in every play or greeting situation – just those in which they become highly excited and/or if they become excited when their bladder is full. If these situations can be avoided by, for example, not returning the dog's greeting at certain times, only greeting it outside where urination is not a problem, or not stimulating the dog further when it is becoming overly excited during play or greeting, a satisfactory solution to the problem may be achieved. This is basically how most owners cope with the problem.

Change of care/maintenance conditions

Not leaving the animal alone for long periods may lower its level of excitement when the owner returns home and – if taken out more frequently as well – its bladder will not be as full at this time as when owner absences are longer. If the owner must work the whole day long, periodic visits during the day by a neighbor who takes the dog out for a walk can help especially if the dog is provided with opportunities for vigorous play during this time.

Cessation of ineffective/undesirable methods

Punishment is not recommended as a treatment for this problem, for it is unlikely that the dog is capable of learning not to urinate in these problem situations. In cases where punishment seems to be effective, this is probably because it changes the dog's emotional reactions to problem situations. Greetings may become times of "mixed emotions" rather than of enthusiastic excitement – an undesirable change in the eyes of most owners.

Training in problem situations

When problem situations are unavoidable, the key to solving the problem may be to elicit and strengthen behaviors in the dog which are if not incompatible with urination, at least lower its probably of occurrence. What exactly the dog should be trained or encouraged to do in potential problem situations varies from case to case. The owner's returning home with the dog's favorite toy which is thrown prior to greeting is one possibility of encouraging the dog's greeting behavior to take a different form. Similarly, one type of game may be deliberately elicited and strengthened and another refrained from when urination occurs in the play setting. Finally, an obedience training approach where the dog is first taught commands and later gradually trained to execute them in potential problem situations can also help change the

dog's behavior and perhaps also the probability of urination in such situations.

Drug therapy

According to Voith (1989), *phenylpropanolamine HCl*, dosed at 0.55 – 4.4 mg/kg bid, increases the tone of the bladder sphincter and helps prevent excitement and submissive urination. Marder (1991) recommends dosages of 12.5 – 50 mg bid-tid. She also states that the tricyclic antidepressant, *imipramine*, dosed at 2.2 – 4.4 mg/kg po sid-bid, was more effective in the few animals for which she "needed the help of drug therapy". (See the "drug therapy" subsection in Chapter 8 for side effects and other important drug-related information.)

Urinary or fecal incontinence

In cases where defecation or urination do not involve normal elimination behavior of squatting while defecating and squatting or lifting the hind leg while urinating – or urinating only when highly excited, submissive, or fearful – the problem requires medical and not behavior-related treatment. In the cases of urinary and fecal incontinence that are occasionally referred to behavior specialists, the specialist is usually called in after the search for a pathophysiological cause was negative. In such cases, the specialist usually can do nothing but confirm the family veterinarians' initial suspicion that the problem is not behavioral and, therefore, suggest that further diagnostic medical examinations are required.

References

Borchelt, P.L., and Voith, V.L. (1985): Punishment. *Compendium on Continuing Education for the Practicing Veterinarian* 7, 780–788.

Burghardt, W.F. (1991): Using drugs to control behavior problems in pets. *Veterinary Medicine* **November**, 1066–1075.

Dunbar, I., and Carmichael, M.: The response of male dogs to urine from other males. *Behav. Neural. Biol.* 3, 465–470.

Fox, M.W. (1963): *Canine Behavior*. Springfield, Illinois, Charles C. Thomas

Marder, A.R. (1991): Psychotropic drugs and behavioral therapy. *Veterinary Clinics of North America: Small Animal Practice* **21**, 329–342.

Mech, L. D., and Peters, R.P. (1977): The study of chemical communication in free-ranging mammals. In D. Müller-Schwarze and M.M. Mozell (eds), *Chemical Signals in Vertebrates*. New York, Plenum.

Neville, P. (1991): *Do Dogs Need Shrinks?* London, Sidgwick and Jackson Limited.

O'Farrell, V. (1992): *Manual of Canine Behaviour*, 2nd Edition. Shurdington, Cheltenham, Gloucestershire, England, British Small Animal Veterinary Association.

O'Farrell, V., and Neville, P. (1994): *Manual of Feline Behaviour*. Shurdington, Cheltenham, Gloucestershire, England, British Small Animal Veterinary Association.

Parker, A.J. (1989): Behavioral signs of organic disease. In Ettinger, S.J. (ed), *Textbook of Veterinary Internal Medicine*, 3rd ed., Philadelphia, WB Saunders.

Reisner, I. (1991): The pathophysiologic basis of behavior problems. *Veterinary Clinics of North America: Small Animal Practice* **21**, 207–224

Voith, V.L. (1989): Behavioral disorders. In Ettinger, S. (ed): *Textbook of Veterinary Internal Medicine*. Philadelphia, WB Saunders.

Voith, V.L., and Borchelt, P.L. (1982): Diagnosis and treatment of elimination behavior problems in dogs. *Veterinary Clinics of North America: Small Animal Practice* **12**, 637–644.

Voith, V.L., and Borchelt, P.L. (1985): Elimination behavior and related problems in dogs. *Compendium on Continuing Education for the Practicing Veterinarian* **7**, 537–549.

18   Miscellaneous Behavior Problems

In addition to the common aggression, fear, and elimination problems discussed in previous chapters, there are a host of other problems with which veterinary or non-veterinary pet behavior problem counselors are often confronted. Commonly these problems are only minor flaws in an otherwise perfectly behaved dog or additional problems in dogs presented for more severe behavior problems. However, this is certainly not always the case. Sometimes they can be as disturbing for owners as any of the other problems discussed earlier.

Uncontrollability during walks

Not coming when called

Three causal factors are often associated with this problem – a potentially very serious one for owners and one of the most common problems of all.

Dog highly motivated to do something else like play with another dog, follow a scent, or chase a small animal.

Variation in whether and how quickly a dog comes when called usually depends on what the dog is doing at the time. When the dog has become disinterested in what it has been doing and nothing else greatly interests or attracts it in the vicinity, it is likely to come immediately. But when other dogs are around and the dog is heading for, greeting, playing with, or threatening one of them, it may be deaf to the owner's commands. Asking owners if their dog comes when called, many answer "only when it suits him" or something similar – an obvious referral to just this sort of situational or motivation-related variation.

Dog has not been well-trained to come when called and/or dog has been inadvertently "trained" not to come when called.

Many owners who have this problem with their dog have simply not made a consistent effort to improve the dog's behavior in this regard using the conventional methods most owners instinctively apply when first training a young puppy – like heaping praise, petting, and baby talk on it when it comes when called. Additionally, some owners have applied the counter-productive method of scolding the dog for not coming sooner when it finally does come, which only makes the problem worse. While owners may realize at some level that they shouldn't do this, they are sometimes too angry or frustrated to do anything else. Then too, owners may think that this method must be effective in the long run due to the dog's behavior when it finally comes: it approaches hesitantly, head down, tail held low, eye contact evasive as if, in owners' words, "he knows exactly that he has done something wrong". Punishment is therefore assumed to reinforce these kinds of „guilt feelings" and therefore make it less likely that the dog will do it again. The dog is, however, only showing signs of fear because it keeps getting punished when it comes after, understandably enough, avoiding coming for as long as possible.

Dominance problem between dog and owner

Many dogs which ignore owners' commands to come also show other signs that they have less than the normal amount of respect for their owners – that is, some kind of dominance-related problem exists. Therefore, it is necessary to question owners closely about possible dominance-aggression symptoms (e.g. does it ever growl at you when you try to take a bone or toy away from it, disturb it when it is sleeping, order it to do something, or brush, bathe, shove, or pet it?) and symptoms of milder dominance-related problems (e.g. is it stubborn, pushy, always slow to obey, or disobedient in other situations?). When there is a problem in this area – as there often is – some of the recommendations from Chapter 10 for increasing

owner dominance should be given along with some of those listed in the box below.

The following sample recommendations box describes one conventional procedure for solving the problem. Various possible problem-solving elements have been combined to produce a maximally effective method for improving obedience in this situation as quickly as possible.

SAMPLE RECOMMENDATIONS

Training a dog to come when called during walks

- Take an ample supply of the dog's favorite food tidbits (i.e. 30 or so pea-sized pieces of cheese, biscuit, sausage, etc.) to use as rewards when going for walks. Unless food rewards are also being used for other training or problem-correcting purposes, don't give it tidbits at any other time.

- For the first few weeks of training, immediately give the dog a food reward every time it comes after being called. Act happy and praise and pet the dog before and after it is given the tidbit as well.

- In the initial stages of training, conspicuously hold out your hand when you call it as if to show it the tidbit. It won't see the object from a distance, but it will see your distinctive body posture and arm gestures and quickly learn what this means.

- Particularly during the first couple of days, only call the dog when you know from experience that at this moment it is likely to stop what it is doing and come. Otherwise, simply wait for such a moment to come or, alternatively, apply the walking-away method described below.

- Always act pleased and generously reward the dog with praise, petting, and tidbits when it comes even if it has taken its good about it and you're furious at having been kept waiting for so long.

- Never punish the dog for not coming quickly enough or having done something wrong (e.g. barked at someone) when it finally comes. Such punishment comes far too late to do any good. Always remember that it is the behavior that the dog is in the act of performing at the time (i.e. coming) which is really being punished. In effect, scolding the dog for being too slow to come essentially trains it to delay coming for long as possible.

- Don't put the dog on the leash as soon as it comes even if it's time to go home. First pet it, praise it, give it two or three food rewards for sitting and staying on command, and then after waiting a bit, put it on its leash and praise, pet, and give it another food reward or two for cooperating.

- After the dog has been reliably coming on command for a few weeks, you can begin slowly phasing out the food rewards by first only occasionally omitting the tidbit and then omitting it more and more frequently. However, it is best to never stop giving food rewards entirely and the dog should always be praised and petted for coming when called.

- In place of food rewards, one can also use something like throwing a ball as an effective reward if the dog really loves chasing it. Always take the ball with you on walks and make it a rule to only throw it as a reward for coming – and as an additional reward for bringing it back after chasing it.

Walking-away method:

- If the dog doesn't immediately come when called, turn and walk directly away until the dog notices this and comes after you. Reward the dog as usual when it comes no matter how long it takes.

(In cases where the problem is symptomatic of a dominance-related problem in the relationship between owner and dog, some of the recommendations for increasing owner dominance discussed in Chapter 10 are also appropriate.)

Not stopping misbehavior on command

Regardless of whether the dog is pulling on the leash, going after a child's ice-cream cone, or barking at someone in a wheelchair, there are often occasions in which normally well-behaved dogs start doing something that they shouldn't do which owners must put a stop to. When owners sometimes have difficulty suppressing minor problems – but overall the dog is not a problem in the sense of the major problems discussed in this book – one of three scenarios is often involved. Owner dominance is not quite as high as it should be, owners are reluctant for ethical reasons to use any kind of authoritarian or punitive measures, or they are unable to do so effectively for personality-related reasons (e.g. particularly soft-spoken or mild-mannered individuals).

In all three cases, the main recommendation is the same: *get tougher with the dog* – which means scolding it or scolding it more severely, possibly accompanied by some other kind of punishing stimulus like giving a sharp jerk on the leash. Not only does this end the problem behavior and, if consistently applied, help train the dog not to behave in this way in the future, it also may quickly and dramatically increase the dog's overall respect for an owner who has been reluctant to react this way in the past. One of the reason most owners have few problems with their dogs is that from puppy age onwards, they have always had the good sense to react with appropriate severity whenever their dog has tried to ignore their "No!" order to stop misbehaving.

For the particular case of pulling on the leash, O'Farrell (1992) briefly describes one possible training method for solving problems which persist in spite of owners repeated scolding and other punitive measures:

"Analysis of the situation usually reveals that the pulling is being rewarded by the walk continuing and therefore by new and interesting sights and smells. This situation can be reversed by the owner turning round and retracing his steps immediately whenever the dog starts to pull. The turning round should be preceded by a command such as 'Heel' so *that eventually the command alone will be enough to stop the pulling."* (p. 113)

Begging/pestering for food, playing, petting, etc.

Although this common problem is often minor, in some cases the behavior of the dog has been allowed to get out completely of hand and its pushy, demanding barking, scratching, nudging, jumping up, or mouthing behavior is driving family members crazy. Theoretically, these problems are easy to solve. Owners must simply make it a hard and fast family rule that the dog should be completely ignored and never given what it wants when it starts begging and pestering for something – an animal learning procedure that is technically referred to as *extinction*. Also taboo are all potentially rewarding distraction measures applied to stop the behavior like, for example, offering the dog a toy to stop it from barking when family members are eating. If the dog is simply too pushy and demanding to be ignored, it should be scolded or otherwise punished with sufficient severity to immediately stop the bothersome behavior. Another potentially effective strategy here is for the owner to get up and leave the room whenever the dog becomes unbearable – a way of ignoring the dog which may also function as a mild punishment.

Every owner suspects that this is how the problem should be handled, but after having tried to react this way they are not so sure. For when the dog is not given what it wants, the pushy, demanding behavior seems to get worse and not better: the barking gets louder or the jumping up more frantic until the owner finally gives in.

One reason for failure is that the owners may be rather childish and lack the kind of self-discipline and basic good sense which most other owners display. They might even find the dog's pushy behavior amusing at times and be basically unwilling to apply the extinction procedure in the kind of across-the-board, absolutely-no-exceptions way which is necessary to eliminate the problem. However, most owners simply lack the necessary confidence in this approach to implement it in the long-term, 100% consistent way which is required. In this case, it is important that the counselor explain in detail the dynamics of this problem from the point of view of the following four animal behavioral science principles. For to be successful, owners must know exactly what to expect at all stages of extinction process:

- In all higher animal species, when the extinction method (i.e. the complete cessation of rewards for a learned behavior that has always, often, or occasionally been rewarded in the past) is applied, animals initially react by *increasing* response frequency or intensity. It is only later, after this more energetic responding has yielded no rewards, that the frequency of the behavior begins to decline.
- The extinction process is aversive for animals. The concept of "frustration" is often evoked to characterize the animal's general reaction to the situation and point out similarities to its behavior in other situations where its access to a desired goal is blocked or prevented in some way. One can compare the dog's agitated, sometimes aggressively demanding behavior at this time to our own behavior when a soft drink dispensing machine swallows our money without given us a can (e.g. trying it again, repeatedly operating the change return level with increasing vigor, banging on the machine with our fist, kicking it, swearing under our breathe, etc.) to help explain to owners what the initial stages of the extinction process might feel like to animals.
- Partial reinforcement produces greater resistance to extinction: that is, responses which in the past were only rewarded sometimes (as opposed to every time) take much, much longer to be abandoned than those which were previously rewarded every single time they occurred. It is as if it takes the animal much longer to become really convinced that the behavior is not going to produce the desired reward if, in the past, it is accustomed to sometimes performing the behavior without being rewarded. In the

above soft-drink machine example, we give up as fast as we do because we have been *continuously rewarded* every time we have operated the machine in the past. However, we don't give up nearly so easily when operating, for example, a one-armed bandit in Las Vegas that only rewards its operator *intermittently* on a random schedule which makes it impossible to predict which depression of the lever will be rewarded.

- The course of extinction is uneven in two respects. First: responding is not regular, but rather occurs in bursts of rapid responding interspersed with pauses in responding lasting various lengths of time. Therefore it is to be expected that the animal will give up after trying hard for awhile, go away, come back and try repeatedly again, then apparently give up again, etc. on a somewhat erratic basis. Second: the animal may stop trying on one day, but begin the next day by responding at a high level. This *spontaneous recovery* (i.e. reappearance of response which was apparently completely abandoned the day before) may occur day after day for some time – with the amount and duration of this renewed responding irregularly decreasing over the course of many days.

Of course, the counselor need not extensively explain all of these technical details to owners. Rather, it is simply a matter of understanding the principles oneself and then using everyday language coupled perhaps with human examples to remind owners of how they too react this way in certain situations. The primary aim here is to convey to them that eliminating behaviors using the extinction procedure can be a long tedious process, with the animal's behavior often being surprisingly persistent and highly variable both on an hour-to-hour and day-to-day basis. This helps owners understand why this method didn't work in the past and what they will have to do to effectively apply it to correct the present problem.

Owners should also be firmly warned against half-heartedly applying this method. Usually ignoring a dog's begging but giving into to it when the dog becomes particularly pushy and intolerable simply trains it to be more pushy and intolerable. In effect, it teaches the animal that in the long run it will get what it wants if it doesn't give up. Thus, either owners are prepared to apply the extinction method correctly, or they better not apply it at all. For inconsistent application will make the problem doubly difficult to correct in the future.

If the extinction method simply does not work in spite of being diligently and consistently applied, the dog is probably motivated to perform the behavior at least partly for reasons unrelated to rewarding consequences stemming from owners behavior. Often, the behavior is self-rewarding. For example, the petting and attention a dog receives by jumping up on family members and guests during greeting may be only part of the reason why this behavior is so persistent in spite of frequent punishment. It may also be a natural expression of the increased activity and excitement aroused by the greeting context. Another possibility is that it is related to the height difference between humans and dogs and the fact that the dog cannot carry out the kind of face-to-face behavioral interactions which are normal among dogs and wolves (e.g. subdominant wolves often lick the snout of the more dominant pack member when greeting it).

In such situations, the extinction method alone may not be enough and a combination of punishment and counterconditioning methods might also need to be applied: that is, ignoring and/or punishing of undesirable behavior (e.g. jumping up) can be combined with a method which uses food tidbits and other rewards to gradually train the animal to perform some acceptable alternative behavior (e.g. sitting quietly) in problem situations (e.g. Askew, 1991). In effect, one teaches the animal a new, effective (for it), but acceptable (to the owner) behavioral strategy for obtaining rewards in this situation.

However, it is best to not get overly complicated if this is unnecessary. In most cases of begging/pestering behavior in dogs, the self-reinforcing element is negligible or minimal and it is therefore sufficient if owners simply make it a hard and fast rule to never reward such behavior again.

SAMPLE RECOMMENDATIONS

Begging/pestering for attention, play, food, etc.

1. Make it a hard and fast family rule never to give the dog what it wants when it begs or pesters in any way. Ignore it entirely every time it starts begging/pestering until it gives up even if this takes several minutes.

2. If the dog becomes so pushy and demanding that it is impossible to ignore (e.g. increasingly loud barking), either get up and leave the room or, alternatively, scold the dog severely enough to immediately stop the behavior.

3. The dog's reaction to being ignored during the first day or two is likely to be to beg/pester much more than usual. This is normal. Its usual strategy isn't paying off so it is naturally inclined to try harder. But it will give up sooner or later if you are stubborn enough not to give it what it wants.

4. You must be 100 % consistent for this method to work. Weakening and giving in to the dog once in awhile will make the problem worse and not better.

5. Be prepared for the fact that the dog won't just simply stop and never beg or pester again: it will stop for a day or so, try it again a few times, give up again, try it again a few days later, and so on.

Unusual attention-getting behavior

Some dogs learn to obtain rewarding owner attention in more bizarre ways. A common scenario is when a dog that has recovered from some illness or injury which impaired normal movement continues to show a version of the impairment after the illness has passed or the injury has been completely healed. So-called "sympathy lameness" where a dog with a previous limb injury still limps after all signs of the physical problem are past is one well-known example. Another is when a dog occasionally or frequently suffers from "attacks" involving apparent breathing abnormalities, muscle spasms, inability to walk, etc. for which medical tests reveal no pathophysiological cause.

The continuation of limping after it has become unnecessary is easy to understand in the sense that the limping behavior during the illness was often rewarded with a shower of owner concern and attention. But how a dog could learn to perform such attack-like behavior is more difficult to account for. One of my cases involved one of two family poodles which had periodic "attacks" which terrified the middle-aged woman owner to such an extent that she continuously watched the dog and became herself close to having an attack every time the dog began exhibiting the pre-attack state of apparent heightened muscle tension. In questioning the owner, it appeared that the first time the attack-like signs occurred was when the dog collapsed into an apparent semi-conscious state which lasted a few minutes after it bumped its head on a stone while racing around with the other dog in the backyard. Theoretically, this could be enough. One could imagine, for example, that the owner might have been more traumatized than the dog by the experience and would be likely to react with alarm if the dog showed behavior (e.g. unusually rapid or irregular breathing, trembling, postural twitching) that even vaguely resembled that which it showed at the time of its injury. This could then provide the basis for unintentional *shaping* (i.e. a technical term for the production of some target behavior through the positive reinforcement of a series of responses representing closer and closer approximations to it) which, over time, could produce a learned attack which closely resembles the kind of one the woman most fears.

The first step in such cases is, of course, to carry out the medical examination and tests required to rule out any medical cause. If this has been done and a purely behavioral cause is suspected, it often makes sense to investigate this possibility further before carrying out more extensive medical tests because it is often relatively easy to confirm the attention-getting behavior diagnosis on the following grounds:

Common owner/home situation profile

Hart and Hart (1985) suggest that such problems are especially common in homes where dogs are "heavily indulged with love and petting" or where there is more than one dog in the family and therefore competition between dogs for the owner's attention. A third common characteristic may be an owner who tends to be a worrier who overreacts and becomes extremely nervous and upset when the dog behaves in an unusual manner.

Past history and present nature of owner-dog interactions consistent with attention-getting behavior diagnosis

A learning-related explanation would lead one to look both for a pattern of gradual development (e.g. increasingly exaggerated behavior, increasing frequency) and some clue as to what started the ball rolling: that is, what happened the very first time that the owner noticed the behavior and became worried. It need not be something dramatic like the injury in the above example, rather only something like the owner having noticed one day that the dog was breathing strangely or twitching a little. Of course, disease processes too may gradually worsen over time producing this same progressive development pattern. Thus, this feature is not decisive in making the disease vs. behavioral origin decision. However, the absence of the kind of gradual development pattern one would expect if learning were involved might be an indication that the problem may be purely physical after all.

Of course, assessing the degree to which a learning-related explanation might account for the behavior also involves carefully considering how owners react to the problem behavior. For example, at first signs of the problem behavior, the owners may tend to become concerned, stop whatever they are doing, and the dog is fussed over, picked up, and offered toys and tidbits to try and stop the behavior or keep it from worsening. In short, this line of inquiry may indicate that from the dog's viewpoint there is an immediate and considerable payoff for behaving in that way.

Occurrence of the problem only in the owner's presence

Hart and Hart (1985) suggest that detective work is required to see if the dog exhibits the behavior when no one is around to observe and reward it. While it may not be possible to do this with behavior which occurs relatively infrequently like the above attacks, with limping, for example, it is easy to arrange a situation where someone hides and can spy on the dog (e.g. through a window or keyhole) when it is alone. Sometimes the difference is dramatic: when alone, the dog walks normally with no signs of the pathetic hobbling it displays in the owner's presence. As Hart and Hart point out, this would be conclusive evidence of attention-getting motivation.

Behavior more common at times when owner is preoccupied with other things and paying little attention to the dog

In the poodle case discussed above, the owner had noticed that the dog was especially prone to having attacks when guests were staying in the home and she was very involved with them instead of showering attention on the dog as was normally the case when she was alone with the two dogs.

Changed owner reaction has dramatic impact on the behavior

When the owner can be persuaded to treat the problem using the approach outlined in the above sample recommendations box for begging/pestering problems – preferably leaving the room rather than scolding or simply ignoring the behavior – improvement may be rapid and dramatic, which would of course support the attention-getting behavior rather than medical disorder diagnosis.

Stereotypies

Stereotypies are repetitive, stereotyped or ritualized (i.e. highly constant in form), apparently functionless acts which animals frequently or almost continuously perform – to the point of self-mutilation in some cases. Examples are flank sucking, chewing feet, self-scratching, lick granuloma, fly chasing (when there is no fly), tail chasing, whirling in a circle, etc. Leuscher et al. (1991) point out, however, that the above definition needs to be qualified somewhat in the sense that (1) some stereotypies (e.g. motionless staring at the wall) are continuous and not repetitive, (2) the form of the behavior may be somewhat more variable than the term stereotypy suggests (particularly when it first begins to develop), and (3) a few stereotypies like, for example, masturbation have an obvious purposeful/functional element.

Leuscher et al. (1991) offers the following classification system for stereotypies in dogs:

Grooming behavior: chewing feet/nails, flank sucking, lick granuloma (acral lick dermatitis), licking objects, self scratching

"Hallucinatory" (where behavior seems to be directed towards some nonexistent object)*:* staring, fly snapping, prey searching/nose to ground, prey pouncing

Eating/drinking: polydipsia, polyphagia, drooling, gravel/dirt eating, stone chewing, wool sucking

*Locomotory (*i.e. movement-related)*:* circling/whirling, pacing, jumping in place, fence-line running, digging, freezing

Vocalization: rhythmic barking, barking at food, growling or snarling at self

Neurotic: vicious biting of feet or tail, unpredictable aggression to humans

Information and ideas from two major fields have had an impact on the approach to treatment of these fairly widespread types of problems in companion animals. The first involves zoo and farm animals. Because some stereotypies can represent major economic problems for farmers, they have been studied much more extensively in farm animals than in companion animals. Fraser and Broom (1990) devote three chapters to the description and treatment of common farm animal stereotypies classified in terms of whether the behavior is directed towards the *individual's own body*, the *inanimate surroundings*, or *other individuals*. Examples in horses, cows, pigs, and chickens are pacing, rocking, swaying, weaving, rubbing the body against something, pawing and stall-kicking, head-shaking or nodding, eye-rolling, bar-biting, drinker-pressing, self-mutilation, licking own hair/wool/feathers, sucking/eating solid objects/litter/earth/dung, overeating, polydipsia, homosexual behavior, and belly-nosing, anal-nosing, milk-sucking, and aggressive behavior directed towards other animals.

Fraser and Broom (1990) suggest that stereotypies "have been shown to be a consequence of ways in which the animals are housed or managed" and are therefore "an indicator of poor welfare". Specific causal factors mentioned by the authors are associated with situations in which individual lacks control over environment, future events are unpredictable for animals, there is a lack of variety in environment, or animals lack movement possibilities, social partners, sexual partners, food, or other resources. Hereditary effects have also been identified and the effects on brain chemistry or functioning due to sensory inputs from repeated activities seem to be an important element in some cases.

Leuscher (1991) too discusses similar causal factors for companion animals. For example, conflict induced by inappropriate environment or management, symptoms of high arousal or vacuum activities resulting from the absence of releasing stimuli or target objects for species-specific behavior, displacement activities, restraint of normal motor patterns, change in social environment (separation from owner), unstable social order (changing dominance re-

lationships), or lack of predictability or controllability in environment.

Thus, both discussions of farm and companion animal stereotypies point to a *problem environment* which is somehow incompatible with or not conducive to the animal's natural behavioral tendencies/repertoire as the primary causal factor. And for both farm and companion animals, the behavior counselor must therefore look either for some important element which the environment lacks or some disturbing, threatening, or stressful element which it contains. Also running through both discussions is the central, still unresolved issue of whether particular stereotypies are functional in the sense of somehow helping the animal cope with the effects of adverse environmental conditions (e.g. via needed discharging of energy, de-arousal, or sensory feedback) or functionless, essentially useless wastes of energy reflecting some kind of central nervous system pathology.

Over and above the many similarities in environmental causal factors, there is one difference in the environment of companion and farm animals which can be crucial in understanding some pet stereotypies. Namely, the intimate, virtually full-time association and intense behavioral interactions between owner and pet – and the resulting potentially powerful rewarding effects of owner attention, petting, and other behavior towards the pet – raises the possibility in particular cases that unintentional owner reinforcement has helped shape and maintain the stereotypy in precisely the same way as with the attention-getting behavior problems considered in the last major section.

The second major field of direct relevance to stereotypies in companion animals is human clinical psychology and psychiatry. Strongly emphasizing the similarity of stereotypies in companion and other domestic animals with *obsessive-compulsive behavior disorders* in human beings (e.g. stereotypic, ritualistic behavior like compulsive hand-washing, hair-pulling, gas jet/lock/light checking), Leuscher et al. (1991) argue that it is "less ambiguous to describe stereotypies as obsessive-compulsive disorders" or OCD, an abbreviation which is then very frequently used along with the term stereotypy throughout the article. Overall (1994) too suggests that the use of the term obsessive-compulsive disorder is appropriate for many stereotypies:

"For a disorder to be considered obsessive-compulsive in human beings, it must be ritualistic and sufficiently invasive, cognitively or physically, to interfere with normal function. These criteria are applicable to canine behavior that includes stereotypic, ritualistic circling, spinning, and pacing; some howling; some hallucinatory and ingestive behaviors; and many self-mutilation/grooming disorders such as acral lick granuloma." (p. 1738)

The importance of this parallel between human obsessive-compulsive disorders and stereotypies in companion animals is twofold. On the one hand, if many stereotypies in companion animals are indeed directly analogous to obsessive-compulsive disorders in human beings, these may serve as an animal model of the human disorder which can be used for the experimental study of the behavioral phenomena, its physiological substrates, and various behavioral and drug treatment possibilities. On the other hand, drugs which have been found to be useful in the treatment of obsessive-compulsive disorders in human beings may be similarly helpful in companion animals – which does indeed appear to be the case.

Treatment possibilities

The stereotypy phenomenon is therefore exceeding complex and wide-ranging, involving not only companion animals but human beings and other domestic animals as well. Although potential causal elements too are diverse and difficult to unravel in particular cases, a few general treatment possibilities can still be derived from the above discussion which are often helpful in companion animal cases. These are presented below not in the form of specific recommendations, but rather as areas which must be explored by the counselor when questioning owners.

- *Does the behavior have an attention-getting element? How exactly does the owner react when the animal shows the behavior? Does the animal exhibit the behavior even when it is alone?*

If the owner attention "payoff" seems to be a major factor, having owners ignore the stereotyped behavior – or better, leave the room every time it begins – may produce dramatic improvements in some cases. As Overall (1992a, 1992b, 1992c, 1994) suggests, it usually makes good sense to investigate and rule out this possibility first before the various drug treatment possibilities are considered.

- *Can the behavior be interrupted by distracting the animal?*

If it can, this kind of interruption can serve as a basis of a behavior modification approach to treating the problem. For example, a stimulus which is regularly used to direct the animal's attention elsewhere and induce it to perform some other, positively-rewarded behavior when it is in the process of performing the stereotypy can later be used to prevent the problem behavior entirely if it is consistently administered just before the behavior begins.

On the other hand, if the behavior cannot be interrupted and the animal must either by physically restrained or allowed to perform the behavior until it stops of its own accord or collapses from exhaustion, the motivation to perform the behavior is too high for behavioral measures alone to be effective and, therefore, drug therapy is indicated. If drug therapy is indeed carried out, the ability to interrupt the behavior can be an important indicator of whether the drug has helped to reduce the severity of the problem to the point where behavioral modification measures can be effectively applied.

- *Is there something important which the animal may lack?*

Social contact with conspecifics and exercise are two likely possibilities. The environment may also be deficient in terms of eliciting behaviors which particular animals are highly motivated to perform like play, exploration, hunting, etc.

- *Does the animal find something about the environment disturbing or threatening or stressful? Is it being left alone for long periods of time? Could the daily family schedule be too erratic and unpredictable from the animal's viewpoint? Does it show fear or avoidance of humans or other animals in the home? Does it show any other signs of reacting negatively to something or someone in the home?*

If so, perhaps some of these kinds of things can be remedied or changed so that they cause the animal fewer problems.

- *Could there be some element of frustration involved? Is the animal in some way blocked or prevented from doing something it seems to want to do? Are certain of its natural behaviors being physically (dog tied up) or otherwise (via punishment) suppressed by owners?*

Where punishment appears in any way to be associated with the problem, owners should be advised to stop punishing their dog in favor of relying on alternative reward-based procedures if control or corrective measures are required.

- *Could the animal be in some kind of motivational conflict situation?*

Common conflicts involve simultaneous tendencies to react aggressively and fearfully towards someone, or to approach (out of friendliness) and avoid (out of fear) human strangers, other dogs, or particular family members.

Although identifying and eliminating any environmental source of stress, fear, frustration, conflict, etc. can obviate the need to treat the problem with medicaments, in many cases this kind of questioning does not turn up anything unusual: the animal's treatment by its owner, its activity, play, etc. needs, and all of its other reactions to detailed features of its present environment seem no different than those of other animals. Basically, drug therapy is indicated after the behavioral approach has been applied to the extent that "the perceived cause of the conflict is removed and it is established that the environment, management, and train-ing methods are no longer conducive to stereo-typies" (Leuscher et al., 1991, p. 410) without resolving the problem.

Medical approach

Of course, medical treatment of physical problems produced by some stereotypies (e.g. acral lick granuloma, severely bitten tail) is often required. And physical response prevention (e.g. covering or in some other way preventing access to parts of the body animals are licking, biting, or scratching) may also be indicated.

In contrast to almost all of the other problems discussed in this book, drug therapy is often the only effective means to treat stereotypies in companion animals. Table 18.1 provides a summary of various drugs which have been reportedly used with some success against stereotypy problems. Most of these drugs are not approved for behavioral treatment and/or use in animals (Burghardt, 1991; Marder, 1991), and their use in many cases has been only experimental with in part wide variations in dosages. The table combines information provided by Marder (1991), Leuscher (1991), Burghardt (1991), and Overall (1992c). The reader is referred particularly to Burghardt (1991) and Marder (1991) as well as the "drug therapy" subsection of Chapter 8 for discussions of side effects and important issues related to the use of drugs in the treatment of behavioral problems.

Destructive behavior

In addition to destructive behavior directly related to separation anxiety (Chapter 16) and fear problems (Chapter 15), other common types of destructive behavior problems are puppy chewing and reactions of older animals whose social/activity/play needs are not being met.

Puppy chewing

The normal behavior of puppies to bite and chew up small objects (e.g. socks, shoes) can

Table 18.1: Summary of drugs and dosages reported to be effective in the treatment of stereotypies in dogs.

Drug	Dosage	References
Amitriptyline HCl	2.2–4.4 mg/kg po sid 1–2 mg/kg po bid or tid 1–2 mg/kg bid 0.25–1 mg/kg	Marder (1991) Overall (1992c) Leuscher et al. (1991) Burghardt (1991)
Naltrexone	2.2 mg/kg po sid or bid	Overall (1992c)
Naloxone	11 to 22 μg/kg IM, IV, or SQ as occasion requires	Overall (1992c)
Fluoxetine	1 mg/kg po sid 1 mg/kg po sid-bid	Marder (1991), Overall (1992c)
Imipramine HCl	2.2–4.4 mg/kg po sid-bid	Marder (1991)
Clomipramine	1–3 mg/kg po sid 1–3 mg/kg split orally every 12 hours (max. dose: 200 mg/d or 3 mg/kg, whichever less; must gradually reach dose).	Marder (1991), Leuscher et al. (1991) Overall (1992c)
Hydroxyzine HCl	2.2 mg/kg po tid 2 mg/kg tid	Overall (1992c) Burghardt (1991)
Buspirone	2.5–10 mg/dog po bid-tid 1 mg/kg po sid-bid	Marder (1991) Overall (1992c)

be corrected using the following measures:

- When unsupervised, confine the dog in a "puppy-proof" room, blocked-off section of a room, or large crate (Voith, 1989) where it is only given access to acceptable objects.
- Make a variety of nylon or rawhide chew toys available to the dog at all times. Do not give the dog an old shoe to chew on thinking that this will prevent it from chewing on new ones, as a surprising number of owners do. To the contrary, this simply strengthens the dog's tendency to attack and destroy – and perhaps even search the home for – shoes of any sort.
- Directing chewing towards appropriate objects should be fostered by often giving these to the dog or using them to play tug of war with it.

- Distracting the dog's attention (e.g. by making some sound) and diverting it to an acceptable toy (i.e. by throwing it) is helpful, but only if the distraction occurs *before* the dog actually starts chewing on an unacceptable object. If it occurs after the dog has begun to bite the object, an owner invitation to play might reward and thereby strengthen the problem behavior.
- When caught it the act, the dog should be punished (e.g. scolded, startled) when it bites objects other than its toys. The effect of such punishment is strongest if the dog is punished just as it begins to take the object in its mouth. Punishment administered more than a few seconds after the dog has stopped chewing on something will have no effect on the problem behavior whatsoever.

- Unacceptable objects which are repeatedly chewed can be booby-trapped by, for example, hanging a few tin cans above and attached to the object in such a way that they will fall and startle the dog when it tugs on it (Hart and Hart, 1985), or by sprinkling something like pepper on it to make it taste bad. Both of these are examples of what Hart and Hart (1985) refer to as *remote punishment* (as opposed to *interactive punishment* such as scolding or handclapping which stems directly from the owner). The main advantages of remote punishment methods are that they are immediate – with a negligible delay between behavior and punishment – and impersonal in the sense that the dog does not associate the punishment with the owner. The disadvantage of interactive punishment is that the dog may simply learn not to chew on objects when the owner is present while continuing to chew on them when no one is at home.

Destructive behavior in an older dog

Most instances of destructive behavior in an older dog when it is left alone involve separation anxiety. Sometimes, however, the behavior occurs in a dog that is not distressed but simply lacks the exercise, play, or social stimulation that it requires. Unlike separation anxiety-related destructiveness which normally begins to occur within a few minutes of the owner's departure, this deprivation-related destructive behavior may occur much later – a few hours after the dog is left alone. Presumably, needed activity or play cannot occur because of confinement and/or lack of eliciting stimuli and this, in turn, may result in general restlessness, attempts to play with new objects in the home, displacement activities (e.g. out-of-context digging, hunting, prey attacking), or frustration-related redirected aggressive behavior in the form of destructiveness. In cases where separation anxiety can be ruled out by the timing of the damage and absence of other symptoms (i.e. vocalization when left alone, following owner constantly when at home), what exactly is eliciting the destructive behavior is often not clear. But in spite of this uncertainty, the recommendations for dealing with the problem are the same:

- Confinement in a room or place where damage cannot or normally does not occur.
- Punishment of destructive behavior or play directed towards inappropriate objects: either interactive punishment as when the owner scolds the dog the instant it takes some inappropriate object in its mouth or remote punishment by, for example, pretreating the object with some bad-tasting substance or booby-trapping it with something like turned-over mousetraps or tin cans which fall with a crash when the object is touched.
- Giving the dog the maximum amount of space in the home.
- Providing the dog with a variety of chew toys whenever it is to be left alone for long periods. Some of these should be available to dogs at other times, and the dog should be encouraged with chase-and-fetch and tug-of-war games to play with these until it is well-accustomed to them. The remaining toys should be normally put away and given only at the time of owner departure, for it is hard to predict whether continuous availability or partial availability will make particular toys more attractive and hence better elicitors of chewing than the owner's shoes, papers, and so on.
- Convincing the owner that the dog *must* be provided with more opportunities for exercise and social interaction during the day by, for example, arranging for someone to come to the home and take the dog out for a long walk at midday is critical in cases where the problem is a sign that the animal is genuinely suffering under this long period of social isolation and forced inactivity.

Excessive barking

Borchelt and Voith (1981) list the following possible etiologies for excessive barking, whining, or howling: *aggression, separation behavior, play, reaction to eliciting stimuli, social facilitation,* and *fear.* Absent from this list is the very common case discussed earlier in the chapter where barking is used by the dog as a means of *begging for* or *demanding* something it wants from its owner like food, play, or attention. Finally, Leuscher et al. (1991) add an eighth possible type of barking problem: *vocalization stereotypies* where dogs "compulsively" bark at their food, "aggressively growl" when biting their tail or foot, or give "a single bark constantly repeated at a fixed interval without any apparent eliciting stimuli" (p.403), which is especially common in dogs that spend a great deal of time outside alone.

This section will focus on only two of these vocalization problems, *reactions to eliciting stimuli* and *social facilitation,* which are not covered in previous discussions on aggression (Chapters 9-14), separation anxiety (Chapter 16), fear problems (Chapter 15), or begging/demanding behavior, stereotypies, and play (considered earlier in the chapter). Although both of these problems may involve situations in which a dog begins to bark after hearing another dog barking, social facilitation is not merely a special case of reactions to eliciting stimuli. When a dog barks at another dog which is barking, then a straightforward reaction to an eliciting stimulus (i.e. the other dog's barking) is involved. Social facilitation, on the other hand, occurs when a dog is stimulated by and joins in with another dog that is barking to bark at some other stimulus (e.g. noise, person, third dog, third dog's barking). Hence, social facilitation is essentially a kind of motivational or arousal effect exerted by stimuli from conspecifics that has the effect of increasing responsiveness to other stimuli. In biological function terms, social facilitation would act to coordinate the behavior and underlying moods/motivations of pack members to, for example, facilitate group defensive displays in which all in the group join forces to bark at an intruder.

Possible causal factors

Species-typical response to eliciting situations

Barking at sudden, unexpected noises or other stimuli which startle the dog or attract its attention is understandable in biological terms. At first, when the source and significance of the stimulus is still unidentified, it would function as a warning to other group members, attracting their attention and causing them to either peer in the direction in which the barking animal is facing or walk over to where it is standing. If and when the source is identified as some unfamiliar conspecific or other undesirable intruder, such barking might be the start of a group threat display as was considered in Chapters 12 and 14. In effect, it represents species-typical defensive behavior which functions basically to help a group protect itself against possible dangers of any sort.

Dogs may also bark at potential prey as can be seen, for example, when a dog stands at the base of a tree and barks up at a squirrel. Here too, the primary function of such behavior may be communicative: to elicit the attention and approach of other group members. This is not, however, as serious a problem for pet owners as defensive barking.

Social facilitation

Both warning or threat barking at some unusual, unexpected, or potentially threatening stimulus and barking at potential prey animals are infectious in the sense that one animal's barking is likely to lead to barking in other dogs that might not have barked if they had been alone. Problems involving this social facilitation effect are most common in the case of two or more dogs in the same home.

Usually high motivation/low treshold

From puppy age onwards, some dogs bark readily at anything and everything while others seldom bark. Therefore, dogs seem to differ greatly in both the likelihood that given stimuli will elicit barking and the intensity and duration of such behavior once it is elicited. While greatly influenced by the various factors discussed below, some of these differences between dogs may well be of genetic origin.

Being fundamentally understandable as a group defensive behavior, it is not surprising

POSSIBLE CAUSAL FACTORS

Species-typical response to eliciting situations
(e.g. natural reaction to unexpected/ unusual/potentially threatening stimuli)

Usually high barking motivation/ low barking threshold
(suspected genetic differences between dogs; possible underlying fear problem)

Unintentional owner reinforcement
(e.g. use of calming/distracting measures to stop barking)

Low owner dominance
(results in lack of owner capability to suppress problem behaviors)

Social facilitation
(e.g. the infectious nature of barking among two or more dogs in the same home)

Environmentally-induced frustration/ conflict/stress
(over-excitement/overreaction due to frustration, stress, or conflict induced by suboptimal environment)

Lack of obedience training
(e.g. to stop misbehavior on command)

Erroneous owner beliefs
(e.g. problem is price that must be paid for a good watchdog)

EXCESSIVE BARKING

- In response to unusual/unexpected/potentially threatening eliciting stimuli or due to social facilitation

POSSIBLE TREATMENT ELEMENTS

Alter care/maintenance conditions
(e.g. provide more opportunities for exercise/contact with other dogs)

Correct owner mistakes
(e.g. stop unintentional rewards)

Conventional obedience training
(to increase owner control/training capability)

Increase owner dominance
(to increase owner control in problem situations)

Correct erroneous owner beliefs
(e.g. convince owner that dog will still be a good watchdog after problem corrected/ brought more under control)

Cessation of ineffective treatment methods
(e.g. delayed punishment)

Training in problem situations
(conventional combination of rewards for acceptable behavior with punishment of problem behavior)

Physical aids
(shock/aversive sound collar in some cases)

that many dogs with low barking thresholds, and those which bark with great intensity and persistence once barking has been elicited, often tend to be somewhat fearful animals. The extent to which barking problems should be regarded and perhaps treated in part as fear problems (see Chapter 15) should be explored in detail during the consultation.

Symptomatic of environment-related frustration/conflict/stress

Some dogs take every noise and other unusual stimulus as an excuse to bark not so much because they are reacting fearfully or defensively, but rather because they simply become more easily aroused than other dogs. Excessive barking can therefore also be an over-excitement problem where the dog is predisposed by various factors to "overreact" to commonly encountered situations. Although this is considered in detail below as a problem in its own right, suffice to say here that such overreaction is often a sign that the dog is living in an environment which it finds "frustrating" (e.g. dog kept on chain physically prevented from running or approaching conspecifics), stressful, or which often arouses conflicting motivations (e.g. dog is both drawn to and afraid of something or someone in its environment). These kinds of factors often emerge during consultation if the counselor deliberately explores areas related to the possibility that the barking is essentially a kind of overreaction problem which might indicate that the dog is living in what for it is a deficient environment.

Unintentional owner reinforcement

The unintentional rewarding of problem vocalization is a major factor in cases where the owner tries to calm down a dog which has begun barking in response to some outside noise by petting it, talking reassuringly to it, or distracting it with playing or a tidbit. Although these measures may stop the barking in particular problem situations, they strengthen rather than weaken the dog's tendency to bark in

similar situations in the future for obvious reasons.

Lack of conventional obedience training

Owners who have trouble getting the dog to stop barking on command usually have problems controlling the dog in other situations as well: the dog often doesn't sit or lie down on command, come when it is called, or stop misbehaving when told to do so. In some cases, this is simply because owners have never bothered to carry out conventional obedience training which also involves an element of training the dog to stop doing whatever it is doing when ordered to do.

Low owner dominance

Disobedience and the owner's related inability to suppress problem behavior are often symptoms of low owner dominance. Therefore, questioning the owner closely about possible symptoms of dominance aggression and milder dominance problems is required in all of these types of cases.

Erroneous owner beliefs

Wrongly thinking that such behavior is inevitable in a good watchdog, owners may have been reluctant to do much against the barking problem for fear that the dog's watchdog function will be jeopardized.

Possible treatment elements

Alter care/maintenance conditions

In cases where the excessive barking occurs in a dog which is left alone outside tied on a chain or confined to a kennel all day long, it should be explained to the owner that the problem is a sign that dog is suffering under this situation. If the dog must to be kept in this way, at least it should be provided with some opportunities for vigorous exercise and contact with conspecifics during the day. Something similar should be recommended in the case of a highly active dog which is kept alone in the home all day without opportunities for exercise or social contact.

Correct erroneous owner beliefs

It is important to emphasize to some owners that it is possible to have a good watchdog without having to suffer under the dog's constant barking at harmless stimuli of all sorts; for many owners fear that correcting the barking problem will lower the dog's value as a protector of family and property. In addition to pointing out that reducing the dog's barking will not significantly lower its tendency to defend family and property against threatening intruders, one can suggest training the dog either to stop barking after the first few barks or to stop barking when commanded to do so. In any case, owners must be genuinely convinced that correcting the problem will not have this undesirable side effect. For otherwise they will have mixed feelings about the recommended treatment and apply it only half-heartedly, which will have little effect on the problem.

Correct owner mistakes

Stopping a dog from barking (e.g. at outside noises) by petting it, offering it a toy, eliciting playing, or offering it a tidbit reinforces the behavior and makes it more probable that the dog will bark in similar situations in the future. The problem is, however, that these problem-coping strategies often work in the situation itself in the sense that the dog does stop barking – which, in turn, rewards the owner's use of them and makes it more likely that the owner will use them again in similar situations in the future. In effect, the fact that these measures do often work in the short-term sense means that it may be difficult to convince owners who at least have this limited kind of control over their dog to abandon them entirely in favor of some other method which at first may not seem nearly as effective or easy to apply. And even owners who understand that it is a serious mistake to "bribe" the dog to stop barking with a tidbit may feel that they have no other choice in situations where the barking is disturbing the whole apartment building.

Cessation of ineffective treatment methods

The most common ineffective treatment method is delayed punishment at times where the dog and owner are some distance apart and therefore the barking cannot be punished immediately. It must be explained to owners that to be effective, punishment must be administered during the problem behavior – at best, just at the moment the punished behavior begins.

Conventional obedience training

One place to start the effort of improving the dog's obedience in the barking situation is by carrying out conventional obedience training using the methods recommended in Chapter 8. This is a valuable lesson for both dog and owner, and it helps lay the groundwork for training in problem situations themselves.

Training in problem situations

As is the case with many problems discussed in previous chapters, the most effective way to train a dog not to engage in some problem behavior in specific situations is to combine immediate punishment of the behavior with positive reinforcement for some specified alternative behavior. The punishment can be simple scolding if this is intense enough to immediately and reliably suppress the punished behavior or, if the dog is not sufficiently impressed with this, something else like operating a noise-making device which startles the dog or which it finds especially aversive (e.g. some kind of compressed air device, the rattling sound made by shaking a tin can containing a few small objects).

The rewarded alternative behavior can be anything which includes the element of the dog's not barking. The dog can be called, for example, and commanded to sit or lie down, and then rewarded with a food tidbit for quietly doing so and perhaps again for remaining that way when told to stay. At first, this procedure can be carried out as soon as the barking is suppressed by the scolding or aversive sound. But later, it may be possible and desirable to elicit the rewarded alternative behavior just before the animal starts barking – at the moment that both dog and owner perceive a stimulus which usually elicits barking. This version of the early intervention method is sometimes very effective not only in helping to control or reduce a problem behavior, but to actually change the overall way the animal perceives and reacts to the situation: after some time, the stimulus which formerly elicited barking may instead come to elicit approaching the owner, sitting without being told to do so, and just generally becoming more interested in the owner and what he/she has to offer than in the stimulus itself.

Hart and Hart (1985) recommend another kind of counterconditioning method to train a dog which barks frequently when left outside when no one is at home to remain silent (assuming that separation anxiety is not involved). One first determines how long the dog will go without barking after the owner leaves. If this is 10 min., for example, the owner is instructed to repeatedly leave during daily training sessions for only 5 or 10 min., either have someone else spy on the dog or use a tape recorder to determine whether the dog barked during his/her absence, and then return and "reward nonbarking behavior" with affection and tidbits if it hasn't barked. This is then repeated many times with the length of the owner's absences being progressively increased over the course of time if the dog remains quiet.

Although this kind of procedure might be effective in some cases, a feature of the Hart and Hart discussion that directly contradicts one of the major animal learning principles which have been stressed throughout the present book is deserving of critical comment. Namely, that "nonbarking behavior" is what is being rewarded. Consider what would happen, for example, if the dog sometimes barked 3 or 4 minutes before the owner came back and sometimes didn't – and accordingly was rewarded or not rewarded later. Is this really the kind of procedure in which the dog will learn to associate nonbarking with reward and barking with not being rewarded? To learn this discrimination, the dog would obviously somehow have to associate its barking with the fail-

ure of a reward to occur 3 or 4 minutes later. But animal learning research indicates that animals have difficulty learning such things even with delays of several seconds. What exactly then is rewarded when the owner comes home? Basically whatever the dog was doing at the time the owner returned – like sitting and quietly waiting by the gate. If this method does work, it is not because the non-behavior of "nonbarking" is being rewarded, but rather because some specific type of acceptable behavior such as silently waiting by the gate is being consistently reinforced.

Increase owner dominance

If disobedience in barking situations appears to be a reflection of a mild owner-dog dominance problem, some of the recommendations for increasing owner dominance discussed in Chapter 10 are also indicated.

Physical aids

The use of collars which deliver an aversive shock or sound are sometimes successfully used to control barking at extraneous stimuli when the dog is alone. These can be bark-activated – and hence function when the owner is away from home – or activated by a remote-control device which the owner can operate from inside the house to punish the dog's barking outside. In discussing shock collars, Hart and Hart (1985) point out several possible problems with them. The collar may be inadvertently activated by the barking of another dog, it may be too loose to provide a shock, it may burn the dog's skin at the point of contact, and there may be a problem ensuring that the dog is being shocked with the lowest intensity which is effective in suppressing the barking (i.e. given that the electrical resistance between the electrodes and dog's skin changes depends on whether the dog is wet or dry). Voith (1989) mentions another problem. Namely, the danger of a vicious circle, shock-bark-shock-bark chain of events which might occur with bark-activated collars without some kind of post-shock delay feature if the animal has a tendency to bark in response to being shocked.

SAMPLE RECOMMENDATIONS

Excessive barking (unrelated to aggression problems)

Scenario A: *dog barks at noised in the hall outside of an apartment and ignores owner's command to stop or come away from the door.*

- Barking should be scolded severely enough to stop it immediately every time. It is also possible to allow the dog to bark two or three times, then scold it if it doesn't immediately stop barking when told firmly to do so.

- If the dog simply ignores your scolding, either you must put more authority behind it or you must find some other way to effectively suppress the behavior (e.g. some sudden loud noise which the dog finds particularly aversive).

- Quiet behavior in potential problem situations where, for example, it hears some sound outside but doesn't bark, or stops barking when firmly told to do so, should always be rewarded with petting, praise, and above all with food tidbits. Don't give the dog tidbits at any other time.

- If consistently applied over several weeks, distracting the dog before it starts barking by making some sound and then rewarding it for doing something else besides barking (e.g. coming when called, sitting on command, etc.) as soon as it hears a noise can also be effective.

- Avoid unintentionally rewarding the barking as when, for example, you try to quiet the dog down when it is barking by petting it, talking to it, or distracting it with something it likes (toys, playing, food). Although doing such things may temporarily quiet the dog down, in the long run they reward barking and therefore train it to bark even more.

Scenario B: *dog left alone outside on a chain or in a kennel barks long and loud at anything and everything.*

- The excessive barking is a sign that the dog finds it stressful and frustrating to be kept so long outside alone with its exercise possibilities so severely restricted. It is necessary, therefore, to drastically reduce the amount of time the dog is kept outside alone and/or find a way to take the dog somewhere where it can run and play with other dogs 2-3 times during the day. (This alone will not solve the problem, but it is a necessary first step to create conditions in which some corrective procedure can be effectively applied.)

(If inability of owner to directly suppress barking is symptomatic of insufficient owner dominance, recommendations from Chapter 10 for increasing owner dominance may be appropriate.)

On balance, it would seem that collars which deliver some kind of aversive sound would be preferable from the point of view of the animal's safety. *In the opinion of all well-known pet behavior problem specialists, shock collars should only be used by experienced behavior counselors – or by clients only under direct supervision of counselors – who are well aware of the potential problems with them and know how they can be avoided.*

Overactivity and excitability

Some dogs are extremely restless and active most of their waking hours. While it is normal for dogs to become excited when visitors first come or when the owner starts making signs that its time to go for a walk, the level of excitement of some dogs rises and remains far above what is normal in these and other situations (e.g. riding in cars). Many factors can play a role in producing problems where dogs become overactive or overexcited compared to most other dogs. As a first step in the treatment of such problems, it is helpful to consider which of the following kinds of factors are or may be involved.

Possible causal factors

Physiological disorder

Overactivity or excitability can be a sign of organic disease like, for example, hyper- or hypothyroidism (Parker, 1989) or hyperkinesis (Hart and Hart, 1989). Disease should be suspected particularly when a lengthy behavioral consultation reveals that there is something unusual about the case and it doesn't seem to fit any of the patterns produced by the common causal factors discussed below.

Age of dog

Some puppies and juveniles are extremely playful and active, and the behavior may seem abnormal particularly to owners who are not accustomed to young dogs and who have difficulty in controlling the animal. In most cases, however, it is a question of the normal play behavior of particularly playful and active individuals.

Normal high activity level

Some adult dogs remain puppy-like in their playfulness and love of physical activity. Walks during which they can romp and play with other dogs are the high points of their day, and at home they may constantly pester owners for play by bringing a ball over and over again and not leaving them a moment's peace until they throw it. Basically, extreme playfulness and a high activity level can be normal "personality" characteristics in some dogs which most owners value positively in spite of the problems caused by the dogs' pestering for play and need to be taken on frequent long walks.

Inadequate care/maintenance conditions

Dogs like those described in the last paragraph essentially need to be far more active than other dogs. If they are not taken out frequently enough, kept always on a leash, have little opportunity to play with other dogs, or spend most of their day imprisoned in a kennel or home, they may become abnormally restless, pester for play or attention, or be overly excitable (e.g. when the time for a walk is approaching, anything out of the ordinary happens, or the dog being taken for one of its occasional rides in the car). Basically, the counselor should always consider the possibility that the dog is a problem in one or more of these ways because it is essentially being continuously deprived of much-needed opportunities for exercise and play.

Conflict, stress, or frustration effects

Dogs can behave in an overactive or overexcitable way when exposed to something aversive or frightening (e.g. low-flying aircraft), placed constantly in a situation in which conflicting motivations are aroused (e.g. motivation to both approach and avoid contact with a feared family member), or physically thwarted from performing some activity which they are highly motivated to perform (e.g. going outside to investigate noises or interact with a dog they see through a window). These other possible environmental effects must also be explored during the consultation.

Owner reinforcement

Questioning owners as to specifically how they react when the dog becomes overactive or overexcited often reveals a pattern of unintentional owner reinforcement. As is the case with so many other dog behavioral problems, coping strategies like petting the dog or distracting it with something it likes may help to control the dog's activity or overexcited behavior at the time, but they also reinforce the problem behavior and are therefore strictly contraindicated.

Possible treatment elements

Veterinary examination

Hart and Hart (1985) suggest that the first step in overactivity/overexcitement cases is to rule out pathophysiological causes. This is particularly important in cases where the problem is especially severe or unusual.

Animal's activity/play needs must be met

Some clients have had less active dogs in the past and unthinkingly assume that the former walk routine should be just as appropriate for their present, much more active dog. In such cases, it is usually sufficient for the counselor to point out that dogs which are more active by nature require much more activity than other dogs. With owners who are simply lazy and resent having to devote so much time to meeting their dog's needs, there is little one can do except warn them that unless they start making a more consistent effort to give the dog what it needs, they will continue having problems with it. Finally, although one can understand that some clients' work schedules may not allow them to take the dog out for long walks during the day, it must be emphasized to them that either they must find some other way to provide the dog more opportunities for play and exercise (e.g. by asking or paying someone else to take the dog out when they are working) or they should consider finding the dog a new home with someone who has more time for it.

Eliminate sources of conflict/stress/frustration

Where such causal factors are identified, it might be possible to do something about them. Fear problems can be treated, family members can be instructed to change their behavior towards the dog in various ways, and dogs can be denied access to parts of the house where they are most exposed to aversive or stimulating outdoor sights and sounds.

Eliminate sources of owner reinforcement

Once it has begun to occur, overactive or excited behavior should be either ignored entirely or mildly scolded to the extent required to stop it. Most owners are insecure what to do here – scold the dog, pet it, ignore it, or give it a toy or tidbit? As is the case with all behavior problems, it is extremely important to advise owners exactly what they should do when the dog starts performing the undesirable behavior. Of course, it might also be necessary to explain to them exactly why the way they have been trying to deal with the problem by distracting the dog with something it likes is counterproductive and tends, in the long run, to make the problem worse.

Basic obedience training

Simple obedience training using food rewards coupled with making a consistent effort to be stricter with the dog in all situations can benefit many owners. Some owners have invested little time in training their dog and are permissive in situations where the dog wants to do something other than what they would like it to do. And for them, the combination of obedience training and being firmer with the dog under all circumstances can prove to be extremely helpful when the time comes to control the dog in situations where it becomes excited and starts jumping up on guests, barking in front of the door, or making problems in the car.

Countercondition acceptable behavior in problem situations

Various types of counterconditioning procedures may be appropriate depending on the specific type of problem. Inappropriate play involving aggressive attacks on owner, destructive behavior, and/or bothersome barking can be redirected towards appropriate objects or reduced by fostering another type of game entirely (i.e. by refusing to play inappropriate games with the dog while eliciting and joining in appropriate ones). Similarly, dogs which jump up onto guests can be gradually counterconditioned using food rewards to sit on command and stay sitting when a guest enters the home. Counterconditioning may also take the form of a behavior therapy method like the one, for example, recommended by O'Farrell (1992):

"The dog is pre-trained to sit on command in the stationary car, if this does not excite it. During a training session it is told to sit in the car and the owner proceeds gradually through a hierarchy of stimuli, the dog being rewarded as long as it remains calm. A typical hierarchy might consist of putting the key in the ignition without turning it, turning on the engine and immediately turning it off again, leaving the engine running for longer periods, eventually driving the car very short distances ... During the period of treatment, the dog should not be taken on real car trips" (p.100).

On practical grounds, such complex procedures should probably be viewed more as an undesirable last resort rather than the method of choice. Many owners are unwilling to persistently devote the time and effort required to carry out such a procedure properly, and there are many kinds of mistakes even the most sincere and highly motivated owners can make here. Similarly, the second of O'Farrell's proposals for dealing with overexcitement in the car by stopping the car every time the dog becomes excited and restarting it when the dog becomes calm is also the kind of procedure which few owners would be willing or able to consistently carry out in real traffic situations. Finally, O'Farrell lists the alternative possibilities of caging the dog, harnessing it so it can't see out of the window, or letting it ride harnessed in front with the owner if being separated from the owner is what seems to excite it. Such simple solutions can sometimes be the most realistic, effective, and above all safest for a potentially dangerous problem like this one.

Sexual behavior problems

This section and the following one dealing with maternal behavioral problems relies heavily on Hart and Hart's (1985) brief but excellent treatment of these topics.

Lack of sexual interest in breeding animals

Hart and Hart (1985) identify the following potential causal factors:

- Male may not be familiar enough with – or comfortable enough in – the breeding environment.
- Male's incorrect orientation during attempted mounting may be a result of insufficient contact and sexual play with other puppies early in life.
- Females show marked preferences for some males over others even when in full estrus, and their lack of sexual interest in a particular male may be understandable in these terms.
- Females which are not receptive may also be showing "silent estrus", a condition where the female "shows the physiological but not the behavioral signs of estrus".
- Males may also be somewhat selective with regard to mating and will mate with some females more readily than others.

Objectionable sexual mounting behavior

Most often this is directed towards human legs or arms, but it may also be directed towards inanimate objects like towels or pillows. Figure 18.1 presents some relevant statistics collected with the owners of both problem and non-problem dogs using the client information form presented in Chapter 6.

Unexpectedly, the difference between the 32 males and 23 females in the normal, non-problem animal sample was small in light of the widespread belief that this problem is much more common in males. Although there was no difference between problem and non-problem females, the relative frequency of mounting among problem males was more than twice as high as among males without serious behavioral problems. Suspecting that this difference might have something directly to do with dominance (i.e. because mounting is often used by dogs to assert their dominance over other dogs and dominance problems are far more frequent in males), the data for the 48 problem males were broken down into those which showed mild to severe dominance problems versus other problem males which showed no problem dominant behavior. Here, 50% percent of the males (n = 30) with either mild or serious

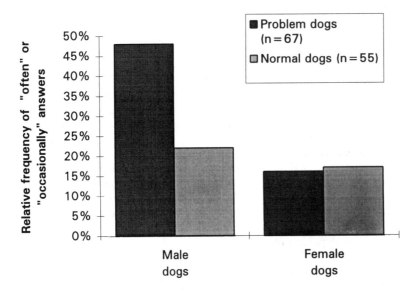

Figure 18.1: Percentage of owners of problem dogs vs. normal dogs answering "occasionally" or "often" to the question "Does your dog show sexual behavior towards human beings?"

dominance-related problems showed at least occasional mounting while this figure was 44% for the males (n = 18) which showed no signs of any dominance-related problem. This appears to indicate that dominance may play a much smaller role with regard to sexual mounting of human beings than is normally assumed.

One possible explanation for the difference between mounting in normal and problem males is that the owners of problem males have more difficulty in controlling the problem behavior than other owners do. Almost all owners find the mounting problem distasteful and discourage it by scolding the dog and pushing it away from the start. The data in Figure 18.1 may therefore represent the percentages of males and females which show the problem either occasionally or often in spite of owner attempts to break them of this habit. Accordingly, the difference between problem and normal males may primarily reflect the lower capability of the owners of problem males to control behavior problems of any sort – either minor ones like this one or the major ones for which the dogs were presented. That a similar effect is not seen in females may indicate that here the

mounting behavior is not as highly motivated and/or resistant to control as in males.

Mounting in puppies

This behavior is common in puppies and often directed towards children. Hart and Hart (1985) suggest that "puppy-play sexual behavior" is involved here, which most puppies outgrow. It can be effectively treated by mildly punishing mounting (e.g. by scolding the dog and pushing it away) every time it occurs.

Mounting in older dogs

Hart and Hart (1985) and/or O'Farrell (1992) identify the following possible causal factors:
• Mounting of human beings may be a sign that the dog was taken away from its litter too early and therefore had too little exposure to other dogs early in life. The redirection of sexual behavior towards the species with which an animal had contact during a brief critical period early in life is a feature commonly associated with imprinting in a variety of animal species where there ap-

Table 18.2: Relative frequency with which males showing sexual behavior towards human beings vs. those never exhibiting such behavior are reported to at least sometimes play with other dogs.

	Normal males	Problem males
Often or occasionally mount human beings	86%	84%
Never mount human beings	73%	62%

pears to be a resulting "misidentification of the species to which it belongs" (Grier and Burk, 1992). If dogs seem completely disinterested in all other dogs, react with hostility when approached by them, or act somewhat awkward and ambivalent with them, these too can be symptoms of this kind of early experience deficit.

As appealing as this hypothesis sounds, however, data collected by asking (with the client information form presented in Chapter 6) the owners of 40 problem males and 29 normal males whether their dogs sometimes (1) played with other dogs and (2) directed sexual behavior towards human beings does not support the simple version of it which assumes that dogs which persist in mounting human beings have imprinted on humans instead of dogs. If this were true, one would expect that dogs which mount humans would tend to be those which never play with other dogs – one of the major symptoms of disturbed interdog social behavior. However, Table 18.2 shows that if anything the opposite is the case: males which often or occasionally show sexual behavior towards humans are more commonly reported to play with other dogs than those which never show such behavior towards their owners.

- Mounting may result in reinforcing attention-getting consequences for the dog. Some owners' attempted scolding of the behavior functions more as a reward than a punishment (e.g. the classic case where a doting owner looks lovingly down at her dog and sweetly says "You bad boy. Mama has told you that's a no-no"). A few owners even find mounting amusing and encourage it, laughing at the dog, tolerating the behavior for some time, and perhaps deliberately trying to elicit it to amuse their friends.

- O'Farrell (1992) speculates that mounting is often "less an expression of bizarre sexual preference than a displacement activity in response to conflict or excitement". She adds that the behavior is often elicited by visitors because of "the conflicts between friendliness and aggression which they may arouse", and children because they are "apt to behave in a more excitable way with dogs, giving them contradictory signals which they find hard to interpret" (p.112). This hypothesis seems plausible and certainly worth considering when increased excitement or probable conflict seem to be a common feature of specific situations in which sexual mounting occurs.

Consistent punishment by pushing the dog away and scolding it severely enough to inhibit it from resuming the behavior is usually effective in reducing or eliminating this problem. Although Hart and Hart (1985) also recommend following this kind of immediate interactive punishment with "social isolation, or at least indifference to the dog for an hour or so", according to experimentally well-established animal learning principles, there is no reason to believe that this type of long-lasting "punishment" would have any direct effect the dog's mounting behavior at all. One punishes a behavior and not the animal, and punishment is effective only if it immediately follows the punished behavior. Therefore it is the act of turning one's attention away from the dog which is punishing, not the hour of ignoring which follows.

Castration or treating the problem with progestins is also reportedly effective in many cases (O'Farrell, 1992; Hart and Hart, 1985). However, seeing that the problem is usually minor and easily eliminated or at least suppressed by punishing it whenever it occurs, there is little justification for castrating animals or prescribing drug therapy merely to correct this problem.

Roaming

Intact males sometimes catch the scent of a bitch in estrus and run away for hours or perhaps days at a time. Castration appears to be an effective treatment in perhaps as many as 90% of cases (Hopkins et al., 1976). Naturally, a castration won't help solve the problem if the dog roams for other reasons like, for example, simple exploration, contact and play with other dogs, or food sources. Most owners have had enough experience with their dogs to feel confident that they understand why their dogs are roaming. Either they have seen how powerful the effects of a female in heat on it are or they have located the dog after it has run away on some occasions and therefore know where it is going and why.

Maternal behavior problems

Nervousness and cannibalism

Mothers may become excessively nervous and attack and perhaps eat their own puppies. In discussing this problem, Hart and Hart (1985) point out that cannibalism of young is seen in many mammalian species, both domestic and wild. In nature, its primary functions are thought to be either to "adjust litter sizes in accordance with environmental conditions and food supply prevailing at the time of parturition" or to remove sickly puppies from the litter before other puppies are infected.

With the exception of the eating of a sickly pup, there seems to be little biological justification, however, for a domestic dog which is well cared for to attack its puppies. Speculating on the causes of this maladaptive behavior, Hart and Hart list without comment common views that this form of cannibalism may be related to immaturity of the mother, lack of maternal experience, hyperemotionality, and environmental disturbances. The authors then hypothesize that (1) some environmental disturbance may be able to trigger cannibalism because the mechanisms which underlie it must necessarily be programmed to respond to the first, subtle abnormality signs (e.g. puppy cold

or inactive) that the puppy is diseased – that is, before it gets so ill that it is likely that other puppies would already be infected – and (2) that at parturition with the expulsion of the placenta, the fall in progesterone levels may "precipitate irritability and aggression towards the young".

A primary theme of Hart and Hart's chapter is that human assistance throughout the domestication process may have allowed maladaptive genes for maternal behavioral problems that are always kept at low levels in wild populations to accumulate. And this in turn implies maternal behavioral disorders such as cannibalism and neglect of healthy pups under favorable environmental conditions may be associated with genetic rather than environmental factors.

Maternal indifference

Hart and Hart (1985) speculate therefore that such domestication-related maladaptive genes or gene combinations may also be the reason why some mothers neglect their pups. However, two other factors may be some kind of hormonal defect in the underlying mechanisms responsible for maternal behavior or, in cases where there is only a single puppy, a lack of the minimum amount of visual, olfactory, auditory stimuli from puppies which are required to maintain maternal behavior – an effect which has been experimentally demonstrated in rats.

Essentially, little is known about the problem beyond the fact that it seems to involve genetically preprogrammed behavior which is not functioning properly for unknown reasons. As is the case with cannibalism, aside from eliminating any possible environmental disturbances, the only thing owners can do is closely supervise maternal behavior and intervene if it becomes inadequate or maladaptive.

Pseudopregnancy

Pseudopregnancy is a well-known and common occurrence where a non-pregnant bitch exhibits maternal behavior like nesting, guarding of enclosed areas, and mothering objects along with related physiological changes like, distended abdomen, engorged uterus, development of the mammary glands, and possible lactation (Voith, 1980). In an excellent detailed article on the topic, Voith (1980) hypothesizes that this is fundamentally a normal canine phenomenon that functions in the wild to turn puppies' aunts into nursemaids which can make a contribution to the puppies' survival – an adaptive mechanism in the wild because of the close genetic relationship between the young and barren female pack members. The author also presents calculated genetic representation figures which demonstrate the considerable potential advantage such a mechanism might have in a wolf-style pack.

While maladaptive from the genetic viewpoint in today's domestic dogs in the sense that it may cause owners to have females spayed, the pseudopregnancy phenomenon is best regarded as an essentially functionless remnant of a mechanism which would be clearly adaptive in the natural, wild-living environment. In effect, the story would be much the same as for preprogrammed hunting behavioral sequences in domestic dogs. This behavior too has been rendered functionless because the dogs' present "unnatural" environment lacks many of the features and requirements characteristic of the environment in which the species' genetically-preprogrammed behavioral repertoire evolved.

Of course, spaying eliminates future pseudo-pregnancy, and both Voith (1980) and Hart and Hart (1985) advise that treatment with *megestrol acetate* dosed at 2 mg/kg po sid will often suppress the symptoms. (See the "drug therapy" subsection in Chapter 8 for side effects and other important drug-related information.)

Ingestion behavior problems

Pica

Some dogs often consume inappropriate materials like stones or other objects which can cause obstructions that require surgical removal (Houpt, 1991). While admitting that the reason for this behavior is unclear, Hart and Hart (1985) hypothesize that it may be an at-tention-getting behavior which has gradually developed as a result of the owner's unintentional reinforcement when the dog picks up, holds, and then perhaps swallows objects (e.g. attention related to concern for the dog's health or chasing the dog, which the dog might enjoy). O'Farrell (1992) speculates that a kind of confusion of different functions of the mouth may be involved: "Sometimes the functions become confused so that the dog ends up by partially ingesting something which it had originally intended only to investigate or remove" (p.108). Why this kind of "confusion" might occur – if it indeed occurs – is uncertain.

In any case, these authors recommend first treating the problem as if it were an attention-getting behavior using either the *extinction procedure,* where all mouthing of objects is scrupulously ignored by the owner, or *remote punishment* where preferred objects are baited with something aversive like hot pepper powder.

If the dog swallows objects when the owner is approaching or in the act of trying to take the object out of its mouth, this practice should be stopped. If objects are dangerous or valuable to the owner, or if swallowing occurs even if the owner ignores the behavior, the dog can be trained to drop objects on command in special practice sessions using food rewards for voluntarily dropping a series of objects which increasingly resemble the objects the dog prefers. The object is given to the dog to hold in its mouth and then the dog is immediately rewarded with a tidbit for dropping it when told to do so. Later, a similar procedure is followed whenever the dog is carrying something in its mouth: the owner shows it the reward and then gives it to it as soon as the object is dropped. O'Farrell (1992) also suggests that owners may intervene just as the dog is seen approaching the object by doing something like clapping their hands to get the dog's attention away from the object, and then calling it and rewarding it for coming by, for example, throwing a ball.

Houpt (1991) suggests that the provision of continuously available food, "attractive but safe toys", and the use of a muzzle are sometimes helpful or required.

If the dog eats grass, Hart and Hart (1985) suggest that this may be an adaptive response to gastrointestinal problems if it provokes vomiting or exerts a laxative effect and, therefore, acts as a "physical purge for intestinal parasites".

Coprophagy

Coprophagy or the eating of feces is very common among domestic dogs. Figure 18.2 shows the relative frequency with which dogs in samples of non-problem (n = 55) and problem animals (n = 67) showed this behavior. Why females appear to show this behavior with greater frequency than males is unknown. As was hypothesized in the section on sexual behavior towards human beings, the fact that problem dogs show this behavior much more frequently may be the result of owners in this population not being able to as effectively control minor types of undesirable behavior as the owners of non-problem animals.

In general, coprophagy has not been experimentally studied and is not well-understood. Hart and Hart (1985) offer the following possible explanations:
- It may be essentially a displacement activity in response to "boredom" – that is, an out-of-context performance of the consumption of fecal droppings of young puppies which mothers are genetically preprogrammed to perform. The observations that the behavior is especially common among females and dogs which are confined alone for long periods would be consistent with this hypothesis.
- It may be an attention-getting behavior which is rewarded by owners as is suspected in the case of pica above. Finding the be-

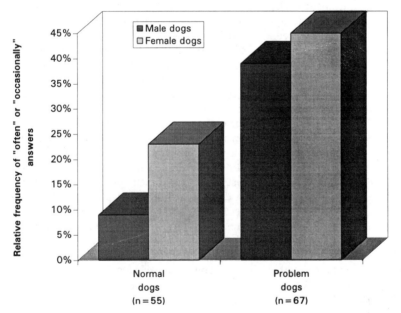

Figure 18.2: Percentage of owners of problem dogs vs. normal dogs answering "occasionally" or "often" to the question "Does your dog eat excrement?"

havior repulsive, some owners react very strongly and immediately to it by calling the dog and distracting it with something like playing or tidbits.

- It may be a response to some sort of unknown nutritional deficiency.
- In very young animals, it may function to establish "an appropriate intestinal flora", or population of desirable, food-digesting microorganisms.

O'Farrell (1992) adds another possibility:

- Like carrion-eating, feces-eating may be an expression of dogs "instinctive preference for food which is decaying".

And finally, Houpt (1991) suggests:

- The ingestion of ungulate feces, especially horse feces which are "enriched by the products of large intestinal fermentation and probably may help to sustain a dog when there is no meat available" (p. 288), is a natural behavior which may be "displaced" to the feces of other animals when no ungulate feces are available.

The other ideas suggested by Houpt (1991) in her list of possible causes that dogs might eat their own feces as an imitation of the "owner's behavior in removing feces" or as a response to "punishment for housesoiling by removing the evidence, especially if the punishment was to rub the dog's nose in the feces" appear to have little to recommend them. Dogs are not imitative in this direct behavior-copying sense and no animal behavioral scientist would agree that dogs are able to behave in this kind of human-like, calculating way.

Treating coprophagy in a dog which eats its own feces when confined alone for long periods of time involves some method of baiting feces with a foul-tasting substance like hot pepper powder which, if consistently applied, can produce a conditioned aversion to feces (Hart and Hart, 1985). Houpt (1991) recommends injecting a hot pepper sauce into the feces so that dogs would not recognize it as quickly as if pepper was simply sprinkled on top.

O'Farrell (1992) suggests that dietary changes can sometimes help to make the dog's own feces less palatable to it. She suggests (1) feeding a high-fiber, high-protein, low-carbohydrate diet, (2) including an iron supplement, (3) adding vegetable oil increased during a period of one week to 15 ml/4.5 kg body weight (a dosage suggestion from McKeown et al., 1988), and/or (4) feeding the dog lesser amounts more often which, like increasing dietary fiber content, may promote a "feeling of fullness" and thereby reduce the dog's appetite. Along these same lines, Houpt (1991) recommends that adding pancreatic enzymes or meat tenderizer to the dog's meal will make the feces taste repugnant. She also raises the possibility of producing taste aversion learning by injecting *apomorphine* into the dog's feces which will cause nausea and vomiting shortly after ingestion. As this kind of learning is often only possible with novel foods, Houpt suggests it might only work if the habit of eating feces has begun relatively recently and the dog has not, therefore, previously learned that feces are a "safe" food. Finally, she cites one case where feeding the dog a diet which produced soft feces solved the problem.

No matter which of these methods are employed, it should always be kept in mind in all of these cases, however, that if the behavior is indeed a displacement activity which indicates that the dog is in some sense suffering under its confinement conditions, changing these conditions themselves is indicated both on ethical and practical grounds. If the dog must be left alone, owners can at least arrange for someone to visit, spend time with, and take the dog out for long walks at intervals during the day.

If the dog eats feces during walks, one can try (1) consistently ignoring the behavior, which might eventually solve the problem entirely if unintentional reinforcement from owners is the primary causal factor, (2) severely scolding the dog every time it shows excessive interest in feces – which is the approach most owners use, often with success – or (3) experimenting with changing or enriching the dog's diet tentatively assuming that some kind of real nutritional deficit is at the heart of the problem.

Anorexia

In the case of anorexia, or lack or loss of appetite, Hart and Hart (1985) cite the following possible causal factors:

- Medical or physiological cause like, for example, a gastrointestinal disorder or food allergy. These authors point out that anorexia is an adaptive response to illnesses, with the loss of appetite in a wild-living animal resulting in its staying "holed up in its den conserving heat to help maintain an elevated body temperature (fever) to combat bacteria and viruses".
- Conditioned aversion to food as result of gastrointestinal sickness resulting from some allergen in food.
- Attention-getting behavior in a dog which has learned that acting anorexic results in increased owner attention. Such an effect may be fairly obvious in cases, for example, where previous to the present anorexic tendencies or interludes, dogs have been becoming steadily more and more fussy about their food, and how they are fed, over the course of months. For example, the dog may refuse to eat anything but specially-cooked and seasoned meat and even then only eat it when the owner is sitting on a stool next to the dog and keeping it company.
- Emotional reasons like, for example, the case cited by Hart and Hart where a dog started acting "depressed" and stopped eating after a young boy who used to play with it lost interest in it and started playing with other children instead. More common are probably situations like those described by O'Farrell (1992) where there is a major change of environment or loss of a person or animal to which the dog is attached – for example, when the dog is boarded in a kennel, moves to a new home, or when someone in the home dies or moves away.

O'Farrell (1992) offers the additional suggestion that by essentially trying to force the dog to eat, worried owners may make the feeding situation aversive for the dog, thereby exacerbating the problem.

Various types of treatments may be appropriate depending on what types of causal factors are involved. When infective illness is responsible, Hart and Hart (1985) suggest that the owners do nothing about the anorexia "during the height of the illness and then help the animal regain normal appetite during the convalescent stage". And when respiratory disease has caused loss of smell which, in turn, produces loss of appetite, placing food in the mouth to activate taste receptors may help stimulate eating.

If an emotional problem is involved, Hart and Hart recommend that the counselor identify and make recommendations to resolve the emotional problem (e.g. advise owner to find another child to play with the dog in the above case example) and/or administer an appetite-stimulating drug (e.g. *medroxyprogesterone*). Houpt (1991) suggests *diazepam*. (See the "drug therapy" subsection in Chapter 8 for side effects and other important drug-related information.)

If owners are trying too hard to get the dog to eat and thereby making the feeding situation aversive for it, O'Farrell (1992) suggests they should offer appetizing food twice daily for 5-10 min., leave the dog entirely alone during this time, and remove the food when the time is over even if the dog hasn't eaten. In extreme cases where owners find this kind of treatment difficult to carry out, a few days in another home with less emotionally-involved persons may help.

A similar sort of approach may be appropriate if the anorexia is basically attention-getting behavior. Although the extinction approach of withdrawing all possible sources of owner reinforcement for the problem will work in the long run, the fact that the problem may temporarily worsen when the attention is first withdrawn implies that owners need to be thoroughly prepared for what to expect when they begin applying this method. Additionally, given that concerns related to possible adverse affects of anorexia on the dog's health are also involved here, ensuring owner compliance can be more difficult than with other attention-getting problems. Dealing with owner anxieties, supporting owners by frequent contact during the early stages of the corrective procedure, and creating favorable conditions for the resumption of eating in the absence of owner attention by maximizing palatability and administering an appetite-increasing drug may all be helpful or necessary here.

Obesity

Houpt (1991) states that this is the most common ingestion behavior problem which involves 20 to 30% of dogs and twice as many spayed as unspayed bitches (because of the decrease in activity and/or increase in intake due to the removal of source of estrogen via ovariohysterectomy). Hart and Hart (1985) suggest that medical disorders like hypopituitarism, tumors of insulin-producing cells, excessive production of adrenal corticosteroids, and cranial tumors which produce pressure on the ventromedial hypothalamus may also lead to obesity.

Both Houpt (1991) and Hart and Hart (1985) cite high palatability of food as a common contributory factor in many cases. Houpt (1991) suggests that obesity is easily controlled by food restriction and the use of commercially-available low-calorie dog foods. She points out, however, that dogs may respond to "calorie dilution" and act hungrier and beg more vigorously for food, which from the owner's viewpoint can be an undesirable side effect. Nevertheless, she remarks that "most owners find it easier to control their pets' weight than to control their own".

However, this type of straightforward approach to the problem often fails. O'Farrell (1991) presents an excellent account of how owners' erroneous views about their dog's need for food and feeding behavior, the pleasure and satisfaction they derive from feeding it, and the emotional difficulty they experience when depriving it of food which it appears to crave make it exceedingly difficult for them to consistently comply with the recommended food restriction/low-calorie food approach. Accordingly, O'Farrell argues that it is important for the counselor to recognize, understand, and discuss these various aspects with owners if compliance is to be achieved. For example, one can explain to owners that a dog's begging for food does not necessarily mean that it is experiencing an uncomfortable hungry feeling the way human beings do. One can also point out that it is natural to enjoying feeding one's pet well and that it is difficult to resist the dog's begging for food even though one knows that this is what should or must be done. In a practical vein, O'Farrell also makes the following suggestions: owners may feed tidbits as before provided the total caloric intake is correct, commercial low-calorie dog foods facilitate precise control, frequent weighing provides helpful feedback which reinforces owner weight-controlling behavior, and giving the dog frequent exercise helps both to control weight and demonstrate to the owner the beneficial effects (i.e. increased fitness) of weight-reduction for the dog.

References

Askew, H.R. (1991): Eine Einführung in Clinical Animal Behavior. Der praktische Tierarzt **72**, 279–284.

Borchelt, P.L., and Voith V.L. (1982): Classification of animal behavior problems. Veterinary Clinics of North America: Small Animal Practice **12**, 571–585.

Burghardt, W.F. (1991): Using drugs to control behavior problems in pets. Veterinary Medicine **November**, 1066–1075

Grier, J.W., and Burk, T. (1992): Biology of Animal Behaviour. 2nd edition. St. Louis, Missouri, Mosby – Year Book, Inc.

Fraser, A.F., and Broom, D.M. (1990): Farm Animal Behaviour and Welfare. 3rd edition. London: Bailliere Tindall.

Hart, B.L., and Hart, L.A. (1985): Canine and Feline Behavioral Therapy. Philadelphia: Lea & Febiger.

Hopkins, S.G., Schubert, T.A., and Hart, B.L. (1976): Castration of adult male dogs: effects on roaming, aggression, urine marking, and mounting. Journal of the American Veterinary Medical Association **168**, 1108.

Houpt, K.A. (1991): Feeding and drinking behavior problems. Veterinary Clinics of North America: Small Animal Practice **21**, 281–298.

Leuscher, U.A., McKeown, D.B., and Halip, J. (1991): Stereotypic or obsessive-compulsive disorders in dogs and cats. Veterinary Clinics of North America: Small Animal Practice **21**, 401–413.

Marder, A.R. (1991): Psychotropic drugs and behavioral therapy. Veterinary Clinics of North America: Small Animal Practice **21**, 329–342.

McKeown, D, Luescher, A., and Machum, M. (1988): Coprophagia: Food for thought. *Canadian Veterinary Journal* **28**, 849–850.

O'Farrell, V. (1992): *Manual of Canine Behaviour*, 2nd Edition. Shurdington, Cheltenham, Gloucesteshire, England, British Small Animal Veterinary Association.

Overall, K.L. (1992a,b,c): Recognition, diagnosis, and management of obsessive-compulsive disorders, Parts 1, 2, and 3. *Canine Practice* **17** (Issue No. 2, 3, and 4).

Parker, A.J. (1989): Behavioral signs of organic disease. In Ettinger, S.J. (ed), *Textbook of Veterinary Internal Medicine*, 3rd ed., Philadelphia, WB Saunders.

Voith, V.L. (1980): Functional significance of pseudocyesis. *Modern Veterinary Practice* **January**.

Voith, V.L. (1989): Behavioral disorders. In Ettinger, S. (ed): *Textbook of Veterinary Internal Medicine*. Philadelphia, WB Saunders.

Part III

Treatment of Cat Behavior Problems

It is now believed that the domestic cat, *Felis silvestris catus*, is descended from the African wild cat or Kaffir cat, *Felis silvestris libyca*, rather than the European wild cat, *Felis silvestris silvestris*. O'Farrell and Neville (1994) cite the results of recent DNA mapping studies which reveal that the domestic cat is "genetically almost identical to the African wild cat" while being clearly distinguishable from the European wild cat.

It is assumed that the process of domestication in cats differs greatly from that of wolves, which were presumably adopted as pups by primitive hunter-gatherer groups, initially used primarily as hunting allies or home-site guardians, and eventually reproduced in captivity while being consciously or unconsciously selected for traits like increased docility, lowered fear, and reduced intragroup aggression. In cats, the process probably involved the *mutualistic* relationship between the two species progressively developing in the direction of increasingly closer and enduring contact. Mutualistic interspecies relationships are those in which two different species derive some benefit from associating with one another (Grier and Burk, 1992). It is assumed that the presence of high rodent pest populations in and around the granaries and rubbish dumps of the villages and towns of ancient Egypt would have supported many cat predators. Given Egypt's grain-based economy, cats would surely have been valued by human residents for their ability to help control rodent populations. During the early stages of this association, selection pressures favoring cats which were less timid with man, or which became more rapidly accustomed to man, would have produced animals that were bold enough or adaptable enough to fully exploit this niche. Once such cats were bearing young in the vicinity of their food sources, and the young were therefore born and raised in close proximity to human beings, the interspecies relationship would have been well on the way towards becoming what it is today.

Like human beings, wolves can hunt cooperatively in groups to bring down prey animals much larger than themselves, which is thought to be one of the primary reasons for the group-living pattern of social organization evolving in both species. The wild ancestors of our domestic cats, however, lived as solitary hunters preying only on animals smaller than themselves. Like other solitary-hunting members of the cat family, they were social only to the very limited extent required to regulate their contacts with other solitary individuals whose hunting territories touched or overlapped theirs and during the breeding season, when males and females must come together to mate and (in some species) care jointly for their young until they were old enough to fend for themselves.

Accordingly dogs and cats are generally contrasted in terms of the degree to which they are social, group-living animals – with dogs being highly social and only at home when living in a stable social group with a clear dominance hierarchy and cats being basically asocial, solitary creatures that do not need or even actively avoid the company of conspecifics. For cats at least, this portrait is a considerable oversimplification. The following represents a brief portrait of cat social organization, the starting point for understanding cat behavior and cat behavior problems. It is based on the combined results of a number of observational studies of feral and farm cat communities which have been carried out during the last two decades.

Cat social organization is extraordinarily flexible, and food availability appears to be the crucial factor in affecting how social cats are –

that is, whether they live in groups or as solitary individuals avoiding contacts with conspecifics and defending hunting/scavenging territories against intruders. Where food is not abundant and cats must hunt for their prey, groups do not form. Under these conditions, the asocial, solitary hunter which avoids contact with other cats and defends its hunting territory against cat intruders is a fair description. Here females have home ranges (i.e. the area each cat regularly uses) which do not overlap, and males have somewhat larger home ranges which may include portions of the home ranges of several females. Although male home ranges may not overlap during most of the year, their sizes increase and they overlap one another during the breeding season. While the female territory size is thought to be determined by food availability, that of males is larger than food considerations would dictate and seems rather to be determined by the availability of females.

However, where food is abundant around human settlement refuse dumps, or when food is regularly and reliably provided by human beings, cats congregate and remain in stable groups of usually up to as many as ten individuals but ranging in some circumstances up to 50 or more. The individuals in these groups engage in a great deal of social behavior with one another and may react aggressively to drive intruders away from the home range core area around nesting areas and food source. Such groups consist mainly of genetically-related adult females and their kittens. The females tolerate one another, react aggressively towards strange females, and jointly participate in caring for the group's young by sometimes nesting together and nursing and supplying prey to each other's kittens. These adult females have considerably overlapping home ranges while sharing the same core area. The fact that prior to systematic observational field studies it was believed such cat groups were mere congregations of individuals around food sources without true social group qualities is revealing. For it suggests the degree to which social interactions between individuals seem to reflect a kind of *mutual tolerance* between individuals rath-

er than the kind of intense mutual attraction characteristic of highly social species such as dogs.

To add males to this picture, it is helpful to conceptualize a community of cats in a rural area composed of several farms. The core area of the home ranges of the members of each farm's group of females is centered around the farmyard or barn where the farm family regularly provides food for them. This form of association between cats and humans is, of course, beneficial to both species. On the one hand, the cats are fed by the farm family because they are helpful in controlling the rodent population which is essentially competing with the farm family for the grain produced for sale or to feed livestock. And on the other hand, food is abundant for the cats both as a result of this feeding and the high availability of rodent prey. In short, the mutualistic character of the interspecies relationship between cats and human beings in the modern farm situation parallels that which is assumed to have formed the basis for the initial domestication of cats in Egypt several thousand years ago.

Such a rural cat community contains males of various ages. When young, males remain with the group in which they were born for some time. As they grow older, they are more frequently attacked by mature breeding males and eventually leave the group and usually emigrate away from their mother's home range. After living a solitary existence for some time, they may then begin challenging the breeding males in the surrounding community and regularly visiting one or more of the female groups in the area. If such female groups are very far apart, or if a single group contains a large number of females, the male may remain with one group most of the time. In this group-living situation too, males generally have much larger home ranges than females, and here again their size and spatial pattern reflects mainly the distribution and sizes of female groups in the area rather than the food supply.

Cat groups do not exhibit obvious, time-stable dominance hierarchies like dogs. However, dominance-like relationships can be observed between pairs of males or in situations in which large numbers of males are congregated around estrous females: during social interactions, one individual may act bolder and more offensively aggressive while the other may become defensive first, crouching down, moving sideways away, and perhaps hissing and striking out with the forepaws. Over time, overt aggression between males in a group may decrease. And in large congregations of males around females, there is less aggression between males that are familiar with one another than towards outsiders that have just joined the group. In general, although some males are more aggressive than others, the resulting "dominance hierarchy" which can be derived on paper using measures such as the number of fights won or number of threats given does not seem to be obviously correlated with rights of prior access to food or receptive females as is the case in dogs. Also revealing are the related facts that cats may eat peaceably together from the same dish and lack the distinct submissive displays (i.e. analogous to the submissive postures and facial expressions exhibited by dogs) which confirm dominance-related status more subtly than by simply moving away, avoiding, or reacting with defense aggression. In effect, all of these observations are consistent with the view that cats do not have true dominance hierarchies in the canine sense.

It has, however, been suggested that dominance is highly relative in cats in the sense of being location- and time-specific (Leyhausen, 1979). When two cats meet on a pathway, for example, the normally more dominant individual may sit down or move to the side and let the other pass by if the location is nearer to the less dominant cat's home area. And regardless of the nature of the apparent dominance relationship between the two animals in other circumstances, the cat that is traveling in an overlapping area of the two animals' home ranges at a time of day other than the one in which it normally does may defer to the other cat in a similar way.

In speculating on the origins of sociality in cats, Bradshaw (1992) poses the intriguing question of how group living developed in the domestic cat given that it would presumably not live in groups at all if it were not for the great abundance of food at refuse dumps and around barns and granaries. He presents the following theory which may be more plausible than he himself argues:

"... virtually all the social groups that have been studied have relied on concentrations of food supplied by man. This raises the unlikely, but not yet disproven, possibility that sociality in the domestic cat has arisen secondarily, as a byproduct of domestication. If, for example, the original reason for domestication of the African wild cat was for rodent control in granaries, man might first have selected individuals that tolerated the close proximity of other cats, because one highly territorial cat would not have achieved the desired result. Subsequently, those cats that displayed affiliative behavior towards people would have been selected from the original, conspecific-tolerant, population. Those affiliative behaviors could have been derived from those shown by kittens towards their mothers, carried into the adult state by a process of progressive artificial neotenization. The process of creating this new animal might have made it even more accepting of members of its own species, so that when some individuals became feral, they were able to use this modified behavior to form independent social groups." (p. 162)

Thus, a two-step process is envisioned. Firstly, selection by man of cats that tolerated other cats – ensuring that large groups rather than single individuals lived around granaries to more effectively control rodents. And secondly, the selection from this new, cat-tolerant population of cats which freely associated with man in a process involving neoteny, evolutionary development in the direction of retaining juvenile behavioral characteristics into adulthood. That neotenous evolutionary developments took place is now revealed in domestic cats by kitten-like behaviors such as lying down to be petted and treading with the forepaws when held as well as their reduced aggressiveness and fear. Although Bradshaw suggests that the complexity of communication between cats and the "lack of correlation between sociability to man and other cats" argues against this theory, there is no reason why this need be the case. Selection pressures for tolerance of other cats could also have involved the modification of ancestral cat-cat communication behavioral systems shown by more solitary individuals at breeding times or between parents and offspring (i.e. neoteny could be involved here too). This two-stage model could also easily incorporate the lack of correlation between sociability to man and other cats as, in effect, the end result of the partially distinct types of selection pressures involved. Essentially, the behavioral mechanisms underlying a cat's tolerance of other cats and affiliative motivation towards man need not be precisely identical.

However, one modification of Bradshaw's hypothesis may be called for. Namely, the evolution of tolerance for other cats – phase one in the two-stage process – need not necessarily be the result of human selection (e.g. farmers killing cats that insist on driving other cats away). Having to constantly defend abundant food sources against other cats is a strategy which would represent a cost in both energy and health-related risk terms for the highly territorial cat which the less territorial, more tolerant cat would not have to pay. And there might not be anything to offset this cost in the sense that if the food source was ample to comfortably support a large group of cats, the territorial strategy would produce little or no additional benefit. Moreover, the fact that cat groups tend to be composed of genetically-related females and their offspring may also imply that the tolerance strategy has the additional payoff (i.e. aside from saving energy and avoiding health-endangering aggression) that by being tolerant, the cat is essentially furthering the welfare of closely-related individuals and, hence, the portion of its own genes which they carry. Essentially, quite apart from any direct human-based selection pressures, there may be others inherent in this highly localized, abundant, and reliable food source situation that would have favored the development of maternal groups of tolerant cats over the solitary/territorial pattern which is obviously most adaptive under natural food availability conditions.

To round out this brief introductory portrait of cat behavior, there is a final element that must be confronted before considering the various cat behavioral problems. Namely, the dramatic and puzzling differences between individual cats in the extent to which they are sociable towards other cats and/or owners. Some cats "like" other cats, others don't. Some cats are playful, others aren't. Some cats like the company of other cats, but don't play with them. Some cats like to be played with and petted by their owners, some only played with, some only petted, and some do not care for either. Studies involving the presence or absence of agreement between the ratings of independent observers of various characteristics clearly indicate that these are stable differences in the "behavioral style" of individual cats – i.e. that cats have something akin to what in humans we term *personality characteristics*. In addition to the degree of sociability towards other cats, such studies have demonstrated reliable differences in characteristics like, for example, activity, curiosity, sociability towards people (friendliness vs. hostility/fear/unfriendliness), and quality of sociability in terms of dimensions such as initiative/friendly (makes initiatives) vs. reserved/friendly (accepts initiatives) and play contact/friendly vs. petting/friendly. As the use of terms like behavioral style and personality suggest, these individual differences seem to be highly stable over time and resistant to change.

As in dogs, one source of such major behavioral differences between individuals lies in the experiences individuals have had when they were young. Much petting and handling by humans between the 2nd and 7th weeks of life tend to make cats more sociable to humans later in life than cats which weren't handled or handled only briefly. Furthermore, handling by a number of handlers during this "sensitive period" tends to produce a cat which is friendly towards all humans as opposed to mainly towards its handler(s), as tends to be the case with cats that were handled during this time by only one person. These are, however, only average tendencies which vary greatly between individuals. Even kittens which are subjected to a great deal of handling by humans sometimes fail to become well-socialized. Similarly, while most cats born into captive colonies are highly sociable towards other cats, others may be noticeably much more solitary in spite of their having been raised in an identical environment.

In general, most writers on the subject of cat behavior are inclined to conclude that while early experience plays a major role, such personality-like differences often seem to have a genetic basis; that is, the factors responsible for these differences can also be inherited. Studies have shown, for example, that friendly-vs.-unfriendly differences between kittens are sometimes positively correlated with similar differences between their fathers with which the kittens have had no direct contact.

Dogs too have what might be loosely termed "personalities" in terms of differing activity levels, playfulness, excitability, fearfulness, and apparent need for physical contact with owners. The fact that there seem to be some reliable breed differences in some of these characteristics implies that genetic factors may also be playing a role (along with early and later experiences) in determining them in dogs as well. But in cats, such differences turn out to be not only more dramatic, but also more puzzling for extremely sociable "pack animals" like ourselves to understand. All dogs are highly sociable towards humans and other dogs if they have had sufficient contact with them throughout their lives. All like petting to some extent, are highly attracted to familiar humans and other dogs if properly socialized, and indeed may appear to suffer when deprived of such social contacts for even short periods of time. But while some highly sociable cats behave similarly, others don't seem to be like this at all. Conspecifics may be treated with hostility or tolerated without the hint of an affiliative motivation. And our cats may gladly accept our food but dislike being touched by us, show no in interest in shared playtimes, and just generally act like our comings and goings and other behavior were of no consequence or interest to them.

In answering owners' questions as to why their particular cat doesn't like petting or playing as much as other cats do – or why one cat persists in reacting negatively to the obviously friendly approaches of another with which it may have shared the same home for years – the behavioral counselor can do little but confirm that such differences in the social behavior and sociability between individual cats are often genetic in origin and thus are basically unalterable; essentially, that such great individual differences are one of the puzzling facts of life that make these animals so fascinating to human beings.

The fact that cat behavior and cat behavior problems are often far more puzzling and difficult to understand than those shown by dogs will be made clear in the following chapters where the uncertainties and related differences in causal accounts given by various authors are considerable. The truth is that many aspects of cat behavioral problems are very poorly understood. Accordingly, popular accounts of cat behavioral problems given by the world's many self-proclaimed experts in this field tend to be gross oversimplifications which are, scientifically speaking, flawed in a number of critical respects.

References

Beaver, B. V. (1992): *Feline Behavior: A Guide for Veterinarians*. 2nd Edition. Philadelphia, W. B. Saunders Company.

Bradshaw, J. W. S. (1992): *The Behavior of the Domestic Cat*. Wallingford, UK, CAB International

Grier, J. W., and Burk, T. (1992): *Biology of Animal Behavior*. 2nd Edition. St. Louis, Mosby-Year Book, Inc.

Leyhausen, P. (1979): *Cat Behavior: The Predatory and Social Behavior of Domestic and Wild Cats*. New York, Garland STPM Press.

O'Farrell, V. (1992): *Manual of Canine Behaviour*, 2nd Edition. Shurdington, Cheltenham, Gloucestershire, England, British Small Animal Veterinary Association.

Robinson, I. (1992): Social behavior of the cat. In Thorne, C. (ed): *The Waltham Book of Dog and Cat Behavior*. Oxford, Pergamon Press.

Thorne, C. (1992): Evolution and domestication. In Thorne, C. (ed): *The Waltham Book of Dog and Cat Behavior*. Oxford, Pergamon Press.

20 Urine Marking

Pet behavior problem counselors are often confronted with the urine marking problem. Figure 20.1 presents some relevant statistics from my case records. Of 86 recent cat problem cases, 38% of the 104 problems reported involved urine marking. Cases which are severe enough to come to the behavior problem counselor may be only the tip of the iceberg, for statistics reported by Hart and Cooper (1984) indicate that approximately 10% of castrated males and 5% of females sometimes spray in the home.

Biologically speaking, urine marking is a normal feline communicative behavior which presumably functions to convey information to other cats about the spraying cat's individual identity, presence in a certain geographical area, when it was last at the sprayed location, and perhaps other information like reproductive status. In a natural setting, it is commonly assumed that such information acts to coordinate neighboring cats' spatial movements in such a way that they avoid face-to-face contacts with one another or, at certain times, to attract potential mates (Beaver, 1992).

When marking, the cat usually sniffs the site first – usually some vertical surface a foot or so above the ground – and then turns around and sprays a small amount of urine backwards onto the spot. The typical spraying posture is standing with the tail held upright and often with its tip quivering. However when marking horizontal objects, cats may squat as in normal urination. In cat problem cases, differentiating urine marking in a squatting posture from normal excretory urination can therefore sometimes be difficult. Here, the nature of the object or surface on which the urination occurs, the cat's urination and other behavior with respect to the litter box, and the presence or absence of marking using the conventional spraying body posture must be considered in detail. In cases of marking using a squatting posture, objects like shoes, old clothes, and plastic bags rather than surfaces (e.g. wall-to-wall carpets) are urinated on, cats continue to use the litter box for excretory urination as before, they show no behavioral signs that they find the litter box aversive, and they may at least occasionally also spray in the home using a standing posture. The amount of urine is not as helpful an indicator in such cases as one might assume, for

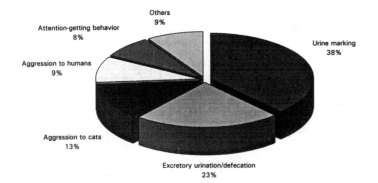

Figure 20.1: Relative frequency of the various cat behavior problems taken from the author's case records for 86 cats

urine marking in cats can sometimes involve relatively large amounts of urine.

In general, urine marking is an extremely serious problem for owners. Repeated marking can destroy valuable furniture and carpets, and the lingering, ever-worsening odor can become so pronounced that neighbors may complain and owners are faced with the choice of solving the problem, giving the cat away, or being evicted from their apartments. In some of the worst cases, walls throughout the home are stained from the tops of tall cabinets down to the floor, carpets are badly discolored in practically every corner of the apartment, and the odor is so stifling that one wonders how it could be possible for human beings to live like this.

Causes of the urine marking problem

In a discussion of the causes of the urine marking problem, Hart and Hart (1985) speculate that the male's "own urine odor probably makes him more self-assured and comfortable... An important cause of spraying is an increase in anxiety or nervousness" (p. 136).

The notions that increased anxiety is a common cause of spraying in domestic cats and that the act of spraying or the urine odor function to reduce anxiety are prevalent in the pet behavior problem literature as the following two recent quotes from other leading authorities suggests:

"Not only does the odor of his own distinct scent provide relief from anxiety..." (Beaver, 1992, p. 78).

"It may therefore be most accurate....to view the function of spraying as increasing a cat's own sense of security in the face of either a territorial challenge or another stressor" (O'Farrell and Neville, 1994, p. 61).

Are cats which show urine marking in the home more nervous or anxious than normal cats?

Figure 20.2 summarizes the replies to four questions from the client information form (see Chapter 6) filled out by a number of owners of urine marking and normal, non-problem cats.

Four aspects of these results are relevant to the present discussion:

- Many cats from the normal cat population which do not exhibit urine marking are also reported to sometimes show fearful and restless behavior to an excessive extent.
- The percentage of marking cats reported to be "nervous" is dramatically higher and the percentages which show excessive restlessness or fear reactions are somewhat higher than the comparable figures for cats from the normal, non-marking population.
- Almost 60% of cats which urine mark in the home are not, however, described by their owners as being especially nervous individuals.

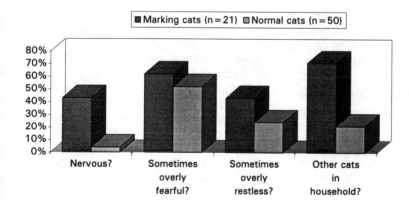

Figure 20.2: Relative frequency of the owners of marking vs. normal cats who responded affirmatively to the question „Is your cat nervous?", answered „occasionally" or „often" to the questions of how often the cat showed „excessive fear reactions" or „excessive restlessness", and reported that there were other cats in the household.

- While there is at least one other cat living in 71% of the marking cats' households, only 21% of the non-marking cats live with other cats.

Although this data can only be regarded as suggestive given the small sample sizes and the fact that subjective owner reports are involved, it provides limited support for the hypothesis that increased, above-normal tendencies towards nervousness and reacting fearfully to environmental stimuli are indeed correlated with the marking problem in some cats. However, the *majority* of cats displaying the urine marking problem in a form which is serious enough to warrant the contacting of a behavioral counselor do not in fact seem to be any more anxious or fearful than other cats. Thus, Borchelt and Voith's (1986) contention that "emotional factors" are involved only in a minority of cases seems to be supported to a limited extent by the present data.

Although the data provides support for the Hart and Hart view that anxiety is often correlated with the problem, this does not necessarily mean that it is causally related to it even in the most nervous or fearful cats. Almost all owners admit to having tried to control the urine marking problem with punishment – in some cases, relatively severe punishment because the problem is so serious for them and they are convinced that this is the only way to solve the problem. It is likely, therefore, that at least some of the nervousness and excessive fearfulness/restlessness referred to in the questionnaire by owners of marking cats may be direct reactions to owner punishment. Such an effect would further reduce the true proportion of urine marking cats whose general levels of anxiety and nervousness appear to be in some way directly related to the problem.

To what extent can anxiety and/or nervousness be considered to be a cause of the urine marking problem?

Obviously, the underlying conception of the Hart and Hart (1985) view is of a cat that is made to feel anxious or nervous by something and then most certainly feels more self-assured, comfortable, or secure after it has responded by spraying and can smell its own urine. This view has had a major impact on theorizing in the field as a whole. Consider, for example, the following quote from a well-known pet behavior problem counselor:

"Cats usually have no need to spray indoors because their lair is already perceived as secure and requires no further endorsement... When such marking occurs indoors it is usually a sign that the cat's lair is under some challenge. The challenge may be obvious in the shape of a recent arrival or a cat or dog, or a new baby, or an increased challenge from a cat outdoors, or it may result from moving or changing furniture, redecorating, family bereavement, having guests to stay, bringing outdoor objects anointed by other cats into the house, bringing novel objects (especially plastic bags) ... Almost certainly such marking is designed to help the perpetrator feel more confident by surrounding him or herself with his or her own familiar smell. Hence cats which spray indoors are trying to repair 'holes' in their own protective surrounds caused by change, the arrival of new objects or the addition of strange smells on new objects, cats or people, or the loss of a contributor to the communal smell that helps identify every member of the den... The home therefore needs to be reanointed in similar manner to the outdoors to identify occupancy and ensure that the resident encounters his or her own smell frequently." (Neville, 1991)

Scientifically speaking, the major problem with such a view is its almost exclusive reliance on circular reasoning. Urine marking is elicited by a challenge, but what is challenging is defined by whether or not urine marking is elicited. There is no independent criteria of what is or is not challenging. An invasion by another cat might rightly be regarded by anyone as a challenge. But what about an invasion by a plastic bag? How does one know that represents a challenge to the cat? According to the logic expressed in the above quote, because the cat marks it. In effect, saying marking occurs in response to challenges, and then defining challenges as things or events which elicit marking, is in fact saying nothing of substance beyond the original observation that these certain kinds of things and events sometimes elicit marking.

A related example of circular reasoning is the implication that some subjective feeling of insecurity is the cause of marking: challenges make cats feel insecure. The urine smell makes cats feel secure. So challenges are marked because the cat feels insecure. And how does one know that the cat feels insecure? Because it marks.

All this explains nothing really. Why might a cat mark in response to a plastic bag being brought into the home? Even if it somehow could be established that the cat feels threatened by the bag and perceives it as a challenge, the behavior remains unexplained, for one must still account for *why* the cat feels this way about the bag and *why* it marks when it feels this way. In effect, any feelings and perceptions the cat might have while marking the plastic bag should be regarded as correlated subjective phenomena which themselves require the same kind of objective, scientifically-sound explanation required for the marking behavior itself.

Do plastic bags make some cats feel insecure? The truth is that we don't know. Sometimes plastic bags do elicit marking. That seems clear. But why do cats mark on them? The bag is a strange new object. But why should strange new objects elicit marking? We really don't know that either. And here is the point where it is tempting to the non-scientist to speculate on what is going inside the animal to try and answer his/her questions. Perhaps the cat is frightened by the bag – because it smells so strange and foreign – and marking on it gives it a familiar odor, which in turn reduces its fear-provoking character. This is only a more elaborate version of the view criticized previously: strange things elicit fear. The bag is strange and therefore elicits fear. Strange things can be made less strange by urinating on them. So the cat urinates on them basically because it is afraid and trying to reduce its fear by reducing the strangeness that causes the fear. Here again, all of this inside-of-the-cat action tells us nothing of substance. We know the cat marks

the bag. We don't however know why. Essentially, such apparent explanations represent little more than unproductive speculations about how marking cats might be feeling at the time which, unfortunately, create more problems than they solve in terms of their standing in the way of a genuinely scientific analysis of the problem.

One final comment on insecurity/anxiety-reduction hypothesis: if marking is a natural response to insecurity which functions to make a cat feel more secure – which would presumably reduce its further motivation to mark – then why tell owners to clean the marked sites thoroughly as all counselors routinely do? According to anxiety-reduction theory, the advice should be the opposite: *Whatever you do, don't clean the marked sites!* By cleaning them, one should theoretically be removing the odor that the cat put there for a good reason and will have to put there again if someone insists on washing it off every time. Thus, according to this view, the urine marking problem should be self-correcting. A cat whose urine marking sites are left untouched should stop or reduce marking there fairly quickly. They don't, however.

Possible causal factors

Hormonal influence

The facts that the overwhelming majority of problem sprayers are males and castration and progestin therapy are sometimes effective treatments for urine marking in males clearly reveals the influence of hormonal factors on the problem. However, many females and castrated males also spray, which indicates that other major factors are involved as well.

Inherited predisposition

Why do some males never spray in the home while others continue to spray in spite of castration, drug therapy, and behavior-oriented treatment measures? We don't know. Many of these cats seem to be more nervous or anxious individuals than the average cat, but that is not

POSSIBLE CAUSAL FACTORS

Hormonal influence
(marking much more common in males;
often effectively treated by castration)

Inherited predisposition
(suspected genetic difference between cats
as reason for individual differences in marking behavior)

Social eliciting stimuli
(e.g. presence of other cats in home; new cat
in home, observation of cat outside in yard)

Other eliciting stimuli
(e.g. visitor or strange object in home;
change in household/family life)

URINE MARKING

• Urine sprayed backwards on vertical sites by a cat in a standing posture or, less
  commonly, deposited on horizontal objects or surfaces by a cat in a squatting posture.

POSSIBLE TREATMENT ELEMENTS

Cessation of ineffective methods
(e.g. punishment long after the fact)

Correct owner misconceptions
(e.g. spraying is abnormal behavior/cat's way
of protesting)

Castration
(for intact males and female that mark
during estrus)

Training in problem situations
(mild punishment when caught in act)

Care/maintenance condition changes
(e.g. find new home for other cat in household; deny cat access to certain rooms;
interrupt cat's view out of windows)

Alter marked sites
(e.g. put food bowls at marked sites; change
marked surfaces; booby trap marked site;
clean marked sites)

Medicaments
(e.g. progestins, diazepam, buspirone,
amitriptyline)

Chemical tracer substance
(to identify culprit in multi-cat household)

Other types of surgical intervention
(olfactory tractotomy/bilateral ischiocavernosus myectomy as last resort)

an explanation, simply an additional fact that
also needs to be explained. It is also insufficient
simply to point out that the spraying-eliciting
effect of other cats in the household may be
more powerful than treatment influences, for
many cats from multi-cat households never
spray. As is the case with most behavioral problems, it is suspected that genetic differences
between cats are in some way associated with
individual differences in spraying behavior.

Social eliciting stimuli

The commonly-reported observation that cats
may sometimes mark in direct response to a
new cat coming into the home or the observation of a cat in the yard through the window,
the statistical information presented above
which indicates that sprayers are much more
likely than non-sprayers to come from multi-
cat homes (71% vs. 21% respectively), and the

widely-accepted view that urine marking is a social behavior which functions to communicate information between cats are all consistent with the view that social stimuli can be important elicitors of urine marking in the home.

Why do particular cats respond to such social stimuli with marking and others not? Although pointing to unknown genetic differences between cats is not at all the kind of explanation that tends to satisfy puzzled owners, it should be explained to them that accounting for why some animal exhibit certain problems and others don't is much like accounting for why some people are more intelligent, aggressive, or excitable than others. In effect, the answer to such questions often lies partly in the inherited genetic makeup of the individuals.

Before leaving the topic of social stimuli from other cats in the home eliciting marking, another interesting possibility should be raised. Namely, Leyhausen's (1971, 1979) hypothesis that one major function of urine marking is to reduce contact between cats in the sense that outdoors cats may use urine mark information to coordinate their behavior with one another in order to avoid the direct, face-to-face contacts which might lead to problems. This could be achieved simply by cats avoiding trails which have been freshly marked by other cats in favor of trails which are unmarked or were last marked long ago. Perhaps therefore the greater prevalence of marking in multi-cat homes should be regarded as a vain attempt of one of the residents to establish a "time sharing system ... which would allow several animals to occupy an area but reduce the chance of conflict between them" (Robinson, 1992) in this extremely confined area.

Other eliciting stimuli

The apparent fact that cats sometimes mark in response to new objects brought into the home, visitors, or major changes in family life that might represent some kind of a problem for them is one of the mainstays of a theory which is popular among "cat people": cats can't talk. They only have limited ways of showing their feelings. And unfortunately, urine marking is one of them. Thus, cats sometimes mark "out of protest", to tell their owners that they are unhappy or dissatisfied about something.

As we have considered, the available scientific evidence appears to indicate that outdoor urine marking does indeed probably function in some way to transmit messages which other cats receive and presumably respond to in the interest of coordinating behavioral movements, territory use patterns, and reproductive behavior. But this is a far cry from "protest spraying", which is based on the anthropocentric proposition that the behavior is being performed for the owner's benefit. The erroneous idea that cats are spraying as a kind of protest often originates with owners themselves. Perhaps the main source of this impression is the cat's spraying posture itself, which may make the cat look bold or confident at the time. Coupled with the fact that the cat sometimes does it practically right under the owners' noses, this is enough to make owners suspect that "maybe he's trying to tell me something". Generally speaking, it is basically a natural owner response to elimination problems of all types to consider the possibility that the cat may feel frustrated or dissatisfied and the behavior is a manifestation of this.

Possible treatment elements

Cessation of ineffective methods

Nearly all owners of urine marking cats have relied heavily on the use of punishment to try and control the problem. Typically, the cat is carried back to the newly discovered damp spot, its nose is held down close to or even touching the spot, and it is punished by being scolded or hit. This may be followed by carrying it back to the litter box and then confining it there for several minutes. Of course, this method has no direct effect on the problem whatsoever. To be effective, punishment must be delivered immediately, preferably just as the cat begins spraying. Frequent and/or severe punishment can also make a cat fear its owner and therefore avoid contact, flee when the owner enters the room, etc.

Correct owner misconceptions

One should explain to owners that the behavior is a normal territorial marking behavior which both tomcats and females perform outside, but that stimuli inside the home are not sufficient to elicit the behavior in most cats. Accordingly, one can emphasize that the problem does not indicate that the cat is behaving abnormally, protesting against something, or that something is wrong with how it is being taken care of. Giving owners some basic understanding of the nature of the problem behavior helps the prospects for successful treatment of almost all behavior problems, for owners' personal theories often stand in the way of their acceptance of and compliance with the counselor's advice. Correction of misconceptions like the cat is spraying out of protest is therefore often indispensable to treatment success.

Castration

Castration is indicated for intact males of any age. Its effectiveness in reducing or solving the problem is estimated to be around 90% regardless of whether the castration is pre- or postpubertal (Hart and Barrett, 1973, Hart and Cooper, 1984, Hart and Hart, 1985). It is also effective against marking by estrous females (Borchelt and Voith, 1986).

Training in problem situations

Mild punishment is appropriate when the cat is caught in the act of marking. Startling the cat by, for example, loud hand-clapping usually interrupts and suppresses the behavior and quickly trains the animal to inhibit marking in the presence of the owner. This in turn can sometimes help to reduce the overall frequency of marking.

Care/maintenance condition changes

Finding a new home for a second cat may help, for the presence of another cat in the home may be a major causal factor in some cases.

Keeping cats away from regularly marked sites can be a completely effective method for eliminating the problem in cases where there are only a few marked sites and preventing access to them is feasible (e.g. by denying cats access to particular rooms).

Borchelt and Voith (1986) report that allowing cats to spend either more or less time outdoors may affect the frequency of marking indoors in some cases. These authors also suggest that covering the lower portions of windows with translucent plastic that interrupts the cat's view of outdoor cats can eliminate marking where this is the primary eliciting stimulus.

Alter commonly marked sites

If marking occurs at only two or three places in the home, converting the sites to feeding locations is one of the most effective treatment measures. It is therefore often recommended to owners that they try this first. Cats are fed out of a food bowl which is placed and continuously kept (even when empty) at the marked site. If there is more than one site, two or more food bowls are used and the cat's meals are divided between them. Another possible approach is to change something else at the site like its surface characteristics (e.g. by covering it with plastic foil) which makes the site less attractive to the cat for marking. Finally, cats can be trained to avoid the site by placing several set, upside-down mousetraps around it so that one will be triggered off when touched, startling the cat. Most cats quickly learn to avoid the site entirely under these circumstances. Other similar possibilities for producing avoidance of the site by making it aversive are placing trays of marbles, pine cones (O'Farrell and Neville, 1994), or carpet tape (i.e. sticky on both sides) around the base of the marked site.

Owners are often initially skeptical with regard to the ultimate effectiveness of these types of measures. It seems only logical to them that if the cat is somehow prevented from marking on one site, it will simply begin marking on another. But this is not always the case. Many cats are quite fussy in this regard, and altering their preferred marking sites or training the cats to avoid them stops the problem behavior entirely.

Of course, thoroughly cleaning marked sites is essential to remove residual urine odors which might stimulate further marking. The use of cleaning products containing ammonia should be avoided because of the chemical similarity of ammonia with urine.

Medicaments

If too many sites are involved, or if the cat always begins marking at new sites when one of the above methods eliminates marking at the old ones, the problem can only be treated with medicaments. The following Table 20.1 provides information about the most common drugs which are prescribed to control the urine marking problem (Hart et. al, 1993; Marder, 1991).

Table 20.1: Drug information from Hart et al. (1993) and Marder (1991) for the treatment of urine marking in cats.

Medicament	Dosage	Reference
Diazepam	1–2 mg/cat po bid	Marder (1991) Hart et al. (1993)
Buspirone	2.5–5 mg/cat po bid-tid	Marder (1991)
	2.5–5 mg/cat po bid	Hart et al. (1993)
Amitriptyline HCl	5–10 mg/cat po	Marder (1991)
Megestrol acetate	2.5–5 mg/cat po for 7 days, then 2.5–5 mg weekly	Marder (1991)
	5 mg/cat po sid for 7 days, then gradually decrease	Hart et al. (1993)
Medroxyprogesterone acetate	10–20 mg/kg SQ, IM	Marder (1991)

According to Hart et al. (1993), *buspirone* and *diazepam* are more effective than the *progestins* with females but not with males, and buspirone has fewer serious side effects and more often a permanent effect (i.e. after drug therapy is discontinued) than diazepam. Hence, buspirone is the drug of choice, with valium second and the progestins third. Marder (1991) suggests that other anxiolytic drugs like *amitriptyline HCl* may also be useful.

If medicaments are prescribed, the cat should be observed closely for possible side effects – particularly the first time the drug is administered. If the drug must be administered on a more or less permanent basis, the dosage should be gradually reduced to the lowest effective dose and the drug should be completely discontinued every few months to make sure that it is still really needed. (See the "drug therapy" subsection in Chapter 8 for side effects and other important drug-related information.)

Chemical tracer substance

Even owners in multi-cat households who rarely see one of their cats spray usually quite confidently single out one of them as being the culprit. When asked why, owners often report having seen this cat marking two or three times in the past, which makes it likely but by no means certain that it is still the one that is marking. However, owners may believe a particular cat is at fault on other grounds. Perhaps it is a male and the other cat is a female, or it might be the most restless and active cat. Here, one must explain to the owner that females too sometimes mark and that there is no way to be absolutely sure which cat is doing the spraying based on personality or other behavioral characteristics.

For behavioral measures like putting food bowls around the base of marked sites, it obviously makes no difference which cat is involved. But if drugs are to be administered, it naturally makes sense to try and identify the culprit first. A chemical marker may be used for this purpose. Hart and Hart (1985) recommend *sodium fluorescein* either as a 0.3 ml SQ injection (10%, equivalent to 100 mg/ml) or orally (0.5 ml of solution, or 6 strips of ophthalmic test paper inserted in gelatin capsules) given in the late afternoon as a marker substance which can be identified later when marked spots are scanned in darkness under ultraviolet illumination.

SAMPLE RECOMMENDATIONS

Urine marking

- Always thoroughly clean the marked sites to reduce odors which might elicit further marking. Do not use cleaning products containing ammonia because of the chemical similarity of ammonia and urine.
- The cat should only be scolded or startled (e.g. by a sudden loud noise) if it is actually caught in the act of spraying. Punishment that occurs more than a few seconds after the cat has marked will have no effect on the problem.

For intact tomcats or marking by estrous females:

- An immediate castration is to be recommended.

Alternative methods for cases where a cat consistently marks at a maximum of 3 or 4 sites in the home:

- Always feed the cat out of food bowls placed directly at the base of each marked site. Leave the food bowls there with a little dry food in them throughout the day and night.
- Place several set, *turned-over* mousetraps around each of the marked sites so the cat will step on one, spring it, and be frightened away when it goes there to mark.
- Drastically change the characteristics of the surfaces which are marked at each site (e.g. by covering them with aluminum foil, plastic, etc.)

If marking occurs on so many places that these site-oriented treatment measures are not feasible:

- Because the cat marks on so many places in the home, the problem can only be treated with drug therapy.

If cat marks in response to seeing outdoor cats through a window:

- Prevent cat from being able to see outside by, for example, covering the lower portions of windows with translucent plastic.

Surgical intervention

In addition to castration, two other types of surgical procedures have been reported to be effective in eliminating urine marking in some cases where neither behavioral nor drug therapy measures has helped. Hart (1981) reports that an olfactory tractotomy was effective in eliminating spraying in 7 out of 12 castrated males and 4 out of 4 spayed females. Komtebedde and Hauptman (1989) report that bilateral ischiocavernosus myectomy eliminated spraying in 5 and reduced in a further 3 out of a total of 10 operated cats. In general, American behavior specialists caution that these types of surgical interventions may reduce the quality of cats' lives and would, therefore, only be ethically justifiable as a last resort to save a cat from being euthanized.

References

Beaver, B.V. (1992): *Feline Behavior: A Guide for Veterinarians*. W.B. Saunders Co., Philadelphia.
Borchelt, P.L., and Voith, V.L. (1986): Elimination behavior problems in cats. *Compendium on Con-*

tinuing Education for the Practicing Veterinarian **8**, 197–205.

Hart, B.L (1981): Olfactory tractotomy for control of objectionable urine spraying and urine marking in cats. *Journal of the American Veterinary Medical Association* **179**, 231–234.

Hart, B.L., and Barrett, R.E. (1973): Effects of castration on fighting, roaming, and urine spraying in adult male cats. *Journal of the American Veterinary Medical Association* **163**, 290–292.

Hart, B.L., and Cooper, L. (1984): Factors relating to urine spraying and fighting in prepubertally gonadectomized cats. *Journal of the American Veterinary Medical Association* **184**, 1255–1258.

Hart, B.L., Eckstein, R.A., Powell, K.L., and Dodman, N.H. (1993). Effectiveness of buspirone on urine spraying and inappropriate urination in cats. *Journal of the American Veterinary Medical Association* **203**, 254–258.

Hart, B.L., and Hart, L.A. (1985): *Canine and Feline Behavioral Therapy*. Philadelphia: Lea & Febiger.

Komtebedde, J., and Hauptman, J. (1990): Bilateral ischiocavernosus myectomy for chronic urine spraying in castrated male cats. *Veterinary Surgery* **19**; 293–296.

Leyhausen, P. (1971): Dominance and territoriality as complemented in mammalian social structure. In Esser, H. (ed): *Behavior and Environment*. New York, Plenum Press.

Leyhausen, P. (1979): *Cat Behaviour: the Predatory and Social Behavior of Domestic and Wild Cats*. New York & London, Garland STPM Press.

Marder, A.R. (1991). Psychotropic drugs and behavioral therapy. *Veterinary Clinics of North America: Small Animal Practice* **21**, 329–342.

Neville, P. (1991): Spraying behaviour problems in cats. Paper presented at a satellite meeting during the BSAVA Congress, Birmingham, England.

O'Farrell, V., and Neville, P. (1994): *Manual of Feline Behaviour*. Shurdington, Cheltenham, Gloucestershire, UK, British Small Animal Veterinary Association.

Robinson, I. (1992): Social Behaviour of the Cat. In Thorne, C. (ed.): *The Waltham Book of Dog and Cat Behaviour*. Oxford, Pergamon.

21 Inappropriate Urination and Defecation

In cases where a cat is frequently urinating in the home, the first task is to determine whether urine marking or normal urination is involved. As pointed out in the last chapter, this can sometimes be difficult because cats may also urine mark using a squatting rather than the typical standing spraying posture. Exploring the following areas usually helps to differentiate between these two different types of urination problems:

- Does the cat always or usually urinate outside of the litter box? If only marking is involved, the cat would continue to use the litter box for normal excretory urination as before.
- Does the cat show signs that urination in the litter box is unpleasant or arouses fear? Cats with normal eliminatory urination problems may run out of the litter box very quickly after urination, or meow and act nervous and hesitant before entering it, shake their paws after contact with the litter, perch on the edge of the litter box as if trying to eliminate in the box without entering it, and fail to show pre-elimination scratching and post-elimination covering.
- Could fear be involved in the sense that the cat has begun urinating in some remote place in the home where it spends much time hiding from another cat it is very afraid of?
- Does the cat frequently, usually, or always defecate outside of the box as well? If so, more than simple urine marking is usually involved.
- Does the cat sometimes show urination in the standing spraying posture as well? Is the urination while squatting usually directed towards particular objects like shoes, clothes lying on the floor, etc. or is it usually next to pieces of furniture, along the base of

walls, or in corners where cats often spray? Or conversely, does it occur out in the middle of a room away from such distinctive landmarks?
- Were there any signs of illness around the time when the problem first appeared? Was the cat examined at that time for feline urological syndrome, cystitis, urethritis, prostatitis, vaginitis, enteritis, and colitis (i.e. common causes of "elimination accidents" listed by Reisner, 1991)?

In practice, there are cases where even after a long consultation exploring every possible source of information, the counselor still cannot be entirely sure which type of urination problem is involved. This is, however, not as critical as it might seem. One can explain the reason for this diagnostic uncertainty to clients, explain why one feels that one diagnosis is more likely than the other, and then recommend treating the problem as such with the provision – clearly echoed in a summary-of-recommendations letter sent to clients a few days after the consultation – that they should call again if the treatment is not entirely effective or if new relevant facts come to light. In such cases, the animal's response to treatment is often just what is needed to confirm or contradict the provisional diagnosis.

There is some disagreement among pet behavior problem counselors as to whether cats which defecate outside of the litter box are sometimes showing a form of marking behavior and, hence, not all cases of failure to use the litter box for defecation can be regarded as inappropriate excretory defecation. Combining the observation that feces from farm cats are sometimes found along trails or at other conspicuous locations in their home ranges well away from core areas with the fact that feces are apparently used for territory marking in some other feline species like the Spanish lynx, some authors have suggested that feces might sometimes be used as a form of marking in domestic cats as well (e.g. Bradshaw, 1992; Robinson, 1992, Beaver, 1992).

However, failure to cover feces well away from the core areas of home ranges may simply reflect the unimportance of burying behavior there. According to Hart and Hart (1985), burying functions to reduce the danger of cats or kittens ingesting parasite eggs or intestinal pathogens through contact with uncovered feces, and it functions to keep feces away from rodent prey which serve as intermediate hosts of tapeworms which may reinfect cats when the rodents are caught and eaten. Away from home range core areas, these advantages of burying may not be high enough to outweigh the effects of energy-economizing selection pressures which act to ensure that every element of the behavioral repertoire of animals is maximally efficient in the sense of only being performed in situations in which they provide some real survival or gene-reproduction benefit.

Although the hypothesis that uncovered feces may sometimes perform a similar territory marking function as urine spraying is plausible, as yet it is only a hypothesis with little in the way of convincing supporting evidence. Uncovered feces may simply reflect the lack of a suitable digging substrate at certain locations, relatively greater proportions of time spent by cats at certain locations, priority of other competing behaviors at such sites (i.e. full attention to surroundings and remaining quiet and inconspicuous to both potential prey and predators), or the fact that uncovered feces have a much higher chance of being discovered by human observers at such conspicuous sites (as opposed to thick underbrush) which are, after all, described as conspicuous because they are conspicuous to human beings.

However, admitting that the feces marking hypothesis is plausible and should be scientifically investigated is one thing, but defining a new category of cat marking with feces as middening and then proceeding to discuss how middening should be diagnosed and treated is something else entirely (e.g. Neville, 1991;

O'Farrell and Neville, 1994). In general, the concept of a middening behavior problem should be regarded as scientifically unsupported, unconventional among pet behavior problem counselors, and accepted by few if any American behavior specialists. Thus, the approach followed in this chapter is the one followed by Borchelt and Voith (1986), Hart and Hart (1985), Olm and Houpt (1988), and many others: namely, to differentiate between urine marking and inappropriate normal urination while regarding and treating all examples of defecation outside of the litter box as inappropriate normal defecation – and thereby tentatively rejecting the contention that there is such a thing as a middening behavior problem in domestic cats until more convincing evidence in favor of it is provided.

As statistics presented in Chapter 20 indicate, 23% of a sample of 104 serious cat behavior problems involved inappropriate urination and/or defecation. In these cases, 7 of the problems involved only defecation, 8 only urination, and 9 both urination and defecation.

Figure 21.1 presents information concerning the identified or suspected causes of inappropriate urination and/or defecation in a sample of 28 cases. The three definite medical problems involved either an intestinal disorder or bladder infection. Of the five suspected medical causes, four involved abnormally dry stools and the fifth a particularly unhealthy cat showing symptoms like blood in stools and a skin infection at the base of the tail. Three of the four event-related cases involved cats which began eliminating outside of the box when left alone for a week or more when owners went on vacation, and the fourth case concerned a cat which began eliminating outside of the box after spending a week boarded in a university animal hospital. The two fear cases fit the pattern described above where a cat was so afraid of another cat that it remained in a hiding place most of the time and began eliminating there rather than come out to use the litter box.

In 14 out of the 28 cases in this sample, no obvious causal factors could be identified. The problem had existed for periods of time ranging from a few weeks to 5 years, with five of the ca-

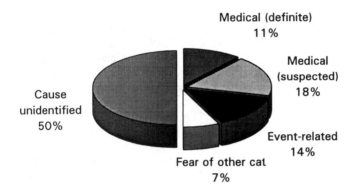

Medical (definite)
11%

Medical
(suspected)
18%

Cause
unidentified
50%

Event-related
14%

Fear of other cat
7%

Figure 21.1: Relative frequency of probable causes of inappropriate urination and/or defecation outside of the litter box in a sample of 28 cases.

ses involving problems that had existed in one form or another for 1 1/2 years or more. When asked if the cat was ill, left alone, or if anything else unusual had happened around the time the problem began, the owners replied that they couldn't remember anything like that. In one of the cases for which the cause was unknown, the cat had been previously treated for the problem with diazepam, which was initially quite effective in eliminating the problem entirely for several weeks. As will be considered below, in cases where fear-related avoidance of the litter box seems to be the main proximate causal factor involved, anxiolytic medication can be a reasonable treatment option – particularly where the problem is of recent origin.

Possible causal factors

Pathophysiological disorder

As mentioned above, disease and other physical problems like dry stools is certainly a common cause and indeed – assuming that some of the 14 cases in the "cause unidentified" category in the above sample of problem cats may have also begun this way – this may be the single most common cause of inappropriate urination and/or defecation problems. Sometimes this is immediately obvious to the veterinarian (e.g. in cases when one of the symptoms which the owner describes along with other illness symptoms is elimination outside of the litter box in a cat which has never done this before). Usually, such elimination prob-

lems require no behavior-oriented treatment. Litter box usage resumes as soon as the illness is well on the way to being healed or stool softeners are administered. In other types of cases, the disease element may not be so immediately apparent. The present author has had several cases where the initial veterinary examination of a cat that had just started eliminating outside of the box failed to reveal any illness. Later, however, disease was discovered as a result of more extensive tests.

Cats that have some kind of medical problem which (presumably) makes elimination painful or uncomfortable tend to start eliminating in other areas besides the litter box. The evolutionary function of this change in behavior is unknown. Extrapolating to a more natural setting, it would result in a cat eliminating in sites other than its formerly preferred one or the communal sites used by, for example, groups of farm cats. To the extent that the germs or parasites responsible are transmitted via elimination products, this change in elimination habits may act in some way to lower the heath-related risks to the animal itself (i.e. through reinfection) or to its genetic relatives (i.e. offspring, siblings). Regardless of function, however, cats with medical problems which affect elimination behave as if they were searching for a new location and/or surface where elimination was not as painful or uncomfortable. If they remain ill, or plagued with some problem like overly dry stools which can also produce discomfort during elimination, cats seem to "try out" new locations/surfaces for a

POSSIBLE CAUSAL FACTORS

Pathophysiological disorder
(disease processes/overly dry stools)

Reaction to major changes in environment
(e.g. new cat in home; cat left alone too long)

Learned aversion to litter box
(e.g. litter box not cleaned often enough; aversion to litter; box poorly sited; cat badly frightened when in box)

Secondary to other behavior problems
(e.g. fear of another cat in home)

INAPPROPRIATE URINATION AND DEFECATION

• Failure to use the litter box for normal excretory urination and/or defecation

POSSIBLE TREATMENT ELEMENTS

Treat related medical problem

Correct owner misconceptions
(e.g. problem not "spite"/"protest" reaction)

Cessation of ineffective methods
(e.g. delayed punishment; confining cat in litter box)

Specific environmental changes
(e.g. clean problem sites; keep cat away from preferred sites; clean litter box more frequently; change litter type; change location of box; alter preferred surface; confine cat to single room/cage)

Treat related behavior problem
(e.g. fear of other cat)

Increase general owner understanding
(problem as learned location/surface preference and/or learned litter box aversion)

Training in problem situations
(mild punishment only when caught in act of eliminating)

Drug therapy
(e.g. anxiolytic medication might help in certain specific cases)

---

short time and then abandon these to go on to others – with the result that over a period of a few weeks, the cat may have eliminated in practically every room and on every kind of surface in the home without developing a stable site preference pattern.

Owners of cats with elimination problems must therefore be questioned closely about the nature of the sites used for elimination and the sequence of sites the cat has used since the problem began. When presenting the problem to a behavior counselor, owners often state that

the cat is eliminating "all over the place". This should not be accepted at face value. Close questioning of the owners of healthy cats usually reveals a distinct *location-related* and/or *surface-related* pattern in the sense that the cat eliminates only in a few specific locations, on a specific type of surface, or a combination of both.

In trying to understand the original cause of why cats have developed well-entrenched and change-resistant habits of eliminating outside of the litter box, some kind of undetected, possibly minor illness that is long since past is therefore a likely candidate. At this stage, however, the matter may be of academic interest only, for it is the cat's residual behavioral habit and not some pathophysiological condition which now must be treated. But an awareness of this causal connection may still be important in these cases as well. Even if the present problem is behavioral and can be solved using the behavior-oriented methods discussed below, owners should be made aware that illness often plays a major role in causing these problems and, therefore, a trip to the family veterinarian is the logical and necessary first step should the problem recur in future.

Learned aversion to litter box

As well as displaying a preference for eliminating at particular locations and/or on particular types of surfaces (e.g. carpets, tiles) outside of the box, cats may also display symptoms that they find something about the litter box aversive. Aside from not entering it to eliminate – which need not indicate an aversion if the cat simply prefers other places more strongly – other symptoms of a litter box aversion in a cat that does sometimes eliminate in the box are the following: the cat runs quickly out of the box after eliminating, no longer scratches and covers in the box (the way it always used to), shakes its paws after contact with the litter, or perches on the rim of the box or squats half in and half outside of it as if trying to eliminate in the box without entering it. If the aversion is very strong, the cat may avoid entering the box entirely and show signs of fear if placed in it.

In a cat that formerly always used the box with its present litter without showing any of these signs, the litter box aversion has obviously been learned as a result of unpleasant experiences the cat has had there. These may be associated with some medical disorder. In effect, discomfort or pain during elimination may become associated with the box through a simple classical conditioning process resulting in a conditioned fear reaction if the cat enters the box which, in turn, causes it to avoid entering it altogether. Theoretically, a similar kind of con-

ditioned aversion could also develop if the cat is badly frightened by something when in the box, or if the box is not being cleaned frequently enough, is used by other cats, or contains runny stools as a result of the cat or another cat in the home having diarrhea.

One related possibility that should not be neglected in these cases is that owners themselves have helped produce the litter box aversion by their ineffective and counterproductive method of carrying the cat to the box (usually just after punishing it while holding its nose close to urine or feces it has deposited outside of the box), putting it in the box, and forcing it to stay there for a few minutes to try to make it understand what it has done wrong and what it should do in the future. This handling and confinement by an emotionally aroused owner may be extremely unpleasant for the cat and, therefore, the danger is great that it will simply add to any aversive qualities of the box, litter, or box location – thereby increasing litter box avoidance in future.

Reactions to major changes in environment

A small percentage of inappropriate urination and/or defecation cases are puzzling in the sense that the origin of the problem does not seem related to any of the above factors. The addition of a new cat to the family, for example, seems to provoke elimination outside of the litter box in some cats. It is not clear why. One could hypothesize that the waste products or odor of a new individual makes the box somewhat aversive to the cat. But why should this be the case? Sometimes this occurs in multi-cat homes where cats are accustomed to sharing the litter box(es) with other cats and have never shown signs that this is a problem. More puzzling still are cases where cats which are left alone for much longer than normal eliminate outside of the box – often on the owner's bed. Why should this happen? Owners always assume that this is a kind of "spite" reaction. Neville (1992) regards this as a form of marking behavior which the cat performs to associate its odor with that of owners, which is particularly concentrated on beds and chairs. And finally,

Borchelt and Voith (1986) regard this reaction as one of the symptoms of separation anxiety in cats where "in a state of anxiety, the cat is attracted to locations that carry an owner's odor". However, none of these explanations are particularly helpful. All essentially point out that the cat is emotionally disturbed in some way at being alone for so long (or having is routine upset), but none gives any kind of plausible account why this should lead to elimination outside of the box. In effect, saying that the cat feels anxious or otherwise distressed by the change does not explain why it eliminates on the owners bed when it feels that way.

In the case of a cat eliminating on the owner's bed when left alone longer than normal, a very different possible explanation is worth considering. Namely, (1) the cat avoids using the box because it becomes unusually soiled (e.g. owner not there at the usual cleaning time, neighbor who is looking after the cat in the owner's absence does not clean the box as diligently as the owner does) and (2) the cat therefore seeks out a new location for elimination which is maximally similar to the litter substrate. Although the resemblances between litter and bed are few, both are soft, depressible surfaces, a similarity that may be critical to the cat. It is possible, therefore, that neither the owner's odor nor the cat's assumed emotionally-disturbed reaction have anything to do with the problem.

Secondary to other behavior problems

One form of excretory urination/defecation problem is not at all puzzling even to owners themselves. Cats that are intensely fearful of other cats in the home sometimes spend almost all of their time in hiding places which they are extremely reluctant to leave. Such cats may eventually start eliminating there presumably because the fear of leaving them is stronger than the forces which attract them to litter box to eliminate. Interesting in such cases is why these cats come out to eat – as most do – but not to eliminate. One obvious answer is that eating is more critical to health and survival than hygiene. But a better one may be that the

behavior of the other cat is much more predictable and the probability of an attack is much lower at feeding times.

Possible treatment elements

Treat medical problem

When the medical problem has not existed for long, successfully treating it will normally resolve the related elimination problem. However, if the medical and associated elimination problems have existed for some time, the animal may have developed a strong aversion to eliminating in the box and/or a strong preference for eliminating at other locations and/or on other surfaces which must then be corrected using the methods described below after the medical condition has been remedied.

Treat related behavior problem

Naturally, a cat which is eliminating in its hiding place will continue to do so as long as the fear of another cat in the home remains acute. Usually this kind of fear problem is highly treatable when it is of recent origin and involves fear on the part of both cats (see Chapter 22). However, when the cat fears an offensively aggressive cat that hunts, chases, and attacks it at every opportunity, the only solution to both the fear and related elimination problem may be to find one of the cats a new home.

Correct owner misconceptions

Most owners entertain the possibility at some point that the cat is eliminating outside of the litter box out of "spite" or as a way of "protesting" against something in the home that is not to its liking. While it may indeed be true that the cat finds something in the home aversive and this may be connected with the problem, this does not mean that the problem is the cat's way of trying to communicate this to the owner. In general, owners should always be dissuaded from attributing human-like motivations and behavioral strategies to cats, for these anthropomorphic beliefs usually stand in the way of the owner's acceptance of the counselor's problem analysis. And if owners don't accept the counselor's explanation, it is unlikely that they will be sufficiently motivated to follow the treatment recommendations either.

Increase general owner understanding

One of the things which owners must understand is that even if the problem is the result of the cat's reaction to something in the home (or about the litter box) which it finds aversive, this does not imply that eliminating this aversive element will be sufficient to solve the problem. Cats which have eliminated frequently outside of the box develop *learned preferences* for eliminating in specific locations or on specific surfaces which can be as strong as the normal house cat's preference for eliminating in the litter box. In effect, by the time the root cause of the problem is discovered and corrected, the cat's habit of eliminating on particular sites outside of the box may be so strong that special methods are required to remedy it. Of course, owners must also understand that a *learned aversion* to the litter box, litter, or litter box location may also be involved, and this too must be reduced along with counteracting learned preferences for other locations/surfaces.

Cessation of ineffective methods

The common punishment method of carrying the cat back to a newly discovered elimination site, putting its nose down close to the spot while punishing it, and then carrying it back to the litter box and forcing it to stay there for a few minutes is objectionable on two grounds. Firstly, punishment more than one or two seconds after a particular behavior like eliminating outside of the litter box will not be associated with the behavior and therefore act to suppress it in future. Such delayed punishments work in human beings, but only because of our symbolic language capability. In effect, there is no way to "explain" to the cat which of the various behaviors is has been engaging in for the last few minutes it is being punished for. What is really

being punished, therefore, is the behavior the cat was in the process of performing precisely at the moment it was set upon by its angry owner. Secondly, carrying the cat to the litter box and confining it there can be very aversive to it and act to strengthen its tendency to avoid using the box in future.

Training in problem situations

Punishing the cat by startling it with a hand clap or other loud noise is only indicated when the cat is caught in the act of eliminating. Of course, this is no solution. Cats quickly learn to delay elimination until no one is around. But it is still to be recommended, for it may act to lower the overall frequency of elimination in a cat which is seldom alone and it facilitates the complete suppression of elimination at times when the cat can be closely supervised.

Specific environmental changes

Successful treatment of these problems generally involves changing various elements of the cat's environment in such a way that it will choose of its own accord to eliminate in the litter box rather than elsewhere. This can be accomplished by increasing the attractiveness of the litter box(es) for elimination while simultaneously reducing the attractiveness of the problem sites or simply keeping the cat entirely away from them.

After the general logic of this approach is thoroughly explained to owners, it should also be explained that it may not be clear from the start which of the following methods for accomplishing the above general objectives will be most effective, and it is possible that a series of two or three combinations of these methods might have to be tried until the right one for the particular problem has been found. Successful treatment often involves the consistent application of the counselor's initial recommendations followed by a progressive modification of these various treatment elements based on how the cat has reacted to them.

- *Thoroughly cleaning problem sites after elimination* is called for because residual odors from elimination products may stimulate further elimination at the site. The use of cleaning products containing ammonia should be avoided because of the chemical similarity of ammonia with urine.

- *Keeping cats entirely away from problem sites* is one obvious way to prevent elimination there. In some cases where the animal's preference for specific sites like on bathroom carpets is strong and there is no concomitant litter box aversion, simply keeping the bathroom door closed to keep the cat out of the room can resolve the problem. Similarly, doing something like placing a large piece of furniture directly over a section of the floor or keeping a little water in bathroom sinks and bathtub is often all that is necessary to resolve problems where cats prefer only these sites to the litter box.

- *Clean litter box more frequently*. Many cats find using a litter box which has not been cleaned for some time aversive. Owners often suspect this on their own when a cat starts eliminating outside of the box at times when they have been especially negligent about cleaning it for several days.

- *Add new litter box(es)*. This is particularly important in multi-cat households where some cats might find it aversive to share a box with other cats or where a single box becomes soiled very quickly. It is also useful in cases where the cat seems to show strong location preferences for two or three different sites in the home. The owner can be advised to initially put new litter boxes at or near all of the preferred locations as a temporary measure that can be gradually phased out once the cat has been consistently using some or all of the boxes for awhile. Finally, using several boxes also allows for a certain amount of experimentation with changes in the type of litter or box itself.

- *Change location of litter box(es)*. Changing the location of the litter box to preferred elimination sites in the home – or putting new litter boxes on these locations as described above – is often a very helpful treatment element. Doing this occurs to most owners, but when the preferred site is in the

middle of the living room they may not be willing to go that far. In persuading them to do this, it helps to point out that this is only a temporary measure. Once the cat has begun consistently using the box at this new site, the box can be gradually moved (e.g. by only a few inches a week at first then by increasingly larger steps later) back to its original location.

- *Experiment with other types of litter*. Most clients have already tried this too, but they may not have gone far enough. In a controlled experimental comparison of the standard commercial clay-based cat litters – which all have particle sizes of around 5–6 mm but vary in terms of deodorants, additives, absorbency, and amount of dust – with other possible litter substances like playbox sand, commercial clay litter with sand-like particle sizes, top soil, and wood shavings, Borchelt (1991) found that the small-grained commercial clay litter was greatly preferred over all of the others. Sand too showed a tendency to be preferred over the larger-particle clay litters and other alternatives. In effect, this experiment confirmed the practice of recommending that owners try materials other than the more or less interchangeable large-particle clay litters – in particular, playbox sand or sand-like commercial clay litters.

One very sensible and productive treatment method is to essentially perform the Borchelt (1991) experiment on a small scale. One can, for example, put several types of litter substances in several makeshift litter boxes (e.g. large plastic containers of any type, cardboard boxes with the sides cut low) and simply allow the cat to chose which it prefers. Appropriate for initial comparisons would be one type of normal litter, the small-particle litter, sand, and perhaps something else like topsoil. When recommending the approach, it is important to point out to owners that this too is a temporary measure. Once the cat is using one or more of the litter boxes consistently again (for several weeks), the new and old litter substances can be mixed together in various proportions (first 90%:10%, then 80%:20%, etc.) to gradually shift back to the originally acceptable and less expensive or inconvenient commercial litter.

- *Drastically alter the nature of preferred surfaces.* In those many cases where a cat strongly prefers eliminating on particular types of surfaces like wall-to-wall carpets, soft throw rugs, linoleum, tiles, or the enamel in sinks and bathtubs – which is clearly seen when the cat eliminates at different locations but always on the same kind of surface – it either must be kept entirely away from this surface or the surface itself must be changed by covering it with some other, very different type of material like heavy plastic foil, cardboard, old carpets, or newspapers. Some experimentation is often required here too before a covering material which inhibits elimination is found. When an effective material has been found, it is kept in place for a few weeks and then later, after the cat has been consistently using the box for some time, gradually removed section by section or by cutting it in strips which are gradually made narrower (and the spaces between wider) over a period of several weeks until it has been removed completely.

- *Confine cat to single room to reestablish litter box use.* Where covering preferred surfaces is impossible or unacceptable – as is usually the case when elimination occurs on wall-to-wall carpets in several rooms in the house – the environment is essentially made more manageable by confining the cat to a single room for a few weeks in which various measures related to the type of surface, box, litter, etc. can be easily manipulated. The cat can be let out of the room as often or for a long as the owner wishes provided that it can be supervised closely enough at this time to entirely prevent elimination. Naturally, much attention must be paid to the cat's social and activity needs, and having the owner schedule several daily playtimes in and outside of the cat's room is one approach to meeting them.

With this confinement approach, the prob-lem is essentially treated in this smaller, more manageable environment precisely as described in the above sections: use of the litter box is reestablished, things are left as they are for several weeks, and then conditions are gradually normalized over the next few weeks by, for example, removing the surface covering material in a stepwise fashion, mixing litter substances in various proportions, and/or reducing the number of boxes. Later, the cat is then gradually given access to the rest of the home – at first only to rooms and at times when it can be kept under close supervision to prevent elimination.

- *Confine cat to cage with floor covered with litter.* In the most extreme cases where the cat's aversion to using the litter box is so strong that none of the above measures prove sufficient to reestablish litter box usage, the cat can be confined for several days to a large cage with the floor entirely covered with litter so that it has no other choice but to eliminate on the litter. Later, the cat's bed can be placed in the cage as well, the proportion of the floor area covered with litter can be gradually reduced, and a litter box of some sort can be introduced. After litter box usage has been reestablished in the cage, the cat can then be given increasing access to the room in which the cage is kept – in which the required surface-covering and box/litter arrangements encourage litter box use – and finally to the other rooms in the home. Here too, the cat must often be let out of the cage, played with, etc. at times when full-time supervision can completely prevent elimination.

One major problem with most of these kinds of recommendations is that owners have already tried versions of them without success, and they may therefore be inclined from the start to be skeptical of whether this kind of approach will be able to eliminate the problem. Remember that owners often suspect that the problem is basically psychological with the cat reacting out of "spite" or "protest" because it is left alone too often or not given enough attention. And when this is the case, convincing owners

SAMPLE RECOMMENDATIONS

Inappropriate urination or defecation outside the litter box

- Punishment of the cat more than a few seconds after it has eliminated outside of the litter box is a completely ineffective way to treat the problem. However, urination or defecation in your presence can be reduced by consistently startling the cat with a loud noise (e.g. clapping your hands) just at the moment it squats to eliminate.
- Never place the cat in the box or force it to stay there. This may have the effect of making it avoid using the box even more.
- Always thoroughly clean the problem sites after the cat has eliminated there to reduce odors which might elicit further elimination. Do not use cleaning products containing ammonia because of its chemical similarity to urine.

Stage 1: prevention of all elimination outside of litter box
(The counselor must decide which of the following alternatives are appropriate for the particular case based on client's description of the problem, position and nature of the sites used for elimination, etc.)

- The cat should not be allowed in the bedroom (bathroom, under the sofa, etc.).
- Place one or more additional litter boxes at other locations in the home.
- Try a box with (without) a hood.
- Place a box directly over the location outside of the litter box where the cat normally eliminates.
- Experiment with using different kinds of litter in the various boxes. In addition to the usual commercial litter products, make sure also to try one of the commercially available litters with extremely small, sand-like particles and/or playbox sand.
- Find a way to drastically change the nature of the surface on which the cat always eliminates by covering it with something very different than the surface itself like thick plastic foil, old carpets, corrugated cardboard, newspapers, etc.
- Temporarily confine the cat along with a litter box to a single room in which it is possible for you to arrange conditions (e.g. covering the entire floor with plastic foil) so that it won't eliminate outside of the box.
- When nothing can be done to get the cat to eliminate in any kind of litter box, keep it for a few days in a cage which has the entire floor covered with litter. After several days, begin providing litter only on a portion of the floor, and as soon as it is regularly eliminating on this rather than the bare floor, place a litter-filled tray in the cage which can later be used outside of the cage.

Stage 2: leave the successful combination of preventative conditions in place for several weeks

- When the right combination of conditions has been found so that elimination outside of the litter box is entirely prevented, don't do anything further for at least another two or three weeks. This will allow the litter box habit to become firmly established.

Stage 3: gradually convert preventative conditions to those which are acceptable on permanent basis
(The following are alternative recommendations corresponding to the various measures used to prevent elimination outside of the litter box)

- After the cat has consistently eliminated in the litter box for several weeks:

  - The material used to cover the floor over the problem sites can be *gradually* removed over a period of several weeks either by taking it away section by section or by cutting it into strips and making the strips a little narrower (and the areas in between a little wider) every week.
  - The number of boxes can be reduced one by one – first at sites where elimination occurred less frequently.
  - The litter can be *gradually* changed to whatever you wish over a period of several weeks by mixing first 10% of the desired litter with that used as part of the corrective treatment, then 20%, 30%, 40%, etc.
  - The litter box can be *gradually* moved to an acceptable location by moving it a little every week (i.e. only a few inches per week at first, then later by increasingly larger steps).
  - The cat can *gradually* be allowed unsupervised access to the rest of the home starting first with rooms in which it has never eliminated.

- If the problem occurs again during this final stage of gradual restoration of normal conditions, you probably have not carried out these changes gradually enough. Go back to the preventative conditions from stage 1, leave them that way for a week or two, and then once again attempt to return to the desired normal conditions, but do so much more slowly and gradually this time.

---

to view the problem as being a kind of "bad habit" which can be entirely resolved by a combination of these environmental-change methods can be problematic.

Of course, owners should also be explicitly warned not to give up too soon. One can emphasize that while this combination of increasing box attractiveness with reducing problem site acceptability may not immediately solve the problem, making a systematic and persistent attempt to combine, recombine, or modify these various kinds of treatment elements – and thinking about what related kinds of concrete steps can be taken to solve the problem using this kind of general approach – ultimately results in the correction of almost all of these problems.

Another warning which should be given to owners is that the cat will never entirely forget its old problem elimination habits, and it is

therefore possible or even likely that the problem will recur now and again in future. If and when this happens and a veterinary examination indicates that there is no pathophysiological problem, the treatment process which led to solution should simply be reinstated. When this is done shortly after the problem recurs, it can usually be quickly resolved, for the cat's more desirable habit of using the litter box is not forgotten so easily either. Generally speaking, it does not bother owners to know that a problem may be recurrent as long as they have an effective solution to apply every time one of these relapses occur.

A final note: one approach that all owners have tried without success is to apply one of the many commercially-available cat repellent substances to the elimination sites outside of the box. The study by Schilder (1991) comparing the repellent effects of several commercially available repellents is consistent with the experience of pet problem counselors that these products are rarely effective.

Drug therapy

As mentioned above, one of my recent inappropriate urination cases involved a cat which had been successfully treated with diazepam for a period of a few weeks. This is consistent with results reported by Hart et al. (1993) for the experimental treatment of inappropriate urination in 9 cats with *buspirone* for several weeks at dosages ranging from 2.5 to 5 mg/cat po bid. Five of these cats (56%) resumed using the litter box and three (33%) continued using it after the drug was gradually withdrawn after 10 weeks of buspirone treatment. Although a very small sample size is involved and the study was uncontrolled in the sense that no placebo group or pretreatment control condition was included, the beneficial effect of this drug in some cases seems clear. Logically, one would expect anxiolytic drug treatment to be most helpful in cases where (1) fear-related avoidance of the litter box is one of the major proximate causal factors and (2) the problem is of recent origin so that no strong preferences for elimination at other locations and/or on other surfaces have as yet developed. Cases where failure to use the litter box do not immediately resolve themselves after some underlying medical problem has been successfully treated would certainly fit this description. (See the "drug therapy" subsection in Chapter 8 for side effects and other important drug-related information.)

References

Beaver, B.V. (1992): *Feline Behavior: A Guide for Veterinarians*. 2nd Edition. Philadelphia, W.B. Saunders Company.

Borchelt, P.L. (1991): Cat elimination behavior problems. *Veterinary Clinics of North America: Small Animal Practice* **21**, 257–264.

Borchelt, P. L., and Voith, V. L. (1986): Elimination behavior problems in cats. *Compendium on Continuing Education for the Practicing Veterinarian* **8**, 197–205.

Bradshaw, J. W. S. (1992): *The Behaviour of the Domestic Cat*. Wallingford, UK, CAB International

Hart, B. L., Eckstein, R.A., Powel, K. L., and Dodman, N. H. (1993): Effectiveness of buspirone on urine spraying and inappropriate urination in cats. *Journal of the American Veterinary Medical Association* **203**, 254–258.

Hart, B. L., and Hart, L.A. (1985): *Canine and Feline Behavior Therapy*. Philadelphia, Lea & Febiger.

Neville, P (1992): Behaviour patterns that conflict with domestication. In J.W.S. Bradshaw: *The Behaviour of the Domestic Cat*. Wallingford, UK, CAB International.

O'Farrell, V., and Neville, P. (1994): *Manual of Feline Behaviour*. Shurdington, Cheltenham, Gloucestershire, UK, British Small Animal Veterinary Association.

Olm, D.D., and Houpt, K.A. (1988): Feline house-soiling problems. *Applied Animal Behaviour Science* **20**, 335–345.

Robinson, I. (1992): Social behaviour of the cat. In Thorne, C. (ed): *The Waltham Book of Dog and Cat Behaviour*. Oxford, Pergamon Press.

Reisner, I. (1991): The pathophysiologic basis of behavior problems. *Veterinary Clinics of North America: Small Animal Practice* **21**, 207–224

Schilder, M. B. H. (1991): The (in)effectiveness of anti-cat repellents and motivational factors. *Applied Animal Behaviour Science* **32**, 227–236.

22   Fear and Aggression Problems

Cats show a variety of fear and aggression behavior problems. Figure 22.1 shows a breakdown of 36 major problems (n = 32 cats) which fall into these two categories. Overall, 26% of the sample of 86 cat cases referred to in the last chapter involved aggression to either humans or other cats as the primary presenting problem. This is in line with statistics from other behavior problem practices which indicate that after elimination problems, aggression is the second most common type of cat behavior problem (e.g. Beaver, 1989a, 1989b).

Fear problems

Fear of particular family members

Fearful behavior is common among cats. According to data collected with the help of the client information form described in Chapter 6, 62 % of 87 problem cat owners and 53% of 49 normal, non-problem cat owners indicated that their animals sometimes showed excessive fear reactions. The most commonly cited fear-eliciting stimuli were strange humans, noises, child-

ren, family members, other animals, riding in a car, and being outside.

Apart from fear of another cat, which will be discussed in the defensive aggression section later in the chapter, the most common fear problem for which owners seek expert advice is fear of particular family members. Although fear of strangers is much more common, this is usually regarded by owners as a form of normal behavior which creates no real problem. The cat hides as soon as visitors enter the home and stays hidden until they leave, and owners simply accept this wariness of strangers as being a feature of their cat's personality.

Fear of particular family members is, however, a major problem for the feared person, the rest of the family, and the cat itself. The cat makes the feared person feel like a monster and, the person assumes, look like a monster in the eyes of other people. It is a problem for all of the other family members who prefer harmony within the family and are uncomfortable or upset when serious relationship problems of any kind exist. And unlike fear of visitors who are only occasionally present and easily avoid-

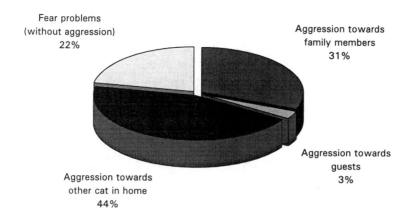

Fear problems
(without aggression)
22%

Aggression towards
family members
31%

Aggression towards
other cat in home
44%

Aggression towards
guests
3%

Figure 22.1: Relative frequency of the major general types of cat fear and aggression problems in a sample of 32 cases.

able, living under the same roof with a feared family member can be a constant source of stress for the cat itself that must adversely affect the quality of its life.

Possible causal factors

Aversive experiences

The most common cause of fear of particular family members is punishment to correct other major and minor behavior problems like housesoiling or destructive scratching. The problem may develop slowly with repeated punishments steadily increasing the cat's underlying fear, or it can appear suddenly which

indicates that such owner behavior can represent truly traumatic experiences for some cats. Other causes besides punishment are less common but nevertheless should be explored during the consultation in cases where owner punishment seems not to be a major factor. For example, the feared person may be the one that operates that horror of all horrors – the vacuum cleaner. Or the person may have been playing too roughly with the cat (e.g. dangling it in the air). It is also common for owners to force contact with the cat, force it to submit to unpleasant petting, force it to stay in certain locations (litter box if there is a housesoiling problem), or young children might force the cat to tolerate having doll clothes put on and being

---

POSSIBLE CAUSAL FACTORS

Aversive experiences
(e.g. owner punishing cat, playing too roughly with it, forcing it to endure aversive petting, confinement, etc.)

Inherited predisposition
(e.g. suspected reason why some cats particularly prone to reacting fearfully/ developing fear problems)

Unintentional owner fostering
(e.g. forcing contact with fearful cat as means of trying to reduce its fear)

FEAR OF PARTICULAR FAMILY MEMBER
• Animal avoids contact with and shows fearful behavior when approached by a particular family member

POSSIBLE TREATMENT ELEMENTS

Correct owner mistakes
(punishment contraindicated)

Cessation of counterproductive methods
(e.g. forcing contact as means of reducing fear)

Drug therapy
(as adjunct to behavior-oriented treatment especially where close contact with feared person inevitable)

Avoid problem situations
(e.g. feared person should avoid closely approaching cat)

Increase general owner understanding
(e.g. best way to have good relationship with cat is to let it determine the time, place, and duration of social interactions)

wheeled around in a baby carriage. Essentially, some cats react passively (i.e. non-aggressively) to these forms of aversive owner treatment, but they escape as soon as they can and avoid the person as much as possible later – clear evidence that such kinds of treatment are aversive for the cat.

Inherited predisposition

There are great individual differences between cats in how sensitive they are to environmental stimuli in the sense of either tolerating or reacting fearfully to aversive environmental events. Some cats can be punished relatively severely without developing any kind of fear problem while others are highly prone to developing such problems and must be handled with great care. When asked, owners can easily describe their cats' "personalities" in this regard. Exploring in the consultation the cat's general tendencies to react fearfully to various kinds of environmental stimuli including those stemming from the owner's behavior is very helpful in developing an understanding of why this particular cat has developed the behavior problem it displays.

That such individual differences often reflect genetic differences between cats is most clearly seen in cases where great differences are observed between cats raised in identical environments, or when cats from the same litter that are raised in different homes develop similar "personalities". Research indicates that the behavioral tendencies or personalities of mothers and fathers appear to be fairly good predictors of some important aspects of the future behavior of kittens like, for example, how social or friendly the animals will be towards human beings and other cats (Turner et al., 1986).

Unintentional owner fostering

Owners often try to actively combat these fear problems by holding the cat against its will, petting it when it doesn't want to be petted, or catching and holding it when it tries to run away as an attempt to show it that this kind of

contact can be pleasant and convince it that their intentions are the friendliest. But such well-intentioned owner behavior only makes matters worse. Even non-fearful cats find this kind of treatment at least mildly aversive, and when the cat is fearful of the person to start with, such contact is doubly aversive. As will be discussed below, only controlled exposure to the mildest of fear-arousing stimuli is to be recommended as a treatment for fear problems.

Possible treatment elements

Correct owner mistakes

Some owners go too far in using punishment to control minor behavioral problems in their cats, and some cats are especially prone to become fearful of anyone in the family who punishes them. Regardless of whether it is a case of overly severe punishment or a hypersensitive cat, the advice is the same: no more punishment – especially by the family member the cat now fears.

Avoid problem situations

Unnecessarily exposing the cat to the fear-eliciting stimuli or situations should be avoided. Basically, the feared person should avoid approaching the fearful cat too closely to the extent that this is possible within the family situation. Of course, some contact is inevitable, but it can often be greatly reduced once the owner realizes that this is called for.

Cessation of counterproductive treatment methods

Naturally, the counterproductive methods of the feared person approaching or catching the cat, forcing it to endure petting, or holding it against its will on the theory that this will reduce the fear by showing the cat that there is really nothing to be afraid of must be abandoned. These will simply make the cat more fearful and thereby increase the severity of the problem.

Increase general owner understanding

Aside from pointing out to owners that their brand of punishment is obviously too severe for their particular cat – and that certain kinds of contact between the feared person and the cat should be reduced – it also helps to discuss with owners the desirability of the general strategy of fostering a good relationship with the cat by letting it be the one that makes all social initiatives. In problem cats as in normal cats, this seems to be the way to maximize a cat's tendency to approach owners and engage in social interactions for longer periods of time (Turner, 1991).

Drug therapy

When fear is particularly intense in a family situation where close contact to the feared family member is unavoidable, a course of treatment with some tranquilizing medicament like *diazepam, buspirone,* or *amitriptyline HCl* may be a helpful adjunct to behavior-oriented measures (see Table 20.1 in Chapter 20 for dosages and the "drug therapy" subsection in Chapter 8 for side effects and other important drug-related information).

Fear of specific environmental stimuli or situations

The basic principles for the treatment of fear of noises, going outside, riding in the car, etc. are the same as in treating fear problems in other complex animal species such as dogs and human beings. They are as follows:

- Avoid exposing the cat to all situations/stimuli which evoke intense fear.
- Draw up a hierarchy of fear-eliciting situations/stimuli ranging from those to which the cat shows only the mildest degree of fear to those in which its fear is extremely intense.
- If it is possible to arrange, expose the cat only to versions of the feared situations/stimuli which evoke only the very mildest fear reactions.
- Repeatedly expose the cat to these as often as possible to habituate it to them to the point that it no longer reacts fearfully.
- If it is possible to elicit positive, non-fearful behavior (eating, playing) in these situations, this can accelerate the habituation process.
- Once the cat's fear to the mildest fear-arousing situations/stimuli has habituated, em-

---

SAMPLE RECOMMENDATIONS

Fear of a particular family member

- Stop punishing the cat.
- Never force contact with the cat. Instead always wait for it to come to you of its own free accord.
- You can give the cat food tidbits, but only when it comes to you of its own free will.
- Always move slowly and calmly around the cat.
- As far as possible, avoid coming too close to the place where it is resting.
- Stop petting the cat as soon as it begins showing even the slightest signs of restlessness or discomfort.
- The feared person should be the only family member to feed the cat or give it food tidbits.
- Other family members should temporarily ignore all the cat's initiatives to elicit playing, petting, and other forms of social contact.
- Someone other than the feared person should take over the vacuum cleaning *(if cat is especially fearful of the vacuum cleaner).*

ploy the same treatment methods with the situations/stimuli to which the cat originally reacted somewhat more fearfully.

- Repeat this process for each of the steps in the hierarchy of fear-eliciting stimuli.
- Do not go on to the next step in the hierarchy until the cat has fully habituated to the last one and no longer shows the slightest trace of fear.
- The temporary administration of anxiolytic medication can lower the level of the animal's fear when exposure to fear-eliciting situations that are too intense to be easily habituated cannot be avoided.
- Gradually reducing the dosage after an effective drug and dosage have been found can help to habituate the cat to these situations/stimuli.

Of course, the specific treatment plan and recommendations depend greatly on the type of fear-eliciting stimulus or situation. For example, attempting to reduce a cat's fear to riding in a car would obviously involve a very different procedure than attempting to reduce its fear of visitors.

That such fear problems are potentially treatable does not mean that they are in fact normally treated. Most cats that are afraid of noises or strangers are simply allowed to hide until the feared situation is past. Cats which are afraid to go outside are not forced to do so. Unlike fear of family members, most of these other fear problems are not problems for owners and only occasionally represent problems for the cat itself. They are therefore usually not regarded as requiring correction. In effect, owners tend to accept the cat's fearful behavior as being part of its personality and react with understanding in the sense of doing nothing to hinder its escape and avoidance behavior.

Fear of litter, litter box, box location

As discussed in Chapter 21, conditioned fear reactions to something having to do with the litter box is a common causal factor in many inappropriate urination and/or defecation cases. Here treatment is essential. The behavioral strategy involves (1) strengthening approach-

eliciting and eliminating-eliciting aspects of litter box characteristics to the extent that these can override the cat's fear-related tendency to avoid eliminating there, (2) reducing the elimination-eliciting features of other sites in the home, and (3) setting up conditions which facilitate gradual habituation to eliminating in the box by arranging things so that fear is minimized (e.g. when box is provided away from its usual location with a new type of litter and then gradually moved back to its original location later). All three treatment elements have parallels in the treatment of fear of particular family members: having feared family member take over feeding and all tidbit-giving would increase approach, having other family members ignore cat would decrease its tendency to approach them when seeking contact, and having the feared person avoid approaching the cat minimizes fear in a way which would favor the required habituation process. In short, similar principles are involved, although the specific form the treatment takes reflects the very different nature of the feared stimulus and behavioral system involved. The suggestion by Hart et al. (1993) that *buspirone* may often be helpful in such inappropriate elimination cases underscores this parallel and adds force to the notion that some elimination behavior problems are basically fear problems.

Fear of another cat in the home

Sometimes owners report that one cat in the family fears another and therefore avoids all contact with it and may spend most of its time hiding in some secure corner in the home. Where such problems involve no aggression on the part of either cat, it is often a case of a younger cat's friendly or playful approaches being intolerable to the other cat which is basically non-aggressive and prefers to run away rather than aggressively defend itself.

In such cases, it is probably best simply to recommend finding a new home for one of the cats. Since the behavior of the cat which is feared is not manageable the way, for example, a fear-eliciting person's behavior is, the problem is essentially untreatable. The friendly or playful cat will simply continue approaching the other in spite of continual rebuffs – and it may even enjoy the resulting running away/chasing game and play it at every opportunity. The problem is, however, that the quality of life of a cat which must spend most of its life avoiding contact and running away and hiding in fear is dismal. And therefore separating it from the other cat may represent the only humane solution.

Aggression behavior problems

Forms of cat aggression

Interestingly, there are major differences between behavior problem specialists in the matter of how many different forms of cat aggression should be distinguished. For example, Hart and Hart (1991), Chapman (1991), Borchelt and Voith (1987), and Beaver (1989) distinguish between 6, 8, 9, and 12 different diagnostic categories respectively. This diversity is revealing, for it reflects something of the uncertainty which is involved in classifying cat aggression problems in terms of the biological function and/or eliciting situation criteria that are more easily applied to dog aggression cases.

Cats are group living only under conditions where abundant food sources provided by human beings are available and cats need not hunt for their food. Such groups lack the co-operative behavioral unit character of the dog pack in which various behavioral mechanisms act to promote group cohesion, coordination, and cooperation in spite of potential competition among group members for limited resources. In comparison to dogs, cats display only rudimentary forms of dominance-submission relationships and no cooperative group defensive or hunting behavior. As a result, meaningful distinctions between intragroup vs. extragroup aggression are more difficult to draw in cats than dogs. And the somewhat asocial nature of cat behavior – which gives the relationship between fellow cat group members an impressional quality more of mutual tolerance than of cohesion and cooperation – makes even the intraspecific versus interspecific

behavior dimension less helpful in understanding various aspects of their aggressive behavior towards each other and towards human beings than in dogs. In short, cat aggression problems require a somewhat different kind of classification system than that which is appropriate for dogs.

At present, the classification systems used for cat aggression problems in the literature are purely empirical. Cat problem case files are, so to speak, sorted into different categories depending, for example, on target, situation, and form-related characteristics. These types of cases are then discussed separately as if they had little or nothing to do with one another. But consider, for example, what are commonly referred to as fear aggression, petting-elicited aggression, pain-elicited aggression, feline asocial aggression, and so-called redirected aggression. Although they differ in context, they are all in some obvious sense purely *defensive* in that they function to in some way drive or keep some threatening or bothersome individual away. On the other hand, other cat aggression problems involve more obviously *offensive* forms of aggression as is the case, for example, with so-called play aggression towards human beings, territorial aggression where a resident cat attacks a new cat in the home, and intermale aggression – a more ritualized form of aggression between males which in wild-living groups results younger males being driven away (and older males being kept away) from cat groups containing breeding females. It seems clear therefore that classification of the various cat aggression problems must start with this defensive-vs.-offensive dimension.

The tolerance concept

Tolerance is a key concept that will be used throughout the following discussion of different forms of cat aggression problems. The tolerance concept and various related expressions like "mutual tolerance" and "lack of tolerance" will be used first and foremost to describe features of the relationship between cats. Simply stated, mutual tolerance exists when two or more house cats can live peacefully in the same home – or two or more farm cats can live peacefully in the same barnyard – without serious fighting. And conversely, an obvious lack of tolerance exists in intercat aggression cases in which the two cats always begin fighting on sight.

The use of the tolerance concept in discussions of cat aggression is not new. Consider, for example, the following quote from Chapman (1991):

> " When territorial aggression is triggered by the introduction of a new cat, it is possible that the cats may learn to tolerate each other over weeks or months. It is also possible that they will never tolerate each other." (p. 318)

Treatment then would presumably focus on building up tolerance for the newcomer in the resident cat, and failure of treatment recommendations would therefore imply failure to reduce the resident's lack of tolerance for the other.

As considered above, the basis of cat sociality is not mutual attraction, group cohesion, and cooperative group behavior as in dogs, but rather in the adult cat's ability to tolerate the presence of adult conspecifics under certain conditions. Basically, cats can peacefully coexist when the environmental conditions facilitate this. Presumably the process of domestication has involved selection pressures to develop further whatever behavioral mechanisms made it possible for predomesticated cats to tolerate each other's presence around abundant, highly-localized food sources like human rubbish dumps and granaries.

The importance of the concept of tolerance to understanding and treating some of the cat aggression problems will be illustrated throughout several of the following discussions. Suffice to say at this point that for many problems involving aggression between cats, the key questions of concern is not, for example, whether the form of aggression is best labeled territorial, fear, feline asocial, feline dispersion, or redirected, but rather how and why tolerance has broken down and/or how tolerance can be established or reestablished.

The simple classification system outlined in the next few paragraphs will be used as a con-

ceptual basis for considering common cat aggression problems. It is quite different than that used to classify dog aggression problems in Chapter 9. Although dogs and cats are both mammalian carnivores, there are critical social behavioral differences between the two species which must necessarily be reflected in the approach taken to understanding aggressive social behavioral problems.

Defensive aggression

Many cat aggression problems involve aggressive behavior which serves some sort of immediate self-protective function. Here, three basic types of scenarios can be distinguished:

- *Defensively aggressive responses to threatening/aggressive behavior* on the part of another cat or human being – for example, when a cat is attacked or seriously threatened by another cat, when it is punished by a human being, or when someone does something to it which elicits pain.
- *Asocial reactions* where the cat behaves aggressively to terminate or prevent unwanted social interactions with another cat or human being. As Beaver (1992) suggests, this is a common reaction of an older cat to the playful advances of a younger one. Also common is the cat's response to either petting by the owner which has gone on too long or the owner's attempt to pick it up and hold it when it is not in the mood for such things. So-called redirected aggression also falls into this category in cases where a cat turns and attacks its owner if disturbed when it is still in an aggressive mood following some kind of aggressive interaction with another cat.
- *Aggressive reactions in competitive situations* as when, for example, a cat growls threateningly when another cat approaches to try and take prey away from it.

Offensive aggression

In the above cases, the cat's aggressive behavior is purely *reactive* – a defensive response to some individual which has approached it, is doing something to it, or is threatening it.

In contrast, cat aggression can also be more *active* or offensive in the sense of the cat initiating aggressive behavior towards another cat or human being which appears entirely unprovoked and therefore cannot be construed as defensive in any kind of proximate, reactive sense.

• *Playful attacks* are naturally most common in younger cats. However, some older cats remain playfully aggressive into adulthood especially if this is fostered or tolerated by their owners. Playful aggression also appears to be the source of so-called instrumental aggression: for example, a cat which springs on the owner's bed and playfully attacks the owner's feet through the blanket may be inadvertently rewarded by the owner's attempt to divert the cat's interest to some other game (e.g. by throwing a toy) or feed it to get it to stop being so bothersome. This, in turn, strengthens the cat's tendency to attack the owner's feet for obvious reasons.

• *Offensive aggression* in the form of unprovoked and sometimes vicious attacks seems to reflect a kind of complete intolerance for the presence of another cat. This form of aggression is most commonly seen in a resident cat's attacks on a new cat in the home. Another common scenario in the home is when the victim behaves fearfully or when it is otherwise behaving abnormally (e.g. when recovering from an operation). Fights between tomcats outdoors also involve this sort of offensive aggression at least in terms of the unprovoked initiation of threats which may lead to serious fighting if one of the males doesn't try and avoid a fight. From a biological viewpoint, the primary function of aggression in these contexts is probably to drive the victim away, and indeed such forms of aggression are often referred to as territorial aggression in the pet problem literature.

Although a somewhat more conventional approach to referring to the various aggression problem scenarios will be followed below, an attempt will be made to analyze and understand the nature and possible forms of each type of aggression problem in terms established by the above discussion.

"Fear aggression" between cats living in the same home

As every small animal veterinarian knows from experience, a fearful cat is a potentially dangerous cat. Behavioral signs that a cat is fearful are easy to detect: pupils are dilated, ears laid back against the head, the cat may crouch with head drawn close to its body and legs tucked under its body, and it may hiss and spit. The classical Halloween cat with ears back and pupils dilated but standing stretched upright, sideways to the threatening stimulus with back arched and fur erect is a threat posture signaling a highly fearful cat's readiness to attack if approached further.

The target of such defensive aggression can be another cat, a dog, or a human being. Distinguishing this form of aggression from others is based on two major features of the cat's behavior. It shows fearful behavior immediately preceding attacks and it only attacks if the fear-eliciting target approaches too closely, attempts to touch it, or – in the case of another cat – threatens or attacks it.

As far as fear-related defensive aggression towards human beings is concerned, this is seldom a problem for owners unless they must approach the fearful cat, for example, to administer some kind of medication. Cats which threaten adult family members or scratch them when fearful are usually simply left alone until they can be approached without eliciting signs of fear. And owners are generally wise enough to find a new home for the cat if the family's toddler is endangered. As a result, most of the fear-related aggression problems which come to the attention of behavior counselors involve aggression between two or more cats in the same home. As the following discussion indicates, there are a variety of forms of this problem which must take into account the behavior and motivation of both cats: not only defensive aggression on the part of a highly fearful cat may be involved, but various forms of offensive or defensive aggression on the part of the other cat as well.

Possible causal factors

Possible genetic/early experience factors

Naturally, cats which tend to be somewhat timid or fearful by nature may be much more prone to reacting fearfully and becoming defensively aggressive than other cats. With this type of cat, the event that precipitated the first severe fight between the cats is usually much less

obvious to the owner than in the other scenarios described below. Insofar as such timidity or fearfulness may reflect the cat's limited early experiences with other cats – rather than genetic factors – potentially this too could play a role in understanding why the problem has developed.

Fear-arousing event

The sudden appearance of a serious aggression problem between two cats which have gotten along well together is often the result of some unusual fear-arousing event like a

---

POSSIBLE CAUSAL FACTORS

Possible genetic/early experience factors
(e.g. possible source of excessive fearfulness in one of the cats)

Fear-arousing event
(e.g. initial fight occurs when one or both cats badly frightened in presence of other)

Fear-arousing social interactions
(e.g. fearful reaction of one cat to approach of playful or offensively aggressive cat, or in response to defensive aggression of asocial cat)

Conditioned fear/aggression
(e.g. mutual threatening/fighting increases fear/aggression)

"FEAR AGGRESSION" BETWEEN TWO CATS IN THE HOME

• Aggression problem appears to directly result from one or both cats' fear of the other.

POSSIBLE TREATMENT ELEMENTS

Avoid problem situations
(keep cats separated to prevent fighting)

Correct owner misconceptions
(e.g. if owner views problem as dispute over dominance)

Increase general owner understanding
(e.g. problem involves cats' normal behavioral reactions to fear-eliciting individuals; underlying fear must be treated)

Behavior therapy methods
(e.g. keep cats in adjacent rooms with net strung across common doorway; keep one or both cats in cage/on leash)

Drug therapy
(e.g. in some cases where fear particularly intense or mild fear problem is of recent origin)

bookcase falling over with a loud crash or the entrance of a strange dog or cat into the home. In one of my cases, the two cats began fighting one morning when all of family members tried on their new, strangely-rustling, high-tech skiwear for the first time. Borchelt and Voith (1987) describe an "accident" scenario where one cat was innocently sitting on a windowsill when the other came charging aggressively towards the window in response to seeing a cat outside in the yard. This sudden aggressive approach immediately frightened and elicited fear-related defensive aggression in the cat that was just sitting on the windowsill peacefully minding its own business.

Fear-arousing social interactions

Neither cat may be fearful at the time the problem began. One common variant is where the problem starts somewhat innocently when a basically playful or friendly cat approaches another which reacts asocially and crouches, hisses, or lashes out, which in turn may elicit fear and/or defensive aggression in the friendly cat and lead to a snowballing of what has become a fear-related aggressive encounter on both sides. Of course, defensive aggression is also often elicited when a cat is boldly threatened or attacked by an offensively aggressive cat.

Conditioned fear/aggression

As a general rule, mutual threatening/fighting tends to increase each animal's fear of the other and therefore the fear-related aggression problem. This can happen very quickly in some cases: one serious fight can result in a cat reacting fearfully and aggressively the next time the other is encountered even though it is not displaying any kind of threatening behavior. In other cases, the problem develops much more slowly. Mild growling in one cat gives way to growling on both sides, then minor skirmishes, then a series of increasingly vicious fights all taking place over a period of several weeks.

Possible treatment elements

Avoid problem situations

Unless the problem appears to be only a relatively mild temporary "misunderstanding" between two cats that is likely to disappear on its own – as many of these problems do – owners are advised to keep the cats separated to prevent the fighting and mutual threatening which tends to increase the severity of the problem.

Correct owner misconceptions

Some owners suspect that the cats are basically fighting over dominance and therefore the problem will resolve itself if the cats are left to fight it out on their own. Of course, such an erroneous view must be corrected, for preventing all fighting and mutual threatening is vital to successful treatment in serious cases.

Increase general owner understanding

It is explained to owners that problems of this kind between cats which have always gotten along well are fairly common and should be viewed as normal behavior for cats which have become afraid of each other for some reason – basically, that the problem is more a fear rather than an aggression problem.

Behavior therapy methods

The logic of the most common *desensitization* method is to allow the cats to only have contact with one another in situations where fighting is entirely prevented and the fear elicited is mild enough to gradually habituate. One very useful method for doing this is to keep the two separated in adjacent rooms with some type of net strung across the common doorway. Each cat can see, smell, and hear the other, and if they wish, they can approach each other closely any time. But if one cat is extremely fearful of another, this allows it to remain safe (behind the net) and far away from the other (at the end of the room opposite the net) whenever and for as long as it likes. This essentially allows both cats to relax in each other's presence and – as fear continues to habituate – come as close to one another as they can comfortably tolerate. The procedure also calls for switching cats and rooms everyday, which presumably helps accustom each to the other's odor. Also, cats are at first fed from food bowls which are far away from the net and, therefore, one does not attempt to use food to coax the cats to go so close to one another that they become fearful – which would retard the habituation process. Only later, when the cats are approaching each other and remaining close to one another on opposite sides of the net of their own accord are the food bowls placed close to the net. And finally, owners may also be instructed to carry out what are basically *counterconditioning* measures to promote positive, non-fearful behavior in potential problem situations. For example, feeding the cats small meals and playing with each several times a day in this situation is assumed to promote fear reduction by eliciting eating and playing behavior which is incompatible with fear.

These measures are applied day after day until the animals become fully accustomed to one another again – which means they often approach each other, eat together next to the net, and sniff each other through the net without showing the slightest trace of fear. Then the net is taken away.

In cases where the fear is of recent origin and not so intense, the problem is usually resolved in this way in a matter of several days. In more severe cases, it can take longer. But this is usually no problem, for these measures can be kept in place for as long as necessary without creating a severe hardship for family members who can, if necessary, attach the net so that it can be easily opened and closed again to allow family members to use the doorway as normal.

Where the physical design of the home precludes this kind of approach (e.g. in one-room apartments), a single cage, two cages, or one or two leashes can be used to create the same conditions. In the sample recommendations box below, for example, an alternative method based on the same principles is described in which one of the cats is housed in a cage for several hours a day, which allows the

other to move about the home at will and accustom itself to the presence of the other without becoming fearful. Another possible variant might be to keep the two cats on leashes on opposite ends of a large room. Here, cats are bound far apart for several days and then the distance between them is gradually reduced over the next several days as they become accustomed to being in the room together without becoming fearful.

A very different method is also worth mentioning. Although rarely recommended by behavior counselors, there may well be certain family/home situations in which would be a fully acceptable and effective approach to the problem. The cats can be kept in cages side by side for several hours a day even though they are very close to and therefore very fearful of one another. If kept like this long enough, fear reactions would be expected to eventually subside and the cats would eventually learn to eat, live, play, etc. in close proximity to one another without being fearful. This is a version of the *flooding* behavior therapy procedure where an animal – cat or human – is continuously exposed to fear eliciting stimuli at their full intensity for a period of time that is long enough for even the most intense fear to subside. To be effective, however, each exposure must last long enough for the fear to decrease considerably, which may well take several hours. Short periods of exposure where the fear is just as strong at the end as it was at the beginning are counterproductive. In the long run, these increase rather than decrease fear. Using a human example, one might well be able to cure an elevator phobia in human beings by having them ride up and down in an elevator nonstop for 6 or 8 hours a day for several days or weeks, but a series of many short trips in which they are as fearful (or more so) when they step out of the elevator as when they stepped into it will simply make the problem worse.

Drug therapy

Anxiolytic drugs may be helpful adjuncts during the initial stages of behavioral treatment in cases where the fear of one or both animals is

SAMPLE RECOMMENDATIONS

"Fear aggression" between two cats in the home

Scenario A: *problem is very mild and of recent origin:*
- At the moment, don't take any steps against this problem. It is possible that the cats will learn to get along again on their own.
- However, if severe fighting should occur which leaves one or both cats extremely fearful, the following treatment method should be consistently applied:

Scenario B: *problem is severe enough to necessitate taking active steps to prevent further fighting:*

Net method:
- Keep the cats separated in different rooms until that each can tolerate being near to the other without showing signs of fear or aggressiveness.
- Close the doorway between the two rooms with a net of some sort (like a fishing or tennis net) so that the cats can see, smell, and hear each other – and approach each other closely enough to touch each other through the net if they wish.
- Change each cat into the other room every day.
- Don't try to bring, force, or entice the two to come close to one another. In the beginning, place food and water bowls far from the net. Only later, when the cats are coming close to one another often and without showing signs of fear or aggression, the food bowls can be put progressively closer to the net. Basically, always let both cats decide for themselves how closely they approach one another.
- Don't take the net away until the cats have shown only normal, peaceful, friendly, etc. behavior when they come in contact with one another through the net – and they approach each other often without showing signs of fear or nervousness – for several consecutive days.

Cage method:
- Keep the less fearful cat in a cage for several hours a day, and allow the other free access to the room and cage area.
- Completely separate the two during times of the day when one of the cats is not confined to the cage.
- Try to feed both cats in the room where one is confined to the cage. If possible, divide the daily food ration into 3-4 small meals distributed throughout the day. However, if the most fearful cat won't enter the room of its own accord, don't force it to. Feed it outside the room but move the feeding location progressively closer to the room and then progessively more and more into the room over the course of several days providing its fear has subsided sufficiently to allow it to enter the room without becoming fearful.
- When the most fearful cat has learned to go fairly close to the cage without showing signs of fear, start keeping the least fearful cat bound to a particular place in the room with a leash instead of in a cage during the several hours per day that the two are allowed to have contact with one another.
- Don't let the cat loose from the leash in the other's presence until the two have essentially interacted normally with one another for several days and it is therefore clear that the fear problem is completely past.

particularly intense. Another possible application is where the fear has just recently appeared (i.e. within the past several days) and is still fairly mild. In this case, drug therapy alone may solve the problem. There are no hard and fast rules or clear guidelines, however, for when drug therapy is or is not appropriate. While the solution of most of these problems does not require medicating one or both animals, the prescription of a temporary course of drug treatment – with a tapered dosage – may be beneficial in particular cases. (See Table 20.1 in Chapter 20 for drugs/dosages and the "drug therapy" subsection in Chapter 8 for side effects and other important drug-related information).

Defensive aggression in response to aversive stimuli

Defensive behavior need not involve conditioned fear. Cats may also simply lash out with teeth and claws when bothered or molested by something – a natural reaction which need not represent any kind of behavior problem if it is possible to avoid doing the things that elicit the aggression.

A basically non-aggressive, non-fearful cat may react aggressively if stepped on or poked at, hit, or has its fur pulled by a young child. Medicating or manipulating a painful area may also cause a cat to lash out with its claws and bite as a defensive response to the pain or discomfort. As Beaver (1989c) points out, this type of pain-elicited defensive aggression should always be suspected when young children are attacked while playing unsupervised with the cat. Naturally, a bite from a playful cat might elicit aggression in another cat for the same reason.

Petting-elicited aggression towards owners is fairly common. Typically, a cat which is lying apparently contented and being petted in the owner's lap suddenly turns around, bites the owner's hand, and then jumps down onto the floor and walks away. Most counselors assume that this is a cat's normal response to petting which has become unpleasant because it has

gone on too long. As Borchelt and Voith (1987) point out, cats vary enormously is the degree to which they like petting and for how long they tolerate petting without finding it aversive.

Although cases of cats reacting aggressively when approached by family members are often classified as fear aggression, sometimes there are no signs that the cat is afraid at all. Therefore, this approach-elicited aggression can be similar to petting-elicited aggression in that the cat is simply signaling "go away" or "leave me alone" to someone who is pestering or bothering it is some way.

Finally, a cat which has become aggressively aroused by, for example, the sight of a cat in the yard outside a window may react aggressively towards the owner if touched or approached closely at this time. An owner who tries to intervene in an aggressive confrontation between two cats in the home also runs the risk of eliciting this kind of aggression. Although many authors refer to this problem as redirected aggression and interpret such behavior psychologically – that is, attacking the owner is implicitly assumed to be a kind of outlet for internal aggressive tendencies aroused by a target which is inaccessible (e.g. outside the house) or no longer immediately present – it may be a simple case of the cat reacting defensively to having its social behavioral interactions with other cats interrupted in this way. Essentially, it may not be a case of aggression which is in some meaningful sense redirected at all.

Two other types of aggression problems are often classified as redirected aggression. Four out of nine problems diagnosed as redirected aggression in Chapman and Voith (1990) involved cats approaching the source of "high-pitched noises" and attacking the person present. And Beaver (1989c) describes the aggressive reactions of cats towards the nearest person upon being released from restraint in a towel or transport cage in a veterinary practice as redirected aggression. While both of these examples may involve the biting of a victim who is not the source of the aversive stimuli, here again the implicit notion of internal aggressive tendencies being "redirected" seems to be speculating too far beyond the interpretations which can be reasonably drawn from these situations. Indeed, one can say little more other than that the cats are reacting aggressively to persons who are in close proximity to aversive stimuli. Why they are doing so is not clear. Perhaps they perceive the nearby individual as the source of the aversive stimuli. Or perhaps this is a kind of asocial defensive reaction of a frightened cat which aggressively lashes out to simply increase the distance between itself and all other individuals under these circumstances.

In all of the kinds of cases discussed in this section, the cat's reaction is an understandable response to stimuli which the cat finds aversive for one reason or another. Rather then implementing some kind of treatment designed to modify the cat's reaction to these situations, the solution to these problems involves counseling owners to simply accept the fact that their particular cat is predisposed to react this way in these situations and take steps to avoid the eliciting stimuli. For example, young children who may mistreat the cat must be kept away from it when unsupervised, the cat must simply be left alone when it is sitting on a windowsill watching cats outside or when it is threatening another cat in the home, and owners must learn to recognize the signs that a cat which is being petted is beginning to find this unpleasant (e.g. twitching of the tail, restlessness, flattening of ears) and stop petting it at this time.

Offensive aggression

When contacted to give advice for cases of aggression between cats in the same home, the initial problem confronting the behavior counselor is to differentiate between fear-related aggression and so-called territorial aggression or offensive aggression indicating a lack of tolerance of one cat in the family towards another. The territorial aggression pattern differs from that of fear aggression in that the aggressor is presumably motivated by something other than fear and indeed may boldly chase, hunt, and attack the other at every opportunity without

showing behavioral signs that it is fearful in any way. At its most serious, the victim spends almost all of its time in some hiding place in the home where it can aggressively fend off the other's attack, and it may be reluctant to come out even to eat or use the litter box.

The problem of distinguishing between this form of aggression and fear-related aggression is particularly acute in cases where it is possible that both cats are fearful but one is much more fearful than the other. For here too, one of the cats may run away quickly when sighting the other, stay hidden most of the time, show much more obvious signs of fear, and be so reluctant to come out of its hiding place that it begins eliminating there.

In these uncertain cases, questioning of the owner should focus on the aggressor and whether or not it too is motivated by fear. In the case of the classical territorial aggression pattern, the aggressor shows no signs of fear prior to attack or chasing the other, and it often appears to be seeking out the other – and waiting in front of its hiding place for it to come out – in order to attack it. When motivated by fear, aggression even in the asymmetrical case where the most fearful cat usually runs away and hides before fighting occurs may have more of a reactive character, with the aggressor always responding to the appearance of the other.

In a few cases, this line of questioning still doesn't allow one to make a definite fear vs. territorial aggression diagnosis. Perhaps one reason for this potential uncertainty is expressed in this quote from Chapman (1991):

"What begins as fearful encounters between unfamiliar cats may develop into territorial disputes." (p. 318)

This raises the interesting possibility that the two forms of aggression can be more closely related to one another than most specialists in the pet problem area assume. As we have considered earlier, the basis of cat sociality is not mutual attraction, group cohesion, and cooperative group behavior as in dogs, but rather cats' abilities to tolerate the presence of conspecifics under certain conditions. As yet, it is little understood why cats sometimes do not tolerate the presence of another cat and are therefore highly motivated to attack it at every opportunity. Certainly this phenomenon is most common when a new cat enters the home – a situation where the fundamental territorial function of the behavior is most apparent. However, the problem often develops between cats which have peacefully lived together in the past. Borchelt and Voith (1987) suggest that the problem usually develops between cats that are between 1 and 3 years old – presumably when the aggressive cat has become behaviorally mature. In one of my cases, however, it seemed clear that the problem began when one of the animals was suffering from eye cancer which resulted in this kind of offensive aggressive behavior in an 8-year-old male that worsened quickly after the ill cat reentered the home after a two-week absence for an eye operation. One might speculate here that the illness-related abnormal behavior of the victim was what originally triggered off the problem – which would certainly be a biologically understandable reaction given that abnormal behavior may often be a sign of an illness which might be contagious.

Another factor which makes it difficult to distinguish between territorial and fear-related aggression in some cases is that to owners it appears as if one cat's fearful behavior elicits the seemingly offensive, territorial aggression in the other. This is open to two interpretations. It may be the fearful behavior of one cat which causes the problem by making it unacceptable to the other. Or conversely, the cat's fearful behavior may be a response to threatening behavior from the other which owners failed to notice. Although the second possibility may seem more likely at first glance, some owners are positive that the fearful behavior came first, and at that time there was absolutely no indication of anything but friendly or playful approach behavior on the part of the other. If this is true, then it would appear that it was one cat's fearful behavior which caused the other to no longer tolerate it. But why should tolerance break down under these circumstances? One possible answer is that for cats too, a fearful cat is a potentially dangerous cat, presumably just as dangerous for them as it can be for human

beings. It might be natural and adaptive, therefore, to simply drive such individuals away rather than having to run the constant risk of being attacked in unexpected circumstances or for behaving in ways that do not normally provoke aggression in other cats.

Rarely, cats may boldly threaten and attack human visitors in the home without showing noticeable fear – apparent offensive aggression towards human beings. In one of my puzzling cases, the cat reacted this way only when several guests were present simultaneously. Over the course of time, the cat also became aggressive to family members, boldly attacking the family's one-year-old child when it came too close or cried on several occasions, and lashing out and scratching the woman when she came too close to its resting place, which suggests that some kind of defensive motivation was involved.

Treatment considerations

The prognosis for successfully treating the classical territorial aggression case where there is a clear, non-fearful aggressor which continually chases, hunts, and attacks a highly fearful victim is so poor that clients are generally advised from the start to find one of the cats a new home (Borchelt and Voith, 1987). In cases where some uncertainty exists in the sense that there is a chance that the aggressor too might be fearful or simply reacting to fearful behavior on the part of the victim, owners can be advised to try treating the problem as if it were a fear-related aggression problem. If the aggression always occurs no matter how long the cats are kept separated, and no matter how gradually and carefully they are allowed to come close to one another and interact again, both the counselor and owner can then be sure that finding a new home for one of the cats is indeed the only solution.

Intermale aggression

While usually placed in a problem category of its own, intermale aggression is also fairly considered to be a form of offensive or territorial aggression. When strange males meet outdoors, ritualized threat behavior may occur which involves standing stiffly with hindquarters slightly raised, staring, ears turned so that the backs face forwards, tilting the head from side to side, growling, and slowly opening and closing the jaws. If one of the cats stops threatening and moves slowly away, fighting may not occur. Under wild or semi-wild circumstances, males are highly territorial and frequently aggressive to one another. Typically, young males are often attacked and driven away from females groups clustered around abundant food sources. Thereafter they tend to remain solitary until they are old enough to aggressively challenge resident breeding males. These observations imply that the ultimate function of such fighting is to settle the matter of access to females for breeding purposes.

Owners of cats which are aggressive to one another rarely report such ritualized threat behavior even when two males are involved. It may be that under conditions of confinement and familiarity, fighting is rarely preceded by the rather extended ritualized threat behavior seen between strange cats outdoors. Or alternatively, it may be that much of this kind of behavior is not accurately reported by owners who, at most, may notice that the cats are growling and intently watching each other.

Treatment considerations

Castration appears to be a highly effective way of treating fighting between two intact toms in the home – or in treating an intact male which is frequently engaging in fights with other cats in the neighborhood. Hart and Barrett (1973) presented data indicating that castration eliminated or reduced intermale fighting in up to 90% of cases. Progestin therapy also seems to be highly effective, but the aggression resumes once the drug is discontinued (Borchelt and Voith, 1987). When a male persists in fighting with other males outdoors even after being castrated, there is no behavioral treatment. Owners are simply advised that keeping the cat inside is the only solution. When the two males live in the same home, the kind of behavioral treatment for the various forms of defensive aggression discussed above can be attempted. If this does not help, the owner is advised to find one of the cats a new home.

Playful aggression towards human beings

Although most common in young cats, playful aggression towards human beings can occur in a cat of any age. The cat may pounce on and bite a family member who walks by, a hand dangling over the edge of an armchair, or a foot moved under the bedcovers at night. Such attacks do not normally cause injuries because bites are usually inhibited and claws retracted. However, some cats bite harder than this and claws are not always retracted. In one of my recent cases, a playfully aggressive cat's scratches often drew blood and the woman contacted me after being scratched in the eye seriously enough to require hospital attention.

The owner's suspicion that the attacks represent a more serious and dangerous form of aggression is a feature of many cases. This in turn may help to account for why the problem has been allowed to develop: for fear of provoking increased aggression, some owners do not punish the cat for behaving aggressively (e.g. by startling or severely scolding it) as most owners who have succeeded in eliminating this problem have done.

Possible causal factors

Inherited predisposition

The playfully aggressive cat is usually young, particularly active, and highly playful in the variety of contexts. However, some older cats too are much more playful or aggressively playful than others. Given the magnitude, stability, and resistance to modification of these individual differences in playfulness and preferences for aggressive types of play, behavior specialists suspect that they may at least in part reflect differences in the animals' genetic makeup.

POSSIBLE CAUSAL FACTORS

Inherited predisposition
(suspected that some cats much more
playful/aggressively playful than others
for genetic reasons)

Victim fostering
(e.g. owner often plays roughly with cat;
trying to hold/push cat away without
punishing it)

Unintentional owner reinforcement
(e.g. throwing toy to stop aggressive behavior)

Inadequate care/maintenance conditions
(e.g. cat lacks opportunities for needed
play/activity)

Erroneous owner beliefs
(e.g. attacks represent serious and
dangerous form of aggression)

Lack of training
(aggressive play not consistently punished/
punished severely enough)

PLAYFUL AGGRESSION TOWARDS HUMAN BEINGS

- Playfully aggressive cat attacks owner when he/she walks by, moves feet under the
bedcovers, dangles hand over the edge of an armchair, etc.

POSSIBLE TREATMENT ELEMENTS

Correct owner misconceptions
(e.g. attacks playful and not dangerous form
of aggression)

Avoid problem situations
(e.g. deny cat access to bedroom if problem
occurs in bed)

Care/maintenance condition changes
(e.g. institute daily play sessions; provide
cat with more play-eliciting objects)

Increase owner understanding
(e.g. the aggression is one normal form of
play in cat with high play/activity motivation)

Training in problem situations
(e.g. punish playful attacks with loud, startling noise; steer playful attacks towards toys
just *before* cat attacks)

Inadequate care/maintenance conditions

Often excessively playful cats are the only cats
the household and left alone a great deal of
the time. In effect, stimuli which might elicit
needed play and physical activity are lacking,
and the playful attacks on owners are therefore symptomatic of a social deprivation effect.

Victim fostering

Often, the victims of the attacks have inadvertently fostered the development of the problem.
Eliciting rough play, for example, accustoms
the cat to playing in this way and is perhaps
responsible for the fact that certain family
members are attacked and not others. And during attacks themselves, the target person may
scream or try to hold/push the cat away which,

if not done in a way which startles or frightens the cat, may stimulate further playing or more aggressive playing.

Erroneous owner beliefs

As mentioned above, owners often suspect that the attacks represent a more serious and dangerous form of aggression – which is the reason why they have not consistently reacted to attacks in a way which is aversive (i.e. punishing) to the cat.

Unintentional owner reinforcement

Owners sometimes use distraction methods like throwing a toy to stop the problem behavior. Although effective at the time, such a strategy may simply reinforce and strengthen the cat's tendency to attack owners in similar situations in the future.

Lack of training

It is unlikely that the cat will continue attacking the owner if the behavior is consistently punished severely enough to stop the behavior immediately. Most owners of playfully aggressive cats have not done this or have reacted too mildly by doing something which the cat may find more rewarding than punishing.

Possible treatment elements

Correct owner misconceptions

For obvious reasons, it is always important to explain to owners that the aggressive attacks are only playful and not some more dangerous form of aggression.

Increase owner understanding

Furthermore, it should be explained to owners that some cats are highly motivated to play and require much more play and related physical activity than others. It should naturally also be pointed out that such aggressive play is entirely normal for many extremely active and playful cats.

Avoid problem situations

As is the case with many pet behavior problems, sometimes the simplest and indeed most sensible "treatment" is to avoid the situations in which the problems occur. For example, a cat which attacks feet under the bedcovers or the owners' legs when they step out of the shower can simply be denied access to the bedroom or bathroom.

Training in problem situations

Two complementary training methods should be employed with such problems. Firstly, playful attacks should be immediately punished every time they occur by scolding the cat severely enough to suppress aggression or by startling it at the moment it attacks by loudly clapping, spraying it with water, or activating some noise-making device that is carried around for a few days in potential attack situations. The intensity of the punishing stimulus must be strong enough to stop the attacks immediately every time they occur, but it should not be so strong that it badly frightens the cat (i.e. makes it hide for awhile and react fearfully towards the owner later). Secondly, playful aggression should be "steered" towards acceptable objects like balls or other toys by encouraging the cat to play with these at other times and, more importantly, by carrying one of these in potential attack situations so that it can be thrown *just before* the cat actually attacks (i.e. when one notices signs that the cat is preparing to pounce). This redirects the attack towards the toy and away from the owner. If the cat has already attacked, however, it is too late to apply this early intervention method. One would then be rewarding the attack by eliciting further playing and thereby strengthening the cat's future tendency to attack in similar situations.

Care/maintenance condition changes

Instituting a few daily play periods in which the owner elicits energetic play from the cat for as long as the cat seems interested in playing, or simply providing the cat with a wider variety of toys (e.g. balls, paper bags, objects

SAMPLE RECOMMENDATIONS

Playful aggression towards human beings

- Every attack should be *immediately* punished by, for example, severely scolding the cat, spraying it with a squirt gun, or making a startling noise (e.g. loud hand clapping or operating some noise-making device like a horn, whistle, rattle, etc. that one can carry around for a few days).
- The punishing stimulus must be strong enough to stop the cat's attack immediately. However, it should not be so intense that the cat becomes very afraid, hides, and stays hidden for sometime afterwards.
- Aggressive behavior must be punished with 100% consistency and the punishment must be delivered immediately (i.e. within 1-2 seconds) after the start of the attack.
- Carrying one of the cat's toys which you can throw to distract the cat's attention towards it *just before it begins to attack* can, if done consistently, help train the cat to direct playful attacks towards toys rather than human beings. However, never do this after the cat begins an attack, for this rewards the cat for attacking and will therefore make the problem worse and not better.
- Your very active, playful cat needs a lot of exercise every day. Making a point to play with it in a way which elicits energetic, active play during a few brief playtimes scheduled throughout the day can help lower its motivation to attack you.
- Provide the cat with more play-eliciting objects or devices like light balls, paper bags, objects suspended from strings, etc. so that it has lots of things to play with when it is alone and feels like playing.

dangled from strings) it can play with on its own, can also be extremely helpful in meeting the cat's play/activity needs and thereby reducing its motivation to direct all play towards the owner.

Instrumental aggression

Sometimes cats learn to use aggressive behavior as an "instrument" or behavioral strategy to obtain rewards from their owners. For example, the cat may come into the owner's bedroom in the middle of the night, jump up on the bed, and repeatedly attack the owner's feet and legs under the bedcovers until the owner finally gets up to feed the cat or keep it company for awhile, or feed it. Such attacks are usually mild and more resemble playful aggression than any of the more serious forms.

The development of these problems is usually traceable to two major factors. One is the owner's use of distraction measures to stop play aggression (e.g. throwing a toy, giving a food tidbit) which have functioned as rewards for the problem behavior. In effect, if playful attacks on the owner's legs in bed can only be stopped by getting up and giving the cat a tidbit, it is natural that the cat will eventually learn that attacking legs is a good way to obtain tidbits. Secondly, aggression may appear for the first time when a cat's meowing or pouncing on the bed to get the owner to get up does not produce the usual payoff. In general, the failure to receive some "expected" reward can be as aversive to other animals as it is to human beings. And it may result not only in an intensification of the instrumental behavior (e.g. cat meows louder), but it could theoretically also lead to the kind of frustration-related aggression which all complex animals sometimes show in such situations. Of course, aggressive behavior is less easy for the owner to ignore than the cat's usual, more purely playful or vocal way of begging, and it is likely therefore that the cat would quickly discover that this is the best way of getting what it wants.

Treatment measures

Since instrumental aggression is treated in much the same way as other kinds of instrumental behavior or "begging" problems, the reader is referred to the lengthy section dealing with these kinds of problems in the following chapter. There is, however, one additional element when aggression – as opposed, for example, to meowing – is involved: since the cat's learned behavioral strategy for obtaining rewards involves being aggressive to owners, if the owner stops rewarding this behavior, it is likely that the cat will initially intensify its aggressive behavior just as it would intensify any other kind of instrumental response when it didn't produce the usual rewards. In effect, owners must be cautioned that solving this kind of problem by eliminating all rewards for the problem behavior is almost certain to initially increase the intensity of the attacks. This in turn implies that additional recommendations should be given to owners of how to deal with this more intense, possibly dangerous aggression by, for example, consistently punishing it or in some way rearranging specific features of the situation so as to avoid eliciting it.

Pathophysiological aggression

Aggression can be associated with a variety of pathophysiological conditions in cats. Some of the disorders mentioned by various authors are neurological disorders related to trauma, infection, and parasite infestations, rabies, arthritic changes, impacted anal sacs, painful oral lesions, FUS, epilepsy, hypothyroidism, hyperthyroidism, tumors, toxins, and feline ischemic encephalopathy (e.g. Borchelt and Voith, 1987; Beaver, 1989c; Reisner, 1991; Voith, 1989). The

effect of such disorders may be direct (e.g. rabies) or indirect (e.g. painful oral lesions) in the sense of a cat which is ill reacting "irritably" with defensive aggression when approached, handled, carried, etc. (Beaver, 1989c). Such medical conditions come under suspicion if other abnormal neurological and physiological signs are present, if close questioning the owner indicates that the aggression does not fit the pattern of one of the categories of normal cat aggression, and/or if the appearance of the problem is especially sudden or puzzling. Obviously, it is the pathophysiological condition and not the aggression which requires treatment in such cases.

Idiopathic aggression

Sometimes family members are attacked by family cats for what appears to be no good reason. Essentially, the aggression does not fit any of the usual defensive aggression or offensive aggression patterns and a veterinary examination has apparently ruled out some pathophysiological condition as a cause of the behavior. Sometimes the attacks are extremely vicious and cause very serious scratch and bite injuries. These baffling attacks which have no identifiable eliciting stimulus are thus often referred to in the literature as *idiopathic* aggression.

Whether or not these attacks really represent another form of aggressive behavior problem is unknown. In theory, they could be a form of one of the defensive or offensive aggression problems discussed earlier which the surprised owner who was attacked for the first time didn't observe closely enough to accurately describe. Alternatively, they could indeed represent some other kind of aggression entirely (e.g. cat's explosive reaction to severe, long-term deprivation, stress, or fear-arousing conditions). Of course, they could also stem from undiagnosed pathophysiological condition, which in the last analysis is the most likely possibility considering that the attack is completely out of character for the animal and nothing of substance has apparently happened to provoke it.

In any case, one must understand the behavior to some extent in order to know how to deal with it. When this is not the case and there is no hint at all of the cat's motivation or the circumstances in which the problem is likely to occur, the problem is basically untreatable – which often means the cat must be euthanized to protect family members. But as Borchelt and Voith (1985) point out, one must be careful before considering euthanasia on these grounds, for most cases which owners initially describe as "sudden, vicious, unprovoked attacks" usually turn out to be some treatable form of defensive aggression.

References

Beaver, B.V. (1989a): Feline behavioral problems other than housesoiling. *Journal of the American Animal Hospital Association* **25**, 465–469.

Beaver, B.V. (1989b): Housesoiling by cats: A retrospective study of 120 cases. *Journal of the American Animal Hospital Association* **25**, 631–637.

Beaver, B.V. (1989c): Disorders of behavior. In Sherding, R. G. (ed): *The Cat: Diseases and Clinical Management*. New York, Churchill Livingstone.

Borchelt, P.L., and Voith, V.L. (1985): Aggressive behavior in dogs and cats. *Compendium on Continuing Education for the Practicing Veterinarian* **7**, 949–957.

Borchelt, P.L., and Voith, V.L. (1987): Aggressive behavior in cats. *Compendium on Continuing Education for the Practicing Veterinarian* **9**, 49–57.

Chapman, B. L. (1991): Feline aggression: Classification, diagnosis, and treatment. *Veterinary Clinics of North America: Small Animal Practice* **21**, 315–327.

Chapman, B. L., and Voith, V. L. (1990): Cat aggression redirected to people: 14 cases (1981-1987). *Journal of the American Veterinary Medical Association* **196**, 947–950.

Hart, B. L., and Barrett, R.E. (1973): Effects of castration on fighting, roaming, and urine spraying in adult male cats. *Journal of the American Veterinary Medical Association* **163**, 290–292.

Hart, B. L., Eckstein, R.A., Powel, K. L., and Dodman, N. H. (1993): Effectiveness of buspirone on urine spraying and inappropriate urination in cats. *Journal of the American Veterinary Medical Association* **203**, 254–258.

Reisner, I. (1991): The pathophysiologic basis of behavior problems. *Veterinary Clinics of North America: Small Animal Practice* **21**, 207–224.

Turner, D. C. (1991): The ethology of the human-cat relationship. *Schweizer Archiv für Tierheilkunde* **133**, 63–70.

Turner, D. C., Feaver, J., Mendl, M., and Bateson, P. (1986): Variation in domestic cat behaviour towards humans: a paternal effect. *Animal Behaviour* **34**, 1890–1901.

Voith, V.L. (1989): Chapter 43: Behavioral disorders. In Ettinger, J. S. (ed): *Textbook of Veterinary Internal Medicine*. Philadelphia, W. B. Saunders Company.

23   Miscellaneous Behavior Problems

Predatory behavior

There are great differences between cats in the degree to which they are motivated to hunt birds and rodents when allowed outside. If a cat is highly motivated to hunt and often brings home dead prey, the owner may wish to try to control this problem. Neighborhood disputes between cat owners and bird lovers are common, and owners may find it distasteful to find feathers or dead mice in the home.

The only completely effective way to control predatory behavior is to keep the cat inside. Otherwise the owner can do little more than put a bell on the cat's collar to help birds escape and perhaps try feeding the cat just before its primary hunting times – which probably won't entirely stop it from hunting but may reduce its hunting motivation somewhat. It may be possible, however, to train a cat not to bring dead animals into the home by making a noise to startle it every time it tries to enter the home carrying prey. As always with punishment methods, the cat must be consistently punished in this way just as it is the act of bringing the dead animal in through the door. Punishing the cat when the prey animal is discovered later in the home is completely ineffective, for such punishment is then no longer closely associated with the behavior which is to be suppressed.

When a cat persists in molesting a caged bird in the home, the best approach is to arrange some kind of booby trap (e.g. a ring of set, turned-over mousetraps placed around the base of the cage) which frightens the cat badly enough when it comes close to the cage to cause it avoid that area in future. If the owner him/herself personally punishes the cat by, for example, making a loud noise which startles it, this is likely to produce avoidance of the cage area when the owner is present, but not when the cat is alone in the room.

Sexual behavior problems

Mounting of other cats

Sometimes a male persists in mounting a female or another male in the household. In some cases, the male is constantly after the other, chasing and attempting to mount it several times a day. The victim may then become fearful, running away and staying hidden most of the time as is often the case with offensive aggression problems. Beaver (1992) suggests that inappropriate mounting directed towards another female or a passive male can also be displayed by females "as a consequence of sexual energy not released during estrus" or by estrous females showing signs of "tension and frustration".

Beaver (1992) maintains that in captive groups in homes or colonies there appears to be no hierarchical social order between most of the cats except for a single dominant male which "walks stiff-legged with raised back and tail, seizing each of the other cats and pushing their backs down with his hindquarters, and mounting each as if for copulation". However, Bradshaw (1992) disputes the generality of this phenomenon by pointing out that Winslow's (1938) observation of this behavior in one laboratory colony – which is the source Beaver (1992) cites – has not been reported by other authors who have observed captive cat colonies.

Finally, Beaver (1992) points out that it is relatively common for a dominant territorial male to mount any cat that enters his territory, whether male or female. She also cites a laboratory study which indicated that when the mounting male is placed in the mounted cat's territory, the situation is reversed in the sense that the formerly mounted cat now does the mounting.

In farm cats, mounting of inappropriate animals like young females, kittens, or other males is most frequently seen in adult "non-breeder" males which spend more time close to food sources where females tended to congregate, but interact with other cats less frequently than "breeders", respond defensively to aggression from breeders – which are more aggressive – mark less frequently, and achieve fewer intromissions. After summarizing these findings, Bradshaw (1992) argues that this high rate of mounting but low rate of breeding success "appears to be of some merit in a strategy of staying close to the adult females and 'sneaking' matings while the breeder males are absent." (p. 150).

Beaver (1992) regards all of the various forms of hypersexual behavior problems in males as indications of some environmental deprivation effect: the lack of normal sexual behavior opportunities results in abnormally lowered thresholds for eliciting sexual behavior so that it may be elicited by other males, anestrous females, kittens, or inanimate objects like cushions or furry objects. She also points out that some of "these behaviors have been linked to specific brain lesions".

Treatment possibilities

Hart and Hart (1985) suggest two possible approaches to treatment with castrated males for which a pathophysiological cause has been ruled out:
- Progestin treatment with medroxyprogesterone acetate or megestrol acetate to attempt to lower the male's sexual motivation and, perhaps, his overall level of arousal as well.
- Punishment of the *victim* whenever it tolerates mounting rather than defending itself against this kind of assault with the usual vocalization, struggling, hissing, and aggressive striking out (Beaver, 1992) characteristic of anestrous females or fearful cats of both sexes. Hart and Hart (1985) suggest that some form of remote punishment like water which is sprayed in such a way that it

doesn't appear to come from the owner is most appropriate. When unsupervised, the cats should be separated.

Based on Beaver's view that the problem is often a symptom of a deficient or suboptimal environment, it might also be reasonable to try giving an inside cat access to outdoors or holding several daily playtimes with it in the home during which it is encouraged to play vigorously.

Lack of sexual interest in males

Sometimes males do not cooperate when it comes time to breed with a receptive female. Hart and Hart (1985) suggest several possible reasons for this:
- The male is uncomfortable in an unfamiliar breeding environment. While some males mate readily in a new environment, others may require a month or two to accustom themselves sufficiently to it to mate.
- The male may mount and thrust but seems incompetent as far as obtaining complete intromission – which the authors suggest might be due to lack of experience "in executing the right movements".
- A hair ring may form around the glans penis (due to collection of hair by the epithelial papillae which cover it) which prevents intromission. Sometimes this is removed by the male himself, but if not, it can be removed by the veterinarian or owner by sliding it over the penis.
- Abnormally low testosterone levels may be responsible. However, Hart and Hart (1985) point out that evidence indicates that this level must be greatly depressed to account for lack of sexual interest, for males will copulate even though levels are half the normal value.
- Seasonal fluctuation exhibited by males may somehow be involved particularly in cases where there is "an otherwise unexplained decline in sexual prowess of a breeding male".

Treatment measures

- Providing inexperienced males with frequent copulation opportunities with receptive females.

- Thoroughly accustoming the male to the breeding environment and the procedures involved in placing the male there, introducing the female, and so on.
- Allowing the male to copulate several times in succession with the female.
- Allowing the female to remain long enough with the male. Hart and Hart (1985) suggest that it can take as long as several hours before the male is ready to mate.
- Using a female which shows very receptive behavior for training purpose. Hart and Hart (1985) suggest bringing the female into behavioral estrus with two SQ doses of 0.25 mg *estradiol cypionate* administered 2 days apart – which will usually produce estrus within 1-2 days after the last injection. (See the "drug therapy" subsection in Chapter 8 for side effects and other important drug-related information.)

Rejection of breeding male by female

Hart and Hart (1985) suggest the following approaches here:
- Restraining the female if the male is an experienced stud which will mate under such circumstances.
- Simply leaving the two together for several hours.
- Trying another male, for females may reject some males and accept others.

Maternal behavior problems

Mothers may neglect kittens to the point where they die or she may attack and even eat them. Hart and Hart's (1985) approach to accounting for such problems is revealed in the following quotation:

"*As with dogs and other domestic mammals, we have taken over some aspects of maternal care by providing food, water, and shelter to kittens when maternal care has not been adequate, leading to the survival of cats whose mothers were lacking in the genetic programming of maternal behavior. Our intervention helps perpetuate the genetic pro-*

gramming for poor mothering. The variety of maternal attitudes among cats is especially evident to managers of catteries. Some cats never seem interested in their own kittens, even after several litters. Others are wildly interested in all kittens they come in contact with." (p. 195)

Basically, it is a case then of genetically preprogrammed behavioral sequences or tendencies which vary enormously from cat to cat and should be viewed essentially as stable individual characteristics which are not modifiable and not fundamentally explainable as reactions to some feature of the environment.

Neglecting kittens

According to one survey cited by Hart and Hart (1985), 8% of kittens which were healthy after birth died, mostly for reasons related to "inadequate or inappropriate maternal care". The details of such cases vary greatly: fetal membranes may not be removed, the mother may not keep newborn kittens close to her, she may lie on and smother them, she may not stay with the litter, or she may not retrieve kittens that are lying outside of the nest.

Aside from warming a hypothermic kitten which has been away from the mother too long before presenting it to the mother again, there is little an owner can do in such cases except observe the mother's treatment of the kittens and intervene when something goes wrong (e.g. put a kitten back in the nest if it is stranded away from the nest and not retrieved).

Summarizing rules developed by Dr. M.F. Stewart of the Glasgow Veterinary School, Hart and Hart (1985) suggest that some of these kinds of problems can be prevented or overcome with the following measures:
- Placing the mother in an individual parturition box at least three days before the kittens are born so that she becomes well accustomed to the surroundings.
- The box should be stable and have sides which are high enough to keep kittens from falling out.
- Mothers should be observed at the time of parturition to make sure they are cleaning

the kittens and the kittens begin suckling soon after birth.

- Mothers which have displayed maternal behavior problems in the past should be watched particularly closely.

Cannibalism

Hart and Hart (1985) suggest that cannibalism is most commonly related to "a larger litter than usual, second pregnancy of a season, and the presence of ill kittens". They also suggest that it is not related to previous experience being a mother. In their brief but excellent discussion, the authors point out that cannibalism can be an adaptive behavior in nature by removing kittens whose inactivity and hyperthermia indicate they are becoming increasingly ill before they infect other kittens or die and the carcasses attract scavengers. The behavior also provides the mother with additional nutrition, which might marginally improve her ability to care for the remaining kittens. Therefore, basically the same reasons which cause mothers to consume fetal membranes and placenta during parturition and ingest stillborn and aborted fetuses (e.g. Beaver, 1992).

Hart and Hart (1985) also speculate that environmental disturbances may lead to cannibalism of kittens which are not in fact behaving abnormally. Beaver (1992) too suggests that environmental stress may be a factor in such cases and recommends "minimization of stress" in the two-week period before the expected littering date (e.g. providing isolated queening area).

Finally, Hart and Hart (1985) point out that infanticide may be exhibited by strange tomcats – as is seen in lions, for example, where coalitions of males that take over a pride normally kill all cubs, which causes the females to come into estrus again. Therefore, the authors support the common breeder practice of allowing resident tomcats access while keeping strange tomcats away from lactating females.

Hand-raising kittens

Although it does not harm and may even benefit kittens to be taken from the nest and briefly handled by owners, Hart and Hart (1985) warn that permanently separating young kittens from the mother can have serious consequences for their later behavior. If separation is necessary due to maternal neglect or the danger of infanticide, it is best to give kittens to another mother with kittens. If this is impossible, the owner should try to provide a young kitten with as much interaction with littermates as possible during the first few weeks of life in cases where it must be separated from the litter for reason of illness, weakness, or material aggression.

Unfriendliness to owners

Cats vary enormously in how much they like petting and other forms of close physical contact to owners. For owners who long to pet and cuddle their cat, a relatively standoffish, independent type of cat which grudgingly tolerates this kind of treatment for a short time and then struggles or bites to free itself can represent a serious problem.

First and foremost in these cases, it must be explained to owners that many cats are like this by nature and there is no way to turn them into cats which love to be held and petted for hours. In effect, owners should be encouraged to view such behavioral characteristics as manifestations of the cat's relatively inalterable personality. However, owners often contribute to making cats as standoffish and unfriendly as they are by constantly approaching them, picking them up, and forcing them to endure being held and petted. This is a serious mistake, for it is aversive to the cat and essentially trains it to react more negatively to human contact.

It is often possible to greatly improve the cat's behavior in the direction of increased friendliness, contact-seeking, and tolerance for physical contact by having owners make it a rule to never initiate contact with the cat. Instead, they should always wait for the cat to approach them, pet it only as long as it seems to enjoy this, and then stop petting it and let is go away when it signals that it has had enough. Always moving slowing and calmly in the presence of the cat, giving it food tidbits now and again, and responding to its play initiatives with games it likes to play for as long as it seems to want to play may help too.

Instrumental behavior problems

The most common and serious problem involving a cat's begging, pestering, demanding, or attention-seeking behavior is when owners are frequently awakened in the middle of the night by its meowing, scratching at the door, or playful behavior on the bed. In such cases, owners must get up and play with it, feed it, or keep it company for awhile before it leaves them alone and allows them to go back to sleep. Such behavior is termed *instrumental* because the cat has learned to use such behavior as an "instrument" or strategy to obtain rewards like attention, food, or playing.

By the time the case comes to the attention of a behavior counselor, the cat's demanding or attention-seeking behavior, and owner's habit of coping with it by giving the cat what it wants, are well-entrenched. Almost all of these owners have tried stopping the cat's pestering with punishment, and they have all tried simply not giving the cat what it wants. But in the long run, neither method has worked. Punishment has resulted in at best a temporary suppression of the behavior problem, and withholding rewards simply causes the cat to intensify its problem behavior.

Treatment measures

There are two treatment possibilities which may be appropriate in these cases. The first is *punishment*. Although owners have tried this, they may not have done so effectively, which means the following:
- Applying the punishing stimulus immediately following the onset of the problem behavior.
- Applying a punishing stimulus that is intense enough to cause immediate cessation of the problem behavior every time it occurs.
- Applying the punishing stimulus every single time the problem behavior occurs.

Typically, owners punish the behavior only sometimes, usually after waiting until it becomes intolerable, and usually with a fairly mild stimulus (e.g. screaming at the cat) which sometimes must be repeated several times before the cat stops. Given that the cat is highly motivated to perform the punished behavior – because it has been so often rewarded for it in the past – a fairly intense punisher is needed here. For example, the dreaded vacuum cleaner can be positioned in front of the bedroom door in such a way that the owner can plug it from inside the bedroom as soon as the cat first starts meowing or scratching. Basically, one has to use something that the cat really "hates with a passion" and not something that it simply dislikes but can to some extent get used to like the thumping from a shoe thrown against the inside of the bedroom door.

The second and most commonly-recommended treatment method is *extinction*, or permanently withholding all rewards for the problem behavior. While this may seem like the obvious method to owners from the start, they have tried it from time to time without success. By the time of the consultation, they therefore have little confidence that this approach is indeed capable of solving the problem. The difficulty here is not, however, with the extinction method but rather that the owners have not applied it correctly: they have not applied it diligently enough and given up too soon when it initially seemed to make the problem worse.

The key to the successful application of the extinction method is not only to explain to owners that they must make it a hard and fast rule to never again give the cat what it wants in problem situations, but one must also explain to them how the cat will react at all stages of the extinction process. The following animal learning principles are relevant here:
- Withholding of the reward will initially produce an *increase* in the intensity and frequency of the problem behavior.
- Not receiving an expected reward is aversive for the cat, and it may cause not only an increase in the problem behavior but also of other, possibly aggressive types of behavior

(or more aggressive forms of the problem behavior).

- Having been rewarded irregularly or after varying lengths of time in the past, the cat is accustomed to not being rewarded sometimes and so it is natural that it will continue the behavior for a long time before starting to give up.
- The course of extinction is always erratic with bursts of responding followed by quiet periods of varying lengths of time when the behavior ceases. Over the course of time, such bursts tend to become shorter and the pauses in between longer.
- The more often the owners have tried extinguishing the problem behavior (i.e. not rewarding it) in the past, and the more diligently and persistently they have done this, the longer it may take to eliminate the problem behavior; for these earlier attempts have basically trained the cat that in the long run it will get what it wants if it never gives up.
- After extinction is apparently complete, the cat will still have a tendency to try the old strategy from time to time – which, like all of these various effects, won't cause owners to lose faith in the treatment method if they know this is normal under such circumstances.

Owners who understand exactly what to expect and are convinced from the start of the potential effectiveness of this method usually have no trouble in eliminating the problem behavior in this way. The only difficulty in some cases is practical: owners need their night's sleep to face the coming working day, and they may therefore have to wait until vacation time before applying the extinction procedure.

Destructive scratching

Approaching, extending the forepaws and claws, and gripping and scratching on a vertical object is a normal cat behavior which probably serves three major functions (Hart and Hart, 1985):

- Pulling off the old, loose outer layers of claw by scratching and thus exposing the new sharp claw growing underneath.

SAMPLE RECOMMENDATIONS

Demanding attention/food in the night

(Example extinction procedure to treat the common instrumental behavior problem of a cat that jumps up onto the owners' bed and wakes them up to be fed or played with in the middle of the night.)

- Always shut the cat out of the bedroom at night.
- To accustom the cat to this as quickly and easily as possible, make it a hard and fast rule to never again open the door when the cat meows or scratches on the door to try to get in.
- When it makes problems outside the door, do not respond to its noises in any way (e.g. by talking to it or making the slightest noise of any kind).
- It is to be expected that during the first few nights the cat will be especially frustrated at not being let in and will therefore make more problems than ever before. This is perfectly normal behavior. You only have to be more stubborn than the cat and weather it through: the cat will give up sooner or later.
- The cat may appear to have given up for a night or two before trying it again. This is also normal and to be expected. It will try it again now and again for some time to come. If you just make sure to *never* give in, these attempts will lessen and eventually disappear altogether when the cat is finally convinced that it's never again going to get what it wants this way.

- Visual territorial marking: objects which are frequently scratched becoming covered with conspicuous scratch marks.
- Olfactory territory marking: secretions from sweat glands in front paws are deposited on the scratched objects.

Both outdoors and in the home, cats typically choose a particular object which they frequently return to and scratch. For a cat which is kept always inside, this is usually the scratching post. However cats can cause thousands of dollars of damage to furniture with their claws. And it is often the case that the behavior counselor is contacted when it comes time to replace the old disheveled sofa with a new one which the owner would like to keep intact. Typically, these cats have always been provided a scratching post which they could never be persuaded to use on a regular basis.

Treatment methods

The logic of the usual treatment method to induce the cat to scratch on a scratching post or board attached to the wall rather than furniture parallels that of methods used to induce it to eliminate in the litter box instead of on the carpet: one tries to make the object which the owner wishes the cat to scratch as attractive to the cat for scratching as possible while, at the same time, taking steps to suppress scratching at the undesirable site.

Making the designated object as attractive to the cat for scratching as possible

If the cat is to be trained to scratch on a scratching post, it is placed directly in front of the piece of furniture which the cat is now regularly scratching – or one moves the piece of furniture away and places the post directly on the same site. Since this may be an undesirable permanent location for the scratching post (e.g. directly in front of the living room couch), it is made clear to owners that this placement is only temporary. Once the cat is fully accustomed to scratching on the post, it can be moved by steps of a few inches every week towards its ultimate preferred location.

As Hart and Hart (1985) suggest that since cats typically prefer to scratch on fabrics with longitudinally-oriented threads which are easily shredded, placing such a material over the more tightly-woven carpet material that is usually provided on commercial scratching posts may make it more acceptable to the cat. Later, as the outer material wears away, the cat will become more accustomed to scratching on the carpet material, which will have taken on the cat's foot pad odor and become more frayed (Landsberg, 1991). Since Landsberg (1991) also suggests that cats tend to stretch and scratch soon after waking up, placing the scratching post – or a second scratching post – near to the cat's bed or usual napping place may help too.

Discouraging scratching at the problem site

It often helps greatly to cover the scratched surface at the problem site with some material which the cat finds unacceptable for scratching. Landsberg (1991) suggests trying, for example, netting, thick plastic foil, aluminum foil, adhesive tape which is sticky on both sides, or some extremely loose fabric in which the claws catch. This material can be gradually removed later (e.g. by gradually reducing the size of the area covered over a number of weeks) once the cat is fully accustomed to scratching on the post.

Another approach is to make the scratched site aversive to the cat by spraying some substance the cat finds aversive (e.g. unscented underarm deodorant) directly in front of its nose several times – without directly spraying it on the nose itself – and then later spraying the same substance on the scratched site.

If these approaches are not feasible because, for example, the cat always shifts to another part of the piece of furniture – or to a similar piece of furniture – scratching can be punished. Loudly clapping, hissing, throwing something, etc. to startle the cat severely enough to immediately interrupt the behavior the instant it starts scratching, or obviously positioning itself to start scratching, is one possibility. However, because this kind of punishment is closely associated with the presence of the owner, cats often learn only to delay scratching until the owner is no longer in the room. Therefore, a better approach is to use some type of remote or impersonal punishment. Landsberg (1991) provides many suggestions for two types of such methods:

- The owner remains out of sight of the cat but observes the cat's behavior in the area of the problem site in some way (e.g. discretely peering around a corner, setting up some kind of mirror system, using video equipment) and then uses some method to punish the cat when required like operating a remote controlled noise-making or water-spraying device, throwing an object like a can full of marbles which makes a loud noise when it hits the floor, or plugging in the vacuum cleaner which is positioned near the site.
- The scratched area is booby trapped with, for example, some kind of electronic device which automatically triggers off the punishing stimulus when the cat begins scratching or comes very close to the scratched surface. Landsberg (1991) describes several commercially available devices which operate on this principle.

Another possibility is Hart and Hart's (1985) mousetrap method (see Chapter 20) for startling the cat when it comes close to the sight. It is not necessary to hang the loaded mousetraps on strings above the marked sites as these authors suggest – and which Landsberg (1991) suggests is dangerous to the cat and impractical in the physical sense. Obviously, placing a few of them at the base of the site where the cat normally must stand to scratch should be equally effective.

Declawing

Surgical removal of a cat's claws from the front feet is a common approach to serious scratching problems in North America. It is illegal in Germany, however, where strict animal protection laws prohibit forms of mutilation simply to make animals more easy to keep as pets. In expressing their support for such legal prohibi-

tions or arguing against the declawing procedure in countries where it is legally permissible, opponents cite three presumed undesirable side effects of the operation: (1) it may lead to other behavior problems like elimination outside of the litter box, (2) declawed cats are more likely to bite their owners, and (3) the cat may not be able to escape a pursuing dog by climbing a tree – or successfully fend off an attack – without its front claws. However, after reviewing a number of studies which looked into these various possible side effects, Landsberg (1991) draws the following, well-substantiated conclusion:

"Although hunting and climbing ability may be reduced marginally, most owners claimed that their cats continued to hunt, climb, and defend themselves admirably following declawing. Declawed cats are no more likely to bite, and there is no increase in inappropriate elimination. Of course, scratching problems are reduced greatly or eliminated by declawing. Most owners of declawed cats are satisfied or have a positive outlook on declawing (96%), and as many as 70% of cat owners report an improved relationship with their cat (bonding) after declawing." (p. 277)

This improved relationship benefit may well be due to the cessation of frequent owner punishment administered for problem scratching.

Landsberg (1991) also argues that the medical side effects of the operation are minimal and that seeing as how a substantial proportion of the owners of declawed cats state that they would not have kept their cat if it had not been declawed, it can be assumed that as many as 40,000 of the 100,000 cats which are declawed in Ontario, Canada, every year have been saved from being euthanized, surrendered to animal shelters, or abandoned far away from the home by the operation.

Landsberg (1991) concludes:

"Declawing should not be performed unnecessarily, because it subjects cats to postsurgical discomfort and the risks and stresses, although minimal, of anesthesia, surgery, and hospitalization. For those owners who are unable or unwilling to correct their cat's scratching problem using re-

training techniques, declawing is an effective alternative." (p. 278)

It is probably fair to state that most other North American behavior problem specialists (e.g. Voith, 1989; Beaver, 1989; Hart and Hart, 1985) share Landsberg's view that declawing is an acceptable "last resort" alternative with few serious side effects.

Other forms of destructive scratching

Destructive scratching as an instrumental behavioral strategy

Cats which were formerly allowed access to the outdoors and now must remain in the home sometimes develop the persistent and destructive habit of scratching the carpet just in front of the front door as if trying to dig their way out. This may also be seen in cats that were formerly allowed into the family bedrooms but are now denied access for some reason. In both types of cases, doors may also be damaged by the cats' repeated scratching.

In some cases, the behavior persists even though it is never rewarded by being allowed to go outside or come into the bedroom. There are three possible ways of accounting for this:
- Using scratching to remove or dig through, around, or under any kind of physical obstacle may be a genetically-preprogrammed behavior in animal species which have the claw equipment to do so effectively.
- The cat is highly motivated to escape, its avenue of escape is blocked, and this in turn leads to the common frustration-situation effect of intensification of the problem behavior.
- There are other sources of reinforcement which are maintaining the behavior: scratching attracts owner attention, and owners may use distraction measures like throwing toys or offering a food bride to stop the behavior.

These may all be involved in many cases, with the first two accounting for the origin of the behavior and the last explaining why it persists in spite of the lack of rewards corresponding to

the apparent goal of the behavior of getting through the door.

As far as treatment is concerned, combining some form of consistent punishment as is recommended for scratching of furniture with the various recommendations for extinguishing begging/demanding instrumental behavior discussed in the previous section will eliminate the problem in virtually all cases.

Destructive scratching related to climbing/ playing/movement

In one case, a cat's habit of playfully scampering up and down living room walls by digging its claws into the wallpaper had ruined areas on two of the walls. Cats may also damage curtains by climbing on them or the smooth surfaces of leather furniture by extending their claws to get a better hold when they spring away from them. One or more of the following methods can help here:
- Altering the surface to make it unattractive or aversive for the cat to touch (e.g. covering it with smooth plastic foil, placing strips of adhesive tape that is sticky on both sides on the surface).
- Consistent punishment for the undesirable behavior using one of the many methods mentioned in the previous section.
- When the cat's exuberant scampering up and down walls or curtains is a sign that it needs more physical activity, owners should be encouraged to integrate regular playtimes with the cat into the family's daily routine during which the cat is encouraged to play energetically in acceptable ways (e.g. with toys, objects dangled or pulled on strings, etc.).

Problems related to ingestion

Anorexia

According to Hart and Hart (1985), possible causes of a cat's refusal to eat are disease, food aversion (e.g. as a consequence of some gastrointestinal upset which occurred after eating a particular type of food), or aversion to feeding at specific location like next to the litter box.

If a sick cat remains anorexic during or after recovery, Hart and Hart suggest either force-feeding to activate the taste receptors – and thereby arouse the cat's interest in feeding – or medication with *progestins*. Beaver (1992) recommends *diazepam* (0.05 to 0.4 mg/kg IV) or *oxazepam* (3 mg/kg po) for this purpose. (See the "drug therapy" subsection in Chapter 8 for side effects and other important drug-related information.)

Naturally, in animals which were not ill, the food aversion and/or site aversion causes can be explored by offering the cat different types of foods and/or at different locations respectively.

Pica

The most dramatic and interesting example of problems with ingestion of non-food objects is wool eating primarily observed in Siamese cats and less commonly in Burmese and cross-bred cats. These cats will suck, chew, and ingest anything wool, destroying sweaters, socks, etc., and this behavior may generalize to cotton and synthetic fabrics. Summarizing the results of a survey by Neville and Bradshaw of 152 fabric-eating cats, O'Farrell and Neville (1994) state that the behavior is equally common in males and females, usually starts occurring at 2–8 months of age, and may occur frequently or only sporadically. Although cats usually experience no ill effects from ingesting fabric, sometimes surgery is required to clear gastrointestinal obstructions.

As possible causes, O'Farrell and Neville (1994) mention genetic factors (supported by high prevalence in Siamese cats), redirected sucking behavior, redirected hunting/prey catching behavior, or the behavior may be a stress-related stereotypy (see following section). These authors suggest the following treatments:

- Remote punishment by spraying water (in such a way that the cat doesn't see the owner doing it).
- Baiting a piece of fabric with menthol or eucalyptus oil (to "neutralize the rewarding effect of chewing").
- Denying the cat access to the material for a few weeks (after which time the cat may not resume chewing again).
- Providing some other "positive outlet for the behavior" by, for example, making dry food available or frequently giving the cat "gristly meat attached to large bones".
- Increasing the fiber content of wet food (i.e. by adding "bran, tissues, or chopped undyed wool").
- Giving the cat unwanted woolen garments to chew – especially at mealtimes.

Beaver (1992) suggests that it is the odor of lanolin or human sweat on the material which may be the crucial factor. She recommends the following:

- Limiting chewing to one permissible object by putting all others away.
- Removing the cat's carnassial teeth to prevent damage from the behavior.
- Feeding the cat a lanolin-containing product.
- *Thyroid hormone* dosed as 0.5 mg/day po.
- Baiting the material with a hot sauce mixture or applying the aversive conditioning technique using underarm deodorant recommended by Hart and Hart (1985).
- Punishing the cat by thumping it on the nose or scolding it (if the problem has just begun).

In contrast to the above authors, Hart and Hart (1985) offer no possible explanation for the problem. They suggest that it usually disappears after a year or so. They also suggest that the only treatment which is successful in some cases is to condition an aversion to the problem material using the method discussed earlier of (1) spraying unscented underarm deodorant in front of the cat's nose a few times and then (2) spraying it on endangered cloth materials once the cat shows signs of having developed a strong aversion to it.

As the diversity of these viewpoints indicate, Hart and Hart (1985) are justified in simply stating without qualification that the cause of this problem is unknown. Voith (1989) states that there is "no reliably effective treatment procedure for this problem" – which indicates that in many cases the problem persists in spite of various methods employed to stop it.

House plant eating

Most cats eat plants from time to time, and this can sometimes become a problem when house plants are involved. A common solution is to provide the cat with potted grass which the cat it allowed to chew while, at the same time, consistently punishing the cat when it approaches house plants by startling it, spraying it with water, or booby-trapping the plant with, for example, set, turned-over mousetraps so that it will be startled and frightened away from the site even when it is alone (Hart and Hart, 1985). These authors also suggest that the conditioned aversion approach (i.e. with deodorant) can be used here as well.

Stereotypies

Stereotypy behavioral problems involve acts which are repetitive, stereotyped in form, and appear to serve no obvious function. Leuscher et al. (1991) list the following kinds of stereotypies (or possible stereotypies) which have been reported in cats:

- *Grooming*: self licking, air licking, hair chewing, lick granuloma
- *Hallucinatory*: staring, air batting, jaw snapping, pouncing, prey chasing or searching, ducking
- *Eating and drinking*: polydipsia, polyphagia, excessive drooling, wool sucking, eating fabrics
- *Locomotor behavior*: sudden body movements like running, jumping, and pacing, head shaking, paw shaking, tail swishing, freezing
- *Vocalization*: crying, howling
- *Neurotic*: aggressive biting and chewing of tail or feet, vicious tearing of the mouth with claws, periodic aggression directed at people

Some of these conditions may not be purely behavioral. Reisner (1991) discusses many pathophysiological conditions that can lead to skin disorders like alopecia, pruritis, and inflammation which, in turn, result in extensive licking or biting (e.g. food hypersensitivity, parasite infestations, metabolic disorders, hyperthyroidism, and many more). Particularly in such self-mutilation cases, a thorough medical examination is obviously required before deciding to treat the problem as a purely behavioral (i.e. stress/conflict-related, attention-getting behavior, etc.). Most are not. Reisner (1991) cites one survey of 800 cats with dermatitis which established that only 4.3% were definitely diagnosed as psychogenic dermatitis – or "self-induced skin conditions occurring in the absence of any physical pathology".

As was discussed in Chapter 18, both general ethological considerations and what is known of situations in which stereotypies occur in farm animals indicate that they are being reactions to what for the animal is a stressful, impoverished, or otherwise deficient environment. In short, these behavior problems are often a sign that the environment lacks something important which the animal requires or, alternatively, the environment contains some sort of disturbing or aversive feature which the animal finds stressful or threatening.

A second major factor which is relevant in many cases is the possibility that unintentional owner reinforcement in the form of attention and distraction measures (trying to interest the cat in playing, food, etc.) which owners use to try and stop the problem behavior may be strengthening or at least maintaining it.

Treatment possibilities

In attempting to treat such problems, the same kind of approach is followed with cats as with dogs (see Chapter 18 for a more detailed discussion). As a prelude to giving specific treatment recommendations, the following areas must be thoroughly explored during the consultation:

- *Does the behavior have an attention-getting element? How exactly does the owner react when the animal shows the behavior? Does the animal exhibit the behavior even when it is alone?*

If owner attention seems to be a major fact or, having owners ignore the behavior – or leave the room every time it begins – can be helpful.

- *Is there something important which the animal lacks?*
  Exercise is one obvious possibility with particularly active cats. If this is the case, playing with the cat several times daily is recommended.

- *Does the animal find something about the environment disturbing or threatening? Could the daily family schedule be somewhat too erratic and unpredictable from the animal's viewpoint? Does it show fear or avoidance of humans or other animals in the home? Does it show any other signs of reacting negatively in any way to something or someone in the home?*

- *Could there be some element of frustration involved? Is the animal in some way blocked or prevented from doing something it seems to want to do (e.g. going outside, playing in an aggressive way)?*

- *Could the animal be in some kind of motivational conflict situation?*
  One possible conflict might involve simultaneous tendencies to approach (seeking contact) *and* avoid (because of past punishment, restraint, or petting against its will) family members. This kind of approach-avoidance conflict might also involve another cat which, for example, reacts aggressively when approached too closely.

These lines of questioning often turn up various possibilities which can then be "tested" by making various kinds of modifications in the way the cat is kept and treated by family members – and, of course, in how specifically they react to its problem behavior.

Medical approach

Medical treatment of physical problems produced by some stereotypies (e.g. severely bitten tail) is often required. Physical response prevention (i.e. preventing access to parts of the body animals are biting) may also be indicated.

Drug therapy is also often effectively used to control stereotypies. However, given the fact that the above behavioral approach alone can eliminate many stereotypies, drug therapy is only indicated after the behavioral approach as been applied without success. Table 23.1 provides a summary of drugs which have been reportedly used with some success to treat stereotypy problems in cats. (See the "drug

Table 23.1: Summary of drugs/dosages which have been reported to sometimes be effective in the treatment of stereotypies in cats.

Drug	Dosage	References
Amitriptyline HCl	5 mg bid po 5–10 mg sid po	Overall & Beebe (1994) Voith (1989)
Hydrocodone	2.5–5.0 mg sid-bid po	Overall & Beebe (1994)
Chlorpheniramine maleate	2–4 mg bid po	Voith (1989)
Diazepam	1–2 mg bid po 1–5 mg bid	Voith (1989), Overall & Beebe (1994) Luescher et al. (1991)
Buspirone	5–10 mg sid po	Overall & Beebe (1994)

therapy" subsection in Chapter 8 for side effects and other important drug-related information.)

References

Beaver, B.V. (1989): Disorders of behavior. In Sherding, R. G. (ed): *The Cat: Diseases and Clinical Management*. New York, Churchill Livingstone.

Beaver B.V. (1992): *Feline Behavior: A Guide for Veterinarians*. 2nd Edition. Philadelphia, W.B. Saunders Company.

Bradshaw, J. W. S. (1992): *The Behaviour of the Domestic Cat*. Wallingford, UK, CAB International

Hart, B. L., and Hart, L.A. (1985): *Canine and Feline Behavior Therapy*. Philadelphia, Lea & Febiger.

Landsberg, G.M. (1991): Feline scratching and destruction and the effects of declawing. *Veterinary Clinics of North America: Small Animal Practice* **21**, 265–279.

Leuscher, U. A., McKeown, D. B., and Halip, J. (1991): Stereotypic or obsessive-compulsive disorders in dogs and cats. *Veterinary Clinics of North America: Small Animal Practice* **21**, 401–413.

O'Farrell, V., and Neville, P. (1994): *Manual of Feline Behaviour*. Shurdingon, Cheltenham, Gloucestershire, UK, British Small Animal Veterinary Association.

Overall, K., and Beebe, A. (1994): *VHUP Behavior Clinic Newsletter* **Summer**. Newsletter of the Behavior Clinic of the Veterinary Hospital of the University of Pennsylvania, Philadelphia, Pennsylvania.

Reisner, I. (1991): The pathophysiologic basis of behavior problems. *Veterinary Clinics of North America: Small Animal Practice* **21**, 207–224.

Voith, V.L. (1989): Chapter 43: Behavioral disorders. In Ettinger, J. S. (ed): *Textbook of Veterinary Internal Medicine*. Philadelphia, W. B. Saunders Company.

Winslow, C. N. (1938): Observations of dominance-subordination in cats. *Journal of Genetic Psychology* **52**, 425–428.

24 Future of the Pet Behavior Problem Field

Worldwide, the developmental trend in the pet behavior problem field seems clear. More and more pet behavior problem counseling practices will be established in the developed countries throughout the world, more veterinary hospitals will begin offering behavior problem consultation services, and many more small animal practitioners will place increasing emphasis on the prevention and treatment of pet behavioral problems in their practices. These developments will both reflect and stimulate developments in the market. Knowledge of the existence of this type of specialized advice and treatment will become more widespread among the population, and consulting one's family veterinarian or a behavior specialist for help in coping with pet behavior problems will become more commonplace than it is today.

In the long run, there will obviously be a need for establishing the kind of regulatory control over the field as is common in veterinary medicine, human medicine, clinical psychology, and related professions. At the present time, however, it is difficult to envision precisely how this aim can or should be realized. Although most people working in this field regard it as appropriate to think in terms of regulating and developing it within the context of veterinary medicine, it is fundamentally an interdisciplinary biological and psychological field rather than a medical one.

As any veterinarian who attempts to specialize in the area soon finds out, becoming a specialist in the treatment of behavioral problems is quite distinctively different from becoming a specialist, for example, in dermatology. The scientific study of behavior within either the experimental psychological or zoological context has a unique developmental history reflecting the unique problems associated with studying and understanding animal behavior.

Correspondingly, many of its principles, technical concepts, and major concerns are also unique and at first seem alien to those from other fields.

The related problem of having to introduce the animal behavioral science perspective and its major concepts, principles, and ways of analyzing and understanding behavioral phenomena to veterinarians who have been trained in a field far removed from the behavioral sciences has resulted in a literature consisting of hundreds of veterinary journal articles which treat the scientific aspects of behavior problems and behavior-modifying treatments at a relatively elementary, sometimes even superficial level. In general, more "depth" is needed in the pet behavior problem field in terms of taking full advantage of what experimental psychology and ethology can tell us about behavioral problems and perhaps also how to more effectively deal with. The field also needs more depth in terms of several major fields of human psychology like social psychology, cognitive psychology, and behavior therapy – not because owners or their animals are neurotic, but rather because solving animal behavioral problems necessitates modifying the opinions, attitudes, and behavior of owners with in part similar kinds of methods employed by some types of psychotherapists or counselors to modify behavior and its underlying cognitive concomitants in human beings experiencing emotional, psychological, or environmental adjustment difficulties. Progress on both fronts basically means going far deeper into the diverse animal and human behavioral science-related aspects of pet behavior problems than is the case in the literature produced by the first generation of workers in the field.

Both in terms of regulation and training, the major implication of this discussion is clear.

Further education of small animal practitioners and the training of veterinary students and non-veterinary counselors should involve much more in the way of extensive training in ethology, animal psychology, and human psychology than is now the case. For competence in the pet behavior problem area and indeed progress in the field as a whole will increasingly require an approach which is based on a deep and up-to-date understanding of these diverse scientific fields.

Research Needs

For a recent article, Askew (1994) compiled a list of 41 pet behavior problem research articles by reviewing most all of the major articles and books in the dog and cat behavioral problem field. Table 24.1 summarizes the result which can essentially be regarded as a portrait of the research basis of this young field.

Table 24.1: Classification of 41 research articles from the pet behavior problem field

Type of article	No. of articles
Relative frequency of behavior problems (statistics from the normal cat and dog populations)	3
Pet behavior problem case statistics	13
Clinical research studies	18
Others (e.g. bite injury statistics)	7

Speaking most generally, the available research in this area is on a very rudimentary level when compared, for example, to the research articles which appear in any animal behavioral science journal. Much of it is purely descriptive – that is, reporting statistical information from surveys of the incidence of behavior problems in the normal pet population (3 articles), statistics concerning the types of problems, animals, etc.

seen in behavior problem practices and veterinary hospitals (13 articles), and other collections of related descriptive statistics such as bite injury statistics taken from hospital or board of health records (7 articles). The remaining 18 articles involve clinical studies of one sort or another. Thirteen of them come from America, three come from Great Britain, and two were published in Germany. Most concern the effect of either castration or drugs on behavioral problems, and some include a behavior therapy element as well.

Taking these 18 clinical research studies together, the animal behavioral scientist is struck by two things. In the first place, only one of the studies included direct observations of the behavior of problem animals (Dodman et al., 1988). The others are all surveys in which the effectiveness of the treatment was assessed by questioning owners after the treatment as to whether and/or to what extent their animals' problem behaviors had improved. In effect, the data of all but one of these studies is entirely composed of owners' subjective impressions of changes or lack of changes in their animals' behavior.

Secondly, only three of these studies (Dodman et al., 1988; Goldberger and Rapoport, 1991; O'Farrell and Peachy, 1990) could be described as well-controlled in terms of conventional scientific standards . Typical of the other 15 studies, one castrates or gives some drug to a group of problem animals and simply reports the "improved" or "not improved" figures obtained by questioning owners at some later time. In fact, not one of the drug studies included a placebo group and only one of the castration studies (O'Farrell and Peachy, 1990) included a control group of non-castrated animals.

From the scientific viewpoint, these are serious shortcomings. On balance, the lack of direct experimenter observations of behavioral change is probably the least serious criticism, for owners' subjective judgments can probably be relied upon as being an imprecise but nevertheless roughly accurate indication of the presence or absence of substantial improvement. In contrast, the lack of the control groups or other control measures (e.g. designing studies so as to use animals as their own controls) required by the modern scientific method is a matter of great concern in light of the fact that the seriousness of particular behavioral problems need not and in many cases does not remain constant over time.

Take 30 problem cats or dogs, have owners put a few drops of some placebo plant extract into their food every day, and by a month later it is likely that as many as four or five and perhaps even more of the owners will tell you that the problem has improved somewhat since treatment began. There are two reasons why. The first is related to the fact that many owners decide to come to counselors for help when the problem is so bad that it "can only get better". And many apparently do spontaneously improve for reasons related to day-to-day, week-to-week, or month-to-month fluctuations in the severity of behavior problems which case experience indicates may be much more common than is usually acknowledged. Indeed, the severity of many behavioral problems seems to vary considerably over the course of time. Rather than remaining constant as the above-mentioned uncontrolled studies have obviously assumed, problems often worsen and improve spontaneously, for reasons which are not understandable to either the client, family veterinarian, or behavior specialist.

This type of variability has a major implication for research in this area: since a considerable number of the problems are brought to the attention of a family veterinarian or behavior specialist in response to some sort of "last straw" problem situation during a phase when the problem is about as bad as it ever gets, a prediction based on purely statistical reasoning (i.e. assuming regression towards the mean) is that only a few of the problems would be expected to worsen, but considerably more would be expected to improve again over the course of the next few days or weeks even if no treatment was carried out.

A second factor which can lead to registering improvements in behavior problems due to factors other than the recommended drug, castration, or behavior therapy treatment is

that the mere fact that a behavior counselor has been consulted and some sort of treatment like drug therapy is being carried out can cause some owners to be attentive to the animal's problem behavior to an unusually high degree. Owners may observe the animal in potential problem situations more closely and, in theory at least, their reactions to problem behavior might be more immediate, intense, or consistent than what would normally be the case. They might also be inclined to react differently in potential problem situations where the animal behaves acceptably, noticing this and perhaps doing something which rewards the animal for its good behavior. Obviously, these sorts of owner behaviors may be another potential source of improvements in problem behaviors which may operate irrespective of whether a placebo or genuinely effective drug is involved.

Thus, the improvement in a particular behavioral problem which an owner observes during the days and weeks following the beginning of treatment may indeed be due to the effectiveness of the drug or behavioral treatment itself. Alternatively, it may be "spontaneous" and/or due to a change in the owner's behavior over and above implementing the counselor's corrective behavioral recommendations. Given therefore that there are grounds to expect temporary improvements in a substantial number of the behavioral problems which have nothing to do with the real effectiveness of recommended drug, castration, or behavioral treatments, particular caution in evaluating the effects of treatments is obviously called for.

Bach flower remedies, dietary changes, many types of behavioral treatment recommendations, castration, progestins, and many types of psychotropic drugs – these are the treatments commonly advocated by American and European pet behavior problem counselors. But do all of these measures really work? And for those that are indeed helpful, to what quantitative degree does improvement occur over and above what would have occurred without the treatment?

Few studies have been designed to answer these most crucial questions. As stated previously, only three of the 18 clinical research studies reviewed were well-controlled. Seven of the 15 remaining studies can be considered as being partially controlled (Cooper and Hart, 1992; Hart, 1980; Hart, 1981a and 1991b; Hart and Barrett, 1973; Hart et al., 1993; Hopkins et al., 1976). Although these studies are not sufficiently well-controlled to accurately assess the true level of effectiveness of the treatments involved, they do yield what most experienced practitioners in this field regard as reasonable results. As for the remaining, fully uncontrolled studies, suggestive evidence is the very best that can be said for them. Certainly the improvement figures given by three of these studies for megestrol acetate (Joby et al., 1984), medroxy-progesterone acetate (Lässig et al., 1992), and castration (Heidenberger and Unshelm, 1990) seem to be greatly inflated compared to what clinical experience suggests is the case. Basically, these latter studies serve as good examples not of projects which yield important data on the effects of the respective treatments, but rather of the extent to which scientifically unsound studies in the animal behavior problem area can lead to erroneous conclusions.

The following kinds of arguments have been offered to defend the obvious methodological shortcomings of clinical research in the animal behavior therapy field:

- Because of the low case intake rate, it is impossible to include enough subjects in studies to allow for the use of control groups.
- It is not feasible to study behavioral problems in the laboratory and therefore owners' observations must serve as the raw data.
- Animals' lives are often at stake – or animals may represent a danger to human beings or other animals – which makes the inclusion in studies of a pretreatment observation or control treatment phase (e.g. administration of placebos) which delay effective treatment unfeasible or unethical.
- Most workers lack sufficient funding to do properly controlled studies, and obtaining grants for behavioral studies is especially difficult.

While these arguments obviously contain much truth, this does not mean that research in this area must necessarily remain as methodologically limited as it has been in the past. Indeed the veterinary profession has just as much cause and right to demand scientifically sound studies from those doing research in the animal behavior therapy field as it does, for example, from the advocates of homeopathic methods. In both cases, the claims that there is something so special about the field that normal scientific standards cannot be directly or fully applied should be vigorously refuted.

In fact, sound clinical research is just as feasible in the animal behavior problem area as in any other branch of veterinary medicine. Studies can be designed to run over a much longer period of time to make sure a sufficient number of subjects are included, or multicenter/multipractice studies can be carried out as is often necessary in the case of medicament research with human patients. Owners can be asked to use such aids as rating forms to help them be more objective and detailed in their assessments of their animals' problem behaviors. The carefully planned use of before-vs.-after comparison methods using each subject as its own control can add a valuable dimension of control to studies in which other kinds of controls are lacking. And in practice, it is usually only in cases involving potentially dangerous animals that the treatment urgency precludes the inclusion of a brief pretreatment control phase on practical or ethical grounds.

Opening up new lines of research

In addition to the need for more methodologically sound clinical research, there is also a need for basic research on the nature and causes of the various cat and dog problems. Two general types of research projects would seem to be most productive in this regard.

Comparative observations of problem and normal animals

The starting point here would be extensively and systematically observing problem animals using video cameras, rating forms, multiple observers, and other aids to objective observations. Such observations could take place both in specific problem situations and in a variety of other environmental contexts. Special test situations and methods could also be devised to gain further information about animals' behavior in their normal home environment and in controlled laboratory settings. The resulting detailed profiles of the various types of problem animals could then be compared with profiles of the behavior of normal, non-problem animals under the same environmental or test circumstances.

The extent to which this approach could be potentially useful is illustrated by the data presented in this book on, for example, dominance aggression and aggression towards human strangers in dogs and urine marking in cats. Although the owner questionnaire approach used should be regarded as little more than a crude pilot project for the kinds of research efforts envisioned above, nevertheless the general approach of comparing problem and normal animals with regard to a number of behavioral characteristics and home situation, owner attitude, etc. variables has been helpful in deriving tentative or suggestive answers to a number of important questions which arise in connection with the various behavior problems.

Comparative observations of owner-animal interactions with problem and normal animals

Owners of problem animals need to be extensively questioned about their general attitudes, personalities, motivations, etc. and their specific attitudes and behavior towards their pets. As O'Farrell (1987) has demonstrated, this approach has great potential for increasing our understanding of the owner-pet interactional dynamics associated with various behavioral problems. Additionally, extensive and systematic observations of owner-pet interactions using the observational techniques mentioned above are also important. Here too, various sorts of tests of owner reactions in various natural environment and laboratory settings might also be devised. The resulting detailed profiles of the various types of owners and owner-pet interac-

tions with problem animals which emerge could then be compared with similar data for normal, non-problem animals and their owners. Finally, owners themselves must be studied not only in terms of such behavioral observations, but also with more specifically "psychological" approaches like that employed by O'Farrell (1987).

Prevention of pet behavioral problems

The small animal veterinarian can do a great deal to prevent the development of many behavioral problems by advising owners to, for example, give their dogs more exercise, thoroughly train them to follow the basic commands, arrange for their dogs to play with other dogs every day, put young dogs in their place when they start growling or snapping at human beings, support rather than interfere with the formation of a stable dominance-submission relationship between two dogs in the same family, hold regular daily play sessions with a cat which seems to need a lot of activity, provide a second litter box when there is more than one cat in the family, bring a cat in for a veterinary examination as soon as it begins urinating or defecating outside of the littler box, never inadvertently reward an undesirable cat or dog behavior by trying to calm or distract the animal with petting, playing, or food, and many more. Not all behavioral problems can be easily prevented, but many can – particularly if owners respond correctly to them early in the course of their development.

Often owners do not think of mentioning such mild behavior problems to their family veterinarians either because they think behaviors such as defending the food bowl and growling at strangers are normal or because it simply doesn't occur to them to raise the topic with their family veterinarian whom they think of solely in terms of medical problems. Veterinarians should therefore encourage owners from the time they bring a newly acquired animal in for the first examination or vaccination to give a brief report on the animal's behavior and any minor problems with it. In addition, waiting-room posters or leaflets like those presented in Figures 24.1 and 24.2 might be used to inform clients of the veterinarian's role as pet behavior counselor and to give them some idea of the kinds of behavior "danger signs" which should be reported.

In spite of the fact that incorporating a strong behavioral problem prevention emphasis in one's practice may cost the practitioner additional time without bringing much additional income, it is still worthwhile for two reasons. Firstly, displaying expertise in the pet behavior problem area fosters a progressive, modern, and genuinely concerned image of the veterinarian in clients' minds. And this, in turn, may attract new clients or avoid losing present clients to colleagues who are more progressive

---

PROBLEMS WITH YOUR DOG?

"Yes"

Does it ever growl or snap at anyone?   ....

Is it sometimes disobedient or hard to control?   ....

Does it sometimes act restless or nervous?   ....

Does it ever have "accidents" in the home?   ....

Do you have to scold or punish it often?   ....

Does it get pushy or demanding sometimes?   ....

Does it make problems when it is left alone?   ....

Does it pick fights with other dogs?   ....

Is it unusually fearful of anything?   ....

Have you noticed any changes in its behavior lately?   ....

If you have answered "yes" to even one of these questions,

ask your veterinarian

Most serious pet behavior problems can be easily prevented if you, the owner, know what to do about them.

Figure 24.1: Sample waiting-room poster designed to encourage dog owners to report minor behavior problems to their veterinarian

in this regard. Secondly, concerning oneself with the behavior of patients is a satisfying and fascinating area in its own right which enriches all of the veterinarian's dealings with the client, the client's family, and the animal itself. To understand behavior, one must know a great deal about the animal, its behavioral tendencies in a wide variety of situations, and the environment in which it lives. And to learn all this, one must go into detail with owners concerning many areas which would not be nearly as directly relevant as far as treatment of the animal's health is concerned: the family's and animal's daily routine, attitudes of family members towards the animal, how they treat the animal in various situations, what it is allowed to do and

---

PROBLEMS WITH YOUR CAT?

"Yes"

Does it ever growl or snap at anyone? ....

Does it ever scratch or bite anyone? ....

Does it scratch the furniture, carpets, etc.? ....

Does it sometimes act restless or nervous? ....

Does it ever have "accidents" outside of the litter box? ....

Do you have to scold or punish it often? ....

Does it make a nuisance of itself sometimes? ....

Does it fight with other cats? ....

Is it unusually fearful of anything? ....

Have you noticed a change in its behavior lately? ....

If you have answered "yes" to even one of these questions,

ask your veterinarian

Most serious pet behavior problems can be easily prevented if you, the owner, know what to do about them.

Figure 24.2: Sample waiting-room poster designed to encourage cat owners to report minor behavior problems to their veterinarian

what not, how family members react when it does certain things, how it usually behaves during walks, with guests, with children, when it wants something, when it is scolded, etc. Such matters become relevant as never before when one focuses on behavior. As any small animal veterinarian who has developed the behavioral side of his/her practice will verify, a genuine concern with behavior fosters a holistic approach to the animal and warmer and more personal relations with clients, both of which can add a great deal to the personal satisfaction derived from a small animal practice.

References

Askew, H.R. (1994): Wie wissenschaftlich ist die Tierverhaltenstherapie? Einschätzung der weltweiten klinischen Forschung über die Wirksamkeit von medizinischen und verhaltens-orientierten Behandlungen auf Haustier-Verhaltensproblemen. *Der praktische Tierarzt* **75**, 539–544.

Cooper, L., and Hart, B. L. (1992): Comparison of diazepam with progestin for effectiveness in suppression of urine spraying behavior in cats. *Journal of the American Veterinary Medical Association* **200**, 797–801.

Dodman, N. H., Shuster, L., and White, S. (1988): Use of narcotic antagonists to modify stereotypic self-licking, self-chewing, and scratching behavior in dogs. *Journal of the American Veterinary Medical Association* **193**, 815–819.

Goldberger, E., and Rapoport, J. (1991): Canine acral lick dermatitis: Response to anti-obsessional drug clomipramine. *Journal of the American Animal Hospital Association* **27**, 179–182.

Hart, B. L. (1980): Objectionable urine spraying and urine marking in cats. *Journal of the American Veterinary Medical Association* **177**, 529–533.

Hart, B. L. (1981a): Progestin therapy for aggressive behavior in male dogs. *Journal of the American Veterinary Medical Association* **178**, 1070.

Hart, B. L. (1981b): Olfactory tractotomy for control of objectionable urine spraying and urine marking in cats. *Journal of the American Veterinary Medical Association* **179**, 231.

Hart, B. L., and Barrett, R. E. (1973): Effects of castration on fighting, roaming, and urine spraying in adult male cats. *Journal of the American Veterinary Medical Association* **163**, 290–292.

Hart, B.L., Eckstein, R.A, Powell, K.L., and Dodman, N.H. (1993): Effectiveness of buspirone on urine spraying and inappropriate urination in cats. *Journal of the American Veterinary Medical Association* **203**, 254–258.

Heidenberger, E., and Unshelm, J. (1990): Verhaltensänderungen von Hunden nach Kastration. *Tierärztliche Praxis* **18**, 69–75.

Hopkins, S. G., Schubert, T. A., and Hart, B. L. (1976): Castration of adult male dogs: Effects on roaming, aggression, urine marking, and mounting. *Journal of the American Veterinary Medical Association* **168**, 1108–1110.

Joby, R., Jemmett, J. E., and Miller, A. S. H. (1984): The control of undesirable behavior in male dogs using megestrol acetate. *Journal of Small Animal Practice* **25**, 567–572.

Lässig, R., Hanschke, S., and Bussian, E. (1992): Möglichkeiten der Behandlung von Verhaltensstörungen bei Kleintieren mit Medroxyprogesteronazetat. *Kleintierpraxis* **37**, 339–341.

O'Farrell, V. (1987): Owner attitudes and dog behavior problems. *Journal of Small Animal Practice* **28**, 1037–1045.

O'Farrell, V., and Peachy, E. (1990): Behavioral effects of ovariohysterectomy on bitches. *Journal of Small Animal Practice* **31**, 595–598.

Index

A

Aggression 96f, 109, 172, 175, 176, 178, 180, 182, 185, 196, 310, 316, 318f, 323f
–, competitive *see* competitive aggression
–, defensive *see* defensive aggression
–, dominance *see* dominance aggression
–, extragroup 98
–, fear *see* fear aggression
–, group-defensive *see* group-defensive aggression
–, idiopathic 180, 324
– in cats 310–325
– –, forms of 310
– – –, classification system 311
– –, tolerance concept 310
– in dogs 96–203
– –, classification 96
–, instrumental 323
–, interfemale 185
–, intermale 185, 189, 319
– –, during walks 191
– –, effects of castration 189
– –, progestin therapy 191
–, interspecific 98
–, intragroup 98
–, intraspecific 98
–, offensive *see* offensive aggression
–, pain-/punishment-elicited *see* pain-/punishment-elicited aggression
–, parental *see* parental aggression
–, pathophysiological causes 182, 324
–, play *see* play aggression (dog)
–, playful *see* playful aggression (cat)
–, predatory *see* predatory aggression
–, redirected *see* redirected aggression
–, self-protective *see* self-protective aggression
– towards other dogs *see* competitive aggression

B

Barking

–, excessive 258, 263
– –, causal factors 258
– –, sample recommendations 263
– –, treatment elements 258
Begging/pestering 247, 249
–, extinction 247
–, sample pestering 249
Behavior 250, 254, 256
–, attention-getting 250 *see also* demanding attention
– –, diagnosis 250
–, destructive *see* destructive behavior
Behavior problems 265, 268f, 343, 327, 331, 343
–, etiological factors 16
– –, lack of required behavioral training 17
– –, past exposure to intense aversive environmental stimuli 17
– –, pathophysiological disorder 16f
– –, present environmental deficiencies/stress 17
– –, restricted early experiences 17
– –, unacceptable forms of species-typical behavior 18
– –, unintentional owner fostering/reinforcement 17
–, ingestional *see* ingestion problems
–, instrumental 331
– –, extinction 331
– –, punishment 331
–, maternal 268, 329
– –, cannibalism 268, 330
– –, indifference 268
– –, neglecting kittens 329
– –, pseudopregnancy 268
–, nature of 16
–, predatory behavior 327
–, prevention of 343
–, sexual 265, 268, 327
– –, lack of sexual interest 265, 328
– –, mounting other cats 327